PREVENTIVE MEDICINE
AND PUBLIC HEALTH

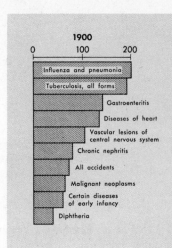

PREVENTIVE

and

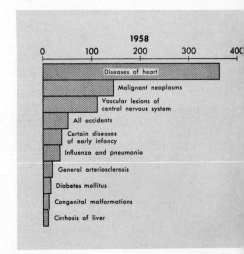

Death rates for the ten leading causes of death in the United States in 1900, and death rates for these same causes in 1958. (*Summary of Health and Vital Statistics of the United States,* U.S. Pub. Health Serv., Pub. No. 600 [Revised, 1960], Washington, D.C.)

The Authors

WILSON G. SMILLIE is Professor Emeritus of Public Health and Preventive Medicine, Cornell University College of Medicine.

EDWIN D. KILBOURNE is Professor and Director, Division of Virus Research, Department of Public Health, Cornell University College of Medicine.

THIRD EDITION

MEDICINE

PUBLIC HEALTH

WILSON G. SMILLIE, *A.B., M.D., D.P.H., SC.D. (Hon.)*

Professor Emeritus of Public Health and Preventive Medicine
Cornell University Medical College, New York, N. Y.

EDWIN D. KILBOURNE, *B.A., M.D.*

Professor of Public Health
Cornell University Medical College, New York, N. Y.

New York   **THE MACMILLAN COMPANY**

MACMILLAN NEW YORK, LONDON

Library of Congress catalog card number: 62-11927

The Macmillan Company, New York
Collier-Macmillan Canada, Ltd., Galt, Ontario
Divisions of The Crowell-Collier Publishing Company

Printed in the United States of America

This text is dedicated to

LEMUEL SHATTUCK

a Boston bookseller, who in 1850 wrote as follows:

Sanitary professorships should be established in all our colleges and medical schools, and filled by competent teachers. The science of preserving health and preventing disease should be taught as one of the most important sciences. It would be useful to all, and particularly to the student in curative medicine.

PREFACE TO THE THIRD EDITION

In the last decade preventive medicine and public health have advanced so rapidly that it has been necessary to make an extensive revision of this text. The primary purpose remains unchanged. This text is planned primarily for the medical student and for the physician who is in the active practice of medicine.

Although the general orientation of the book is global, emphasis has been placed on the newly emerging problems of disease in technologically advanced countries. The discussions of public health administration and medical care have special reference to practices in the United States.

The present edition comprises three parts:

The Introduction is concerned with the basis, language, and techniques of public health;

Book One considers broadly the parasitism of man and its containment, as well as new hazards of the environment and genetic determination of disease;

Book Two provides more specific consideration of the practice of preventive medicine and public health and the services available to the practitioner.

Dr. Edwin D. Kilbourne, Professor of Public Health and Director of the Division of Virus Research at Cornell University Medical College has become co-author of the book. His research interest is in infectious diseases, and his special responsibility has been the writing of all material relative to this subject in the text. He has also contributed the new chapters on air pollution, other chemical hazards of the environment, and human heredity and genetic determinants of disease.

Dr. Irwin Bross has revised the chapter on biostatistics and has added an important section on interpretation of statistical data in medical research.

The promotion of mental health has been given extensive consideration. The increased importance of occupational health has warranted increased emphasis on this topic.

The chapters on preventive aspects of chronic illness have been extensively revised, with special emphasis on rehabilitation of patients who suffer from disability due to chronic illness. The need for realignment of community facilities for care of the aged has been discussed. We have reintroduced Dr. Austin Flint's term "conservative medicine" as a suitable descriptive designation of this important component of medical practice.

The broad field of medical care cannot be fully covered in this text. We have not attempted to present a full discussion of community responsibility for adequacy of medical care, but have concerned ourselves with the responsibility of the practicing physician for the provision of comprehensive medical care, and we have outlined his relationship to the community in these matters. We have also emphasized the joint cooperative efforts that must be employed in future planning for adequate services and facilities that will be needed to provide for changing conditions and new concepts.

We wish to express our appreciation to all those who have given us aid in planning the revision of this text, particularly to Dr. Franklin Foote for his aid in revising the chapter on conservation of vision and to Mrs. Eleanor H. Thomas and Mrs. Edwin D. Kilbourne for their invaluable contribution in the preparation of the manuscript.

The valuable comments of Prof. William T. Ingram on the air pollution chapter and of Dr. Alexander G. Bearn on the chapter on genetic determinants of disease are acknowledged with gratitude.

W. G. SMILLIE
EDWIN D. KILBOURNE

PREFACE TO THE FIRST EDITION

This text on preventive medicine and public health is planned as an introduction of medical students to a *point of view*. The book is not planned for health officers, epidemiologists, sanitary engineers, or others who engage in public health as a career. It is prepared for medical students who are planning to practice clinical medicine and who are interested primarily in the diagnosis and treatment of disease.

The major thesis of the text is that the physician who is in practice has the obligation to his patients and to his community to prevent illness and to promote family and community health. It is his obligation to keep the well person well.

Much material has been omitted in this text that has been taught traditionally by departments of public health. A review of the textbooks on "Hygiene" of twenty-five years ago reveals that two thirds of the pages are devoted to a consideration of environmental sanitation, and particularly to the sanitary engineering aspects of public health. Such topics as the sanitation of water supplies, the construction of public sewers, domestic plumbing, the installations for illumination and ventilation of public buildings and private homes, and the construction of houses and factories are presented in detail. The intricacies of dairy sanitation and the minutiae of inspections for meat and other foods are emphasized.

Readers may be dismayed by the paucity of material upon these subjects in this text. My concept is that a physician should know the general principles of environmental sanitation but need not be familiar with the details, since he will not have the responsibility for their administration. If he should enter the public health field as an administrator, he must take special training to prepare himself for that career.

I have made a distinction between *preventive medicine*, which I consider a function of the individual in promotion of personal and family health, and *public health* as a community function. The author may be accused of hairsplitting sophistry, since there is an obvious overlapping of these functions with no clear-cut distinction between them. But I believe that the distinction is a valid and useful one, and that it will be found to be most practical in organizing the instruction of the students and in planning teaching programs with departments of clinical medicine.

Vital statistics has been dealt with in a very elementary manner. Many teachers of public health will feel that I should have given a more elaborate discussion of this topic. For example, I have not included a discussion of coefficients of correlation, nor have I presented those techniques that a research worker may employ in the interpretation of his data. My opinion is that physicians who undertake clinical investigations must familiarize themselves with various statistical techniques in order to make a sound evaluation of their work. I have not attempted to give this instruction. The purpose in the chapter on vital statistics has been: first, to indicate the importance of every physician as a collector of accurate vital data; second, to show the importance of the analysis of these vital data by competent vital statisticians; third, to teach the medical student to read his medical literature with a critical eye. He is shown the common pitfalls and errors in statistical presentation of clinical data and learns that the data may be evaluated satisfactorily if certain simple statistical criteria are applied to them.

I am fully aware of the limitations of this text in the presentation of matters relating to the influence of social and economic factors in production of illness and the promotion of health. I offer no apology for introducing this subject to the medical student, for the department of public health represents the *community point of view* in all faculty and student discussions. Thus the social aspects of medicine is a subject that should be presented by this department in a judicious and unbiased manner. But the subject is so vast that we have given only a bare indication of the potentialities for teaching in this field.

The consideration of adequacy of medical care in the community, a discussion of the responsibility of government in providing medical services to the indigent, the consideration of such questions as prepayment plans for medical care — in fact, the whole broad field of the social aspects of medical care has been presented most inadequately.

One reason is that these matters are still a fluid concept that is not ready for presentation in textual form. We believe that they should be presented by the department of public health, each teacher guiding the students in accordance with his philosophy and his convictions.

The author wishes to emphasize the fact that a textbook is intended simply as a guide to further reading and investigation. Any standardization of teaching in preventive medicine and public health, particularly in this present period of rapidly changing social concepts, would be most undesirable. Uniformity of schedules of teaching and of content of courses must be avoided as the worst of plagues.

The content of the text brings out the fact that teaching of preventive medicine will be most effective if it is integrated with the teaching of clinical medicine. Thus the members of the departmental staff in preventive medicine should have clinical appointments and should teach their subject not only from a textbook but at the bedside, in the clinic, and in the home.

The departmental teaching should also be integrated with the work of the official health services of the community. The continuity of instruction in those methods that may be employed in the home, for prevention of illness and promotion of health, can best be presented to students of medicine by the public health nurse, the social service worker, the epidemiologist, the school physician, and other health department personnel, since they are in the position to follow the individual situations from the home, through the clinic, to the hospital, and back again along the same path. Thus the department of preventive medicine acts as a liaison between intramural and extramural medical teaching, and establishes in the minds of the physician of the future a new and evolutional point of view of the interrelationship of preventive medicine with clinical practice.

This text has been dedicated to a most remarkable man, Mr. Lemuel

Shattuck. Mr. Shattuck was a Boston bookseller who developed an interest in preventive medicine and public health through his intitial studies in vital statistics of New England. He was a member of the Massachusetts State Legislature and secured an appointment as member of a sanitary commission which made an extensive study of the public health of Massachusetts. His report was published as a legislative document in 1850.*

This report has become a foundation stone for public health and preventive medicine in America. Shattuck's insight was so keen and his concepts were so broad that the plans recommended by him nearly one hundred years ago might serve admirably today as a suitable community program for health protection. It seems most fitting that the quotations at the beginning of each section of the text should be selected from appropriate parts of this great public health classic.

I wish to thank all those who have given so generously of their time and counsel in the preparation of this book. No author can be well informed in all fields, particularly when the subject is so varied as this one. Thus, whatever of intrinsic value is encountered in the discussions of the more specialized topics of this text is due to the contributions of my associates. I wish to express special appreciation to the following persons who aided in preparation of the manuscript and to indicate the subject to which they contributed:

Dr. E. L. Stebbins, who annotated the manuscript with most detailed, careful, and constructive criticism; Dr. Hugo Muench, "Vital Statistics"; Mrs. C. Luther Fry, "Population Trends and the Public Health"; Dr. Franklin M. Foote, "Environmental Sanitation"; Mr. Paul B. Gillen, "Housing"; Dr. Herbert R. Edwards, "Control of Tuberculosis"; Dr. Samuel R. Berenberg and Dr. Myron E. Wegman, "Child Health Protection"; Dr. Leona Baumgartner, "School Health Services"; Dr. Caroline B. Zachry and Dr. Alexander Reid Martin, "Child Guidance"; Dr. Oskar Diethelm, "Mental Hygiene"; Dr. Norman Jolliffe, "Malnutrition and Its Prevention"; Dr. George T. Pack and Dr. Jacob Furth, "Control of Cancer"; Dr. Russell L. Cecil, "Preventive Aspects of Arthritis"; Dr. Horace S. Baldwin and Dr. Mary E. H. Loveless, "Preventive Aspects of Allergic Conditions"; Dr. Thomas A. C. Rennie, "Preventive Aspects of Alcoholism"; Miss Katharine Faville, "The Public Health Nurse"; Miss T. H. Soule, "Medical Social Work"; and to many others who contributed various suggestions and data for the text. I extend my most grateful appreciation to Miss May McKean for her untiring efforts and unflagging interest in preparation of the manuscript.

W. G. SMILLIE

Cornell University Medical College
New York City

---

*Shattuck, Lemuel, *Report of a General Plan for the Promotion of Public and Personal Health*. Dutton and Wentworth, State Printers, Boston, 1850.

CONTENTS

Book One

PUBLIC HEALTH AND THE PARASITISM OF MAN
WITH A NOTE ON NEWER HAZARDS

SECTION I
Infectious Hazards of the Environment   97

SECTION II

The Control of Infectious Diseases Acquired from the External Environment 129

SECTION III

*Man as an Infectious Hazard to Man (The "Contagious"
or "Communicable" Infections Transmitted Directly from Man to Man)* 169

SECTION IV

The Control of Infections Directly Transmissible from Man to Man 219

SECTION V

New Hazards to Man and New Problems of Environmental Sanitation 257

$\mathcal{B}ook\,\mathcal{T}wo$

PROTECTION, PREVENTION, AND CONSERVATION
IN PUBLIC HEALTH

SECTION I
Child Health Protection

SECTION II
Accident Prevention

SECTION III
Conservative Medicine

SECTION IV
Public Health Administration   501

SECTION V
Comprehensive Medical Care   559

INTRODUCTION

An eminent physician (Dr. Edward Jarvis) has recently said: "Our education has made our calling exclusively a curative, and not a conservative one, and the business of our responsible lives has confined us to it. Our thoughts are devoted to, our interests are concerned in, and our employments are connected solely with, sickness, debility, or injury,—with diminution of life in some of its forms. But with health, with fullness of unalloyed, unimpaired life, we, professionally, have nothing to do." Though this may be generally true, professionally, yet the intelligent physician "can see arrows of disease, invisible to any one else; watch their havoc, and know whence they come, and how they may be stayed"; and there are many eminent medical men, who have, as individuals, nobly used the means which their superior position and knowledge have placed within their control, in the prevention of disease, and in the promotion of public health. And we wish to increase the number of such professional men.

LEMUEL SHATTUCK

1. INTRODUCTION

Medicine Is a Social Science

In the preface we have indicated that the purpose of this text is to present a *point of view*. This point of view is, basically, that medicine is a social science.

We are confronted at once with a demand as to our interpretation of the meaning of the term *social science*. Some physicians may even argue that the field of sociology is not a true science at all. Our concept of a science is: a body of knowledge of facts and laws that are obtained, and verified, by a series of exact observations and by correct thinking on these facts. Our concept of a social science is one which observes and studies the individual and his family in his relationship to the community as an aggregate body.

Former Surgeon General Leonard A. Scheele of the United States Public Health Service, in his discussion of opportunities in the teaching of preventive medicine, has emphasized the importance of social science in medical care.(1)

Social factors are the very core of preventive medicine and public health. One cannot discount the relationship of poverty and disease, nor yet the responsibility of the public agencies and the medical profession for attacking both social and physical pathology. I wish to emphasize that when we are talking about the social aspects of medicine, we are concerned with the total health care of an individual in society. We are talking about whether or not a community has the facilities to provide proper and adequate service to all classes of patients. We are talking about whether or not a man's occupation influences his disease, and if so, can he be rehabilitated or can a more salubrious occupation be found? We are talking about whether or not chronically ill patients can be taken care of adequately in their homes – both for the medical benefits that may result and for the more efficient use of hospital beds. We are asking: How can prolonged illness be linked with restorative services, including general education for the children and vocational rehabilitation for the adults?

It is such thinking that projects the concept of preventive medicine and public health far beyond the narrow confines of "isolation and quarantine" for acute infectious diseases. It is such thinking that projects the teaching of preventive medicine far beyond the confines of its present status.

3

The trend of thought in all centers of medical education during the past half century has been that medicine must be founded on the "exact" sciences, particularly on physics and chemistry. It is quite true that the extensive improvements that have been made in understanding of body function and structure, the gains that have been secured in recognition of disease and its treatment, have been achieved, in great part, through the application of new knowledge gleaned from the fields of physiology, biological chemistry, pathology, bacteriology, and pharmacology. These "applied" sciences have their foundation, for the most part, in physics, chemistry, and mathematics.

We have become so completely absorbed in this approach to medicine that many of us have half forgotten the fact that our subject of study — man — is a social being, a unit of a family, and a member of a community. He cannot be taken out of his environment and considered as a thing apart. He is subject to certain social laws and is part of a social structure. If he is removed from this environment, then only a partial and incomplete understanding is possible. This point is developed very effectively by Dr. Harry Richardson in *Patients Have Families*.(2)

Incorporation of Preventive Medicine as an Integral Part of Medical Practice

The most important concept of this century in the field of medical care is that preventive medicine is an integral and essential part of the everyday practice of medicine. It is not a separate body of knowledge to be understood only by a skilled technician who has been highly trained in this field. There is no "specialty" of preventive medicine as there is a specialty of surgery, radiology, or pediatrics. There is, of course, a specialty of public health, which is a well-organized body of knowledge and requires a high degree of skill. But preventive medicine must be interrelated with diagnosis, treatment, and rehabilitation. These are the four basic elements of every physician's continuous progressive plan for medical care for each of his patients.

The great physicians of all times have understood and have followed the principle that the practice of medicine is not simply an exercise in diagnostic acumen nor a test of therapeutic skill, but requires a complete understanding of an individual as a person who is a member of a family, and who lives in an environment that has a profound influence, for better or for worse, upon his health. They have also understood and followed the principle that he is entitled to the benefits of preventive medicine as an essential part of his medical care.

We shall attempt to show, in subsequent pages, that social laws play a tremendous part in the proper conduct of adequate medical care. We shall show that prevention of disease and promotion of individual and community health constitute, for the most part, a social science. Furthermore, it will become clear that the diagnosis of illness, and often the adequate treatment of the individual who is sick, is dependent upon our understanding of social and economic factors that influence his life. Oftentimes the application of this knowledge is just as important as the application of our knowledge of physiology and biological chemistry.

We do not, for one moment, wish to suggest that we as physicians should minimize the value of the *exact* sciences in the proper interpretation of body structure and function. But it is also unwise to underestimate the importance of social science as a factor in the promotion of our whole concept of provision of adequate medical care to the person who is sick, to the person who is well, to the family of which each of us is a part, and to the community as a whole.

Public health and preventive medicine have not been of great concern to the medical profession as a whole. The student of medicine of the past decades has shown slight interest in these subjects because he felt that they had little application to his future career, since they bore no practical relationship to the practice of medicine.

Dowling and Shakow(3) have made an interesting analysis of the allocation of time spent by internists in their medical practice. Diagnosis and treatment require 55 per cent of time, 26 per cent is devoted to preventive medicine, and 19 per cent to health education, which included efforts toward rehabilitation. As chronic disease increases, it is predictable that more internists' time will be devoted to rehabilitation activities.

The practice of pediatrics devotes more than 50 per cent of the time to the field of preventive medicine.

In recent years students of medicine have realized that they must be fully alive to the social implications of medical practice and have become actively interested in the relationship of preventive medicine to clinical medicine.

This book is addressed primarily to medical students, and its purpose is fourfold:

First, we shall emphasize the concept that disease as it occurs in the individual is inextricably linked with infection or disease in the community and that the health of the community is linked in turn with its total environment.

Second, we shall discuss our concept of the responsibilities of the community, and particularly the official agencies of the community, for the protection and promotion of the health of its people. This is a subject of great import to the physician, for public health is, in a broad sense, participation by the whole community in medical affairs.

Third, we shall attempt to indicate to the student of medicine the methods that may be utilized for the incorporation of preventive medicine in the practice of clinical medicine.

Fourth, we shall demonstrate the peculiar and most important functions of the practicing physician, which relate to the health protection and health promotion of the people in the area in which he conducts his practice. It will become clear that these community responsibilities are an integral and inherent part of an effective community-wide health program, as well as an essential part of medical practice.

This book is entitled *Preventive Medicine and Public Health.* What is meant by the term "preventive medicine"? And what is "public health"? To many workers in these fields, the terms are almost synonymous and interchangeable. We believe a real distinction may be made between these terms. The difference lies not in purpose nor in the results achieved. The difference rests in the allocation of responsibility for carrying out the activities required for consummation of a satisfactory community-, state-, and nation-wide health program.

Public Health. What then is public health? Public health encompasses those activities undertaken for the prevention of disease and the promotion of health, which are primarily a community responsibility. These activities may be carried on by an official department of public health, by voluntary health promotion agencies, by departments of education, by state or county medical societies, or by other community agencies.

The physician should be thoroughly familiar with the need for these activities. He should participate in them, but they are not his direct responsibility.

Preventive Medicine. What is preventive medicine? Preventive medicine encompasses those activities that are the direct responsibility of the individual in the prevention of disease and in the protection and promotion of the health of himself and his family.

Who is responsible for the proper conception and execution of these activities? They fall, for the most part, upon the family health adviser. Usually this person is the private physician, who aids and guides all members of the family in all matters pertaining to individual health protection.

Preventive medicine, then, represents individual responsibility for activities that are carried out for the family as the unit. Public health represents a community responsibility which is carried out for community benefit. In the first instance, the family is the unit; in the second instance, the community is the unit for consideration.

As in all attempted definitions of matters with wide social import, this distinction seems rather artificial and pedagogical. Certainly the objectives are the same in each instance. Health promotion is a joint and interrelated enterprise. Any activity that is undertaken for promotion of the health of the individual benefits the whole community. Any activity that is undertaken on a community-wide basis for health protection of all the people obviously will benefit the individual, and the family units as well.

This point is readily granted, but we must re-emphasize the fact that the difference lies not in the activities themselves, but in the assignment of responsibility for carrying out each activity. The foundations of our democracy are based on the principle of individual obligations. An individual is responsible for the welfare and for the protection of his family. He will employ physicians to aid him in carrying out the health protective functions. It is the physician's duty to prepare himself to meet this obligation.

We shall attempt throughout the text to point out the manner in which preventive medicine and public health may be correlated and integrated. Due attention will be given to the *principles* of public health, but the practices of public health will not be presented in all details. These matters are most appropriately presented to the graduate student in public health who plans to make this field his life career. The clinical aspects of preventive medicine and public health will be emphasized throughout the various chapters. Special emphasis will be placed upon that part of the general plan that should be assigned to the physician, in fulfillment of the community-wide design for health protection of all the people.

The Ebb and Flow of Public Health in the United States

It is customary to think of public health as a steadily advancing force which started in a small way many years ago and gradually built up tremendous power. Such has not been the course of events. Rather, there has been an ebb and flow of the public health movement in the United States. At times the tide has come in with great rapidity, driving all before it, only to be followed by a period of recession, great loss of impetus, and real discouragement.

One reason for this is that public health administration is but one small segment of the complete political framework. It is dependent upon and must conform to the general governmental design, which in turn is dependent upon the social conscience of great masses of people. In order to bring about advancement, it is necessary for the people to have a greater appreciation of the purposes and responsibilities of self-government. Thus, public health can move only as fast and as far as public opinion moves, and each modification in procedure must be integrated with changes in other governmental activities.

The *pioneer period* in the development of public health in the United States may be considered to be the era from earliest Colonial times through 1800. In this early period, public health was essentially an attempt to control contagious disease. The philosophy of the times was that the individual should provide for himself and his family; his responsibility included the provision of food, shelter, and clothing, and care in case of illness. The community responsibility was to protect the individual and his family against illness that might be due to communal life. Not much emphasis was placed upon community cleanliness and sanitation, but the principle of the communication of illness from the sick to the well was understood. This resulted in rigid public health measures, which included the isolation of the sick, quarantine of the family, sometimes quarantine of the community, and—most important of all—quarantine of one country from another by means of ship quarantine.

This period was marked by the great epidemics of smallpox in the seventeenth century extending through the eighteenth, and by dominating epidemics of yellow fever in the eighteenth century. Other great epidemic diseases, such as cholera and plague, were not important factors during this period.

Quarantine as a measure of protection failed, in part because of a lack of understanding of the epidemiologic principles of the carrier and his relationship to the spread of infection, and also because the modes of transmission, the incubation periods of disease, and the periods of communicability of infection were not well understood.

The period from 1800 to 1850 represented the *dark ages* of public health in America. It was distinctly a period of ebb tide. This was due in considerable part to the influence of a very important and distinguished physician, Benjamin Rush, who in turn had been greatly influenced by Noah Webster. Physicians of this period did not believe in the contagious nature of disease, although they never were able to get away from the obvious communicability of smallpox. All other diseases, in their theory, were due to outside causes, some as remote as stardust or earthquakes, together with other environmental factors near at hand, such as bad odors from decaying animal and vegetable matter.

There were no national departments of public health, no state departments, and practically no municipal departments. The little local health service that did exist had been organized for the prevention of contagion by the removal of community debris, the abatement of nuisances, and the disposal of dead animals; unfortunately, the community did not assume great responsibility in these matters. One factor of importance was emphasized: cleanliness of the environment.

The period from 1850 to 1875 represented an *awakening of public health* in the United States. Health conditions had become so notorious and control so mishandled that the country was ripe for a rebirth of the simple principles of community responsibility for health protection. Certain young men were responsible for giving impetus to this movement: Stephen Smith with his interest in housing and his horror over the terrible situation in the nursing care of the sick at Bellevue Hospital in New York; Wilson Jewell, who organized in Philadelphia the First National Sanitary Convention; Lemuel Shattuck and his extraordinary insight into the needs for proper public health administration—these were notable leaders in this awakening.

The Board of Health of New York City was so incompetent during this period that Fernando Wood, while mayor in the 1850's, refused to call it into session during the epidemic of cholera, declaring that "the Board of Health was more to be feared than pestilence."

The tide had gone out, but in the early 1850's there were a few faint signs that the inflow had begun. However, the leading physicans still believed that environmental factors were all-important and that a clean city meant a healthy city; they were still under the influence of Benjamin Rush and did not understand the contagious nature of disease.

The period from 1875 to 1900 represents a *golden era of communicable disease control* in the United States. Practically all the basic information upon which our present system of communicable disease control depends was discovered and developed during this period. There came a time of feverish activity in public health affairs. Every leading physician of the day was interested in and took some part in public health matters.

And then the tide went out. During a period around the year 1900, public health administration languished. For a time, important positions in national, state, and municipal official health services became part of the political spoils system. Incompetents were appointed for reasons of political preferment. Trained public health personnel was nonexistent. Public health officers received scant consideration and respect from their fellows; they were the failures and incompetents of the medical profession.

At this time a new philosophy of community responsibility developed, partially as a reaction against the inefficiency and incompetence of the official health services. This philosophy related to the importance of *community action in the protection of the health of the individual.* This was not a concept of the official health services but of the voluntary agencies.

Growth of the Voluntary Health Agencies. The voluntary health agency system had been devised before 1900. The earliest agencies were the visiting nurse associations, but there were many other pioneer associations which eventually developed into nation-wide voluntary health organizations. The emergency plan for feeding the poor in the panic of 1876 produced the baby milk stations, and from these have grown all the well-baby clinic services. Tuberculosis prevention was built almost entirely on the basis of the work of the voluntary associations; the same was true in the prevention of venereal disease, the prevention of hookworm disease, and the promotion of mental and dental hygiene—in fact, practically all the present public health activities that relate to the promotion of the health of the individual were inaugurated by voluntary agencies.

Another phenomenon appeared that proved to be quite unique in the world—the formation of great foundations set up from private fortunes for the purpose of promoting public health. These were followed by a variety of smaller foundations.

The theory behind all this voluntary health work was that these agencies should develop, by the experimental method, certain procedures—usually in a special field—to prevent illness and improve the health of the individual, and thus promote the health and happiness of the community. These plans were largely on a demonstration basis, the theory being that as soon as the value of the work had been demonstrated to the community, then the official agencies would appreciate the results and gradually assume the tasks so beneficial and necessary for satisfactory community life.

There are inherent dangers in this type of philanthropy. They are: (a) the unbalanced program; (b) the development of a vested interest; (c) the unwillingness to surrender successful work; and (d) unintelligent leadership. Each of these defects was later realized, time and again; but nevertheless the voluntary health agencies made a great contribution to the life of the nation, reaching flood tide of their influence about 1925.

The Tide Is Now Going Out. Due to many factors such as higher income and inheritance taxes, the work of these private organizations has diminished. The money that formerly had been devoted to philanthropic purposes by private individuals is now being transferred to the other pocket, and government itself is conducting the health enterprises that have been demonstrated to be so successful by voluntary agencies.

Nationalization of the Public Health in the United States

Beginning in 1925 and extending through the present time is the extraordinary phenomenon of the nationalization of the public health. The public health was, for generations, a community affair, administered under local self-government with some slight degree of state government supervision. Public health has now become a subject of nation-wide interest and importance. Although some communities had excellent local health services and highly satisfactory facilities for care of the sick, other areas were very poorly supplied with these facilities and were not able to provide them from their own local resources. The whole nation has awakened to the necessity for universal distribution of modern facilities and general utilization of modern techniques for protection against illness and promotion of the health of all the people. Whether we like it or not, and whatever our social philosophy may be, it is obvious that the present trend is toward the centralization and nationalization of public health. The reason for this is that the people of the nation have begun to understand the importance, from the community point of view, of health promotion of the individual since the ill health of the individual is a direct menace to the economic security of the community.

The principal risks to economic security that arise from ill health are:

1. The danger of impairment of individual capacity for productive work.

2. The loss of earnings that results from disabling illness among employable age groups.

3. The cost to the community of medical, nursing, and hospital care for preventable illness.

The community has sought in a great many ways to meet the menace to economic security of ill health. Some have believed that if sound provision is made by the community for economic security, then the individual will solve his own problems of ill health. Suggested methods are:

1. Unemployment compensation.
2. Wage increases.
3. Old-age pensions and annuities.
4. Stabilization of employment.
5. Direct relief to the unfortunate.

These methods of meeting the risk to economic security from ill health can have but an *indirect effect* on health promotion since they do not strike at the basic source of illness.

Certain general techniques have been developed by community effort, and whenever they have been systematically applied they have had some effect on the prevention of disease and have influenced community-wide health in a favorable manner. Examples of the methods of approach are:

1. Slum clearance and housing programs.
2. Popular education in the general principles of personal hygiene.
3. Provision for an adequate food supply.
4. Education of all the people concerning the nutritional requirements of the body.
5. Development of community facilities for healthful recreation and physical training.
6. Suitable methods of population control.

These methods are all valuable, and each has its particular importance, but here again the community efforts represent an *indirect attack* upon the basic problem of ill health and its relationship to the economic security of the community.

Three major methods have been employed by the community in a direct attack upon ill health and its attendant economic and social consequences:

1. Standard public health procedures. This includes all those measures of proved effectiveness which may be undertaken by organized community effort to reduce disease and promote mental and physical health *on a community-wide basis.*

2. Medical, nursing, and hospital care of the indigent and other groups in the community who are unable to obtain these benefits from their own resources.

3. Sickness insurance. This method is essentially a comprehensive plan for the distribution of the costs of any illness for any given individual or family over a period of time and among large groups of individuals in the community.

These three methods are now being developed simultaneously, and to a considerable degree they are developing independently throughout the United States. The first has had the longest period of systematic development and has met with a reasonable degree of success. The second method has also been developed extensively throughout the United States, both by voluntary and official agencies. Only recently, however, have the local community, the state, and the nation assumed interest in or responsibility for adequate medical care of all the people.

The comprehensive problem of the distribution of the cost of illness among large groups of individuals has not been solved in any degree. Some attempts have been made to distribute the costs of hospitalization, but it is now quite clear that no plan has yet been devised which is applicable on a nation-wide basis to meet all our community needs and which will fit into our social philosophy. The tide of nationalization of the public health is probably just beginning to come in.

World Health Organization

World-wide promotion of health and welfare is the special province of the World Health Organization—an official agency of the United Nations. Its head office is in Geneva, Switzerland. This organization has enjoyed exceptionally fine leadership and continues to exert a powerful and effective influence on health promotion and protection—particularly in underprivileged nations of the world.

The Problems

It will not be possible in this brief introduction to a very broad and rapidly expanding field to present a comprehensive discussion of the influence of social and economic factors upon illness. The adequacy of medical care, the local, state, and nation-wide programs for better distribution of medical facilities and realignment of the system of medical practice in the nation are matters which must be left for future discussion. The whole field of preventive medicine and public health is so vast, the problems so varied, and the development of plans for the future so fluid and so inspiring to the creative imagination, that we have attempted only to present the available experience and concepts of those who have devoted their lives to these matters and to point the way for future development to those who will take up the torch of progress when we relinquish it.

REFERENCES

1. SCHEELE, L. A.: *J. A. Am. M. Coll.*, 1950, **25**:241.

2. RICHARDSON, H. B.: *Patients Have Families.* The Commonwealth Fund, New York, 1945.

3. DOWLING, H. F., and SHAKOW, D.: *J.A.M.A.*, 1952, **149**:628.

2. POPULATION TRENDS AND
THE PUBLIC HEALTH

A pragmatic consideration of population trends* would suggest that this subject might have some slight significance to the public health worker, but certainly it is not the concern of the practicing physician. Obviously, a study of the trend of population in the nation lies in the fields of economics and sociology. The students of population have insisted, however, that the public health officer has a real responsibility for, and a direct concern with, the whole subject of population trends, and they have indicated that the physician in practice also has a personal interest and responsibility in this matter. Their reasoning follows:

If public health measures are successful, one of the end results will be a lower crude mortality rate and, particularly, a lower infant death rate. But economists have pointed out that a lowering of the death rate may result in community disaster.

If community resources remain static, and if the death rate is reduced, and if the birth rate should remain constant, the results that may occur are:

1. An explosive increase in population.
2. A reduction in the quality of the racial stock because of disturbance of the laws of natural selection, with increased preservation of the mentally and physically crippled and the weaklings of society.

In a rigorously competitive social structure, where resources have not increased commensurately with population increase, these handicapped and dependent individuals would perish, and this would be of great advantage to the state. If this challenge of the economist is valid, it is clear that the potential dangers to society that would be produced by any disturbance in natural selection through the application of the sciences of public health and clinical medicine require

*The student who is particularly interested in population trends is referred to the Population Reference Bureau, Inc., 1507 M St., N.W.; Washington, D.C.

thorough consideration by those who are in charge of health services (see Chap. 21).

Increase in Population in the United States

The growth of the nation through the pioneer period was slow. By 1830 there were about 10,000,000 people in the United States who were living, for the most part, under a rural economy. The death rate was high; there was a correspondingly high birth rate. No effective public health work had been instituted, and there was little immigration. From 1830 to 1960 the nation increased in population from 10,000,000 to more than 175,000,000 people. The trend line is almost straight from 1850 to 1920, when it begins to flatten out. Immigration played a considerable part in this growth, not so much in the actual numbers of immigrants, but because the immigrants were young adults: the women were of childbearing age and came from areas in Europe where large families were traditional. The major increase in population, however, was in the families of the native born and was due to a decrease in the death rate without a corresponding decline in the birth rate.

The growth of the country coincided with the industrial expansion initiated early in the nineteenth century. We have no exact records of vital data for the nation as a whole for that period, and can only make rough estimates from the information obtained from some of the large cities, from census reports, from immigration indices, and from church records.*

It has been estimated that the average expectation of life, at birth, in 1800 was 35 years, and the average woman of childbearing age had 8 children born to her(1). By 1960 these ratios had changed to life expectancy at birth of approximately 70 years. By 1960 also, the average woman who had passed the childbearing age had had 2.3 children instead of 8. The crude death rate during the same period, 1830 to 1950, dropped from 25 (estimated) to the vicinity of 10, and the birth rate from an approximate 55 in 1800 to about 24 in 1960.

This revolutionary change in the population trend was an integral part of the industrialization of the nation. It was produced by many interrelated factors; one of the most important was the development of sanitary science and the mass application of the principles of preventive medicine to community life. The reduction in the death rate

*Lemuel Shattuck's initial study of vital statistics, *Census of Boston*, was not published until 1845, and was based almost completely on records of church sextons.

was phenomenal, but even more important has been the decline in the *infant death rate*. This change was almost miraculously precipitated from an approximate rate of 200 for many parts of the nation in the latter part of the nineteenth century to a rate, 60 years later, of 20 or less in many states (20 deaths of infants under one year of age per 1,000 live births).

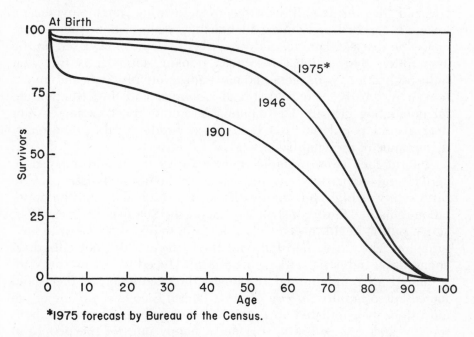

*1975 forecast by Bureau of the Census.

Figure 1. The lengthening life span.

During the past century, the social structure of the nation has been profoundly changed from a rural to an urban civilization. In 1830 practically all the people were living under an agricultural and pastoral economy. By 1960 more than 60 per cent of the population were living under urban conditions; less than 20 per cent were actually living on farms.

Urbanization lends itself well to application of mass methods for prevention of illness. Consequently, this social change has had a great influence upon reduction in the death rate. In fact, at one period in our history (about 1920) a child born in the large urban center had a better chance to survive to adulthood than a baby born under the apparently ideally healthful surroundings of a farm, with every opportunity for abundant and nutritious food and a perfect physical environment. The chief reason was that the application of public health measures in rural areas had not kept pace with urban sanitation.

The Vital Balance

It is obvious that a reduction in the death rate without a lowering of the birth rate must result in a rapid growth of population. If unchecked, the result will soon be: overcrowding, unemployment, a lowered standard of living, bad housing, malnutrition, increase in epidemic disease, famine, and war. This hypothesis is based on the assumption that national resources remain static. It is true that industrialization, with increased mechanization, research, and invention, may greatly increase national resources and thus compensate for population growth. The danger lies not so much in increase or decrease in population but rather in a sudden and revolutionary disturbance of the vital balance.

Puerto Rico is an example. For centuries the island enjoyed an agricultural and pastoral life and an almost medieval civilization. The birth rate was high, but the death rate was high also, and the population remained fairly constant. Following the Spanish-American War, active public health measures were instituted by the American government. The death rate fell, and the birth rate did not fall correspondingly. Industrialization was not introduced to any extent. With a limited area and limited resources, the population of the island increased so rapidly in 50 years that Puerto Rico became one of the most densely populated areas on the whole globe. The result, both socially and economically, was not a happy one for the people of Puerto Rico.

The problem was attacked by:

1. Extensive emigration to the United States.
2. Establishment of new industries in Puerto Rico.
3. Education of the people concerning the advantages of planned parenthood, including instruction in techniques of contraception.

Industrialization and resulting urbanization will, for purely economic and social reasons, inevitably produce a birth rate that is lower than the rural rate. Each new child that is born in an urban home is an increasing financial liability instead of an asset. In fact, as the family increases, the cost of housing, clothing, food, medical care, and other essentials increases almost in direct ratio to each new member of the family.

As the United States became urbanized, the birth rate fell to such a degree that in 1940 it passed the replacement level (0.98) for the nation as a whole. Dublin(2) has pointed out that the vital balance was below 1.0 even before 1940. It is true that in 1933, for example, the birth rate of the nation (16.6 per 1,000 population) exceeded the death rate of 10.7, so that the national increase of the population was 750,000. But this simple approach is misleading, since the margin of births over deaths in any one year is not a true indication of maintenance of population over a whole generation.

"The immediate result of a declining birth rate," says Dublin, "is to give the present population a larger proportion of persons at the reproductive ages than the current fertility and mortality would yield in the long run."

Analysis of the true rates of national increase, corrected for the *temporarily* large concentration of the population in the reproductive ages, showed that in 1933 the *net* reproduction rate was 0.94, and that we were not, in reality, maintaining ourselves over the generations, even though the actual annual increase was three fourths of a million.

This was not true of all parts of the country. The rural areas still had a vital balance well above 1.0, but the larger cities did not, and thus rural areas supplied the urban areas from their surplus population.

During World War II and directly thereafter, there was a great increase in marriages and also an increase in first births. In 1947 the birth rate soared to 27. Thereafter marriages declined and first births also declined, second births remaining constant, With the continuing trend toward small families, it seems certain that the net reproductive rate will in the near future again approximate 1.0. This trend may be interrupted, however. In 1962 larger families are more and more prevalent.

The net reproductive rate is determined by tracing 1,000 girl babies from birth to the end of their reproductive period, with due allowance for deaths that would occur. For example, in 1950, using current age-specific death rates, 973 of these girl babies that are born would survive to a reproductive age of 17 years. In this manner it is possible to calculate the ratio of births of daughters in two successive generations, which is based on established birth rates and existing survival rates. If the net reproductive rate remains greater than 1, the population increases. At the current status of mortality, fertility, marriage, and childless marriage, about 2.8 children are required per mother to secure a stationary population.

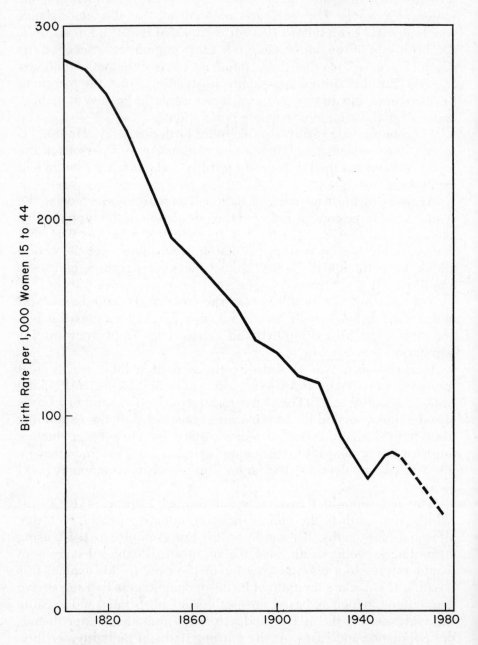

Figure 2. Decline in the birth rate, United States, 1800-1980.

Selectivity of the Lower Birth Rate

The reduction of the birth rate has been quite selective in relation to social groups. Roughly classified, in 1960, the lowest birth rates were encountered in families of:

1. Wealthy people living in large industrial centers.
2. Intellectuals and the social groups that comprise college graduates, the learned professions, and particularly university teachers and others in the teaching and professional fields.
3. The "white collar" class of industrial workers.
4. Skilled workmen in industry.
5. Rural landowners, where mechanization of agriculture has resulted in living conditions that are an approximation to those of urban life.

The average number of children per family in 1960 was in inverse ratio to this social classification. All were close to or below the maintenance level.

The large families in the United States in 1960 were limited, for the most part, to:

1. Families of first-generation immigrants.
2. Urban families of native stock from the lowest economic and social levels.
3. Rural families of low economic and educational status, particularly tenant farmers, and notably the Negro families of the rural areas of the South, and the Mexicans and Indians of the Southwest.

Thus the maintenance of the vital balance of the nation in 1960 was secured by replacement of the population from families of the lowest economic, intellectual, and social levels.

It is not our province, perhaps, to argue whether or not this is a serious matter. This is a question for the sociologist to determine. It seems unfortunate that the families of the wealthy and socially elect do not have sufficient children to perpetuate their own group, but this is not a matter of great importance since they comprise so small a proportion of the total population. But in groups 3, 4, and 5 of the first list lies the nucleus of our national strength. The real virility of the nation is found in the great central mass of the country. Satisfactory leadership and healthy social growth cannot be derived from a small ruling class, but from those leaders who emerge from the central core of society.

Influence of Infant Mortality on National Development

The infant mortality rate is the most delicate and most important index of the degree of the sound development and the measure of the cultural level of any community. The newborn healthy baby is the community's greatest asset. Thus the reduction of infant deaths in the United States during the past 60 years brings justifiable satisfaction. The neonatal rate has not declined to correspond with the decline of the death rate in children from 1 month to 1 year of age. A considerable proportion of neonatal deaths is not regrettable, however, since the death of many of the babies under 1 month of age is caused by congenital physical defects and crippling conditions that would have rendered the survivor a burden upon society.

It is true that a reduction of the infant death rate does, to some extent at least, protect weaklings, and preserves some physically and mentally defective babies that otherwise would have died under the law of natural selection. We nurse and coddle them so that some of them survive to reach maturity and to become a burden to their families.

Lowering of the infant death rate has great advantages, however, which more than counterbalance this obvious and inherent disadvantage. Unfortunately bacteria and viruses, as well as other agents of destruction of mankind, make no distinction between the intelligent child and the dull child, the potential inventor or genius and the potential criminal. Disease is not selective* in its attack on mankind, sparing the finest human material and destroying the poorest. Thus it is necessary to apply health protective measures to all mankind, with the assurance that there is no evidence as yet available that a lowering of the infant death rate has resulted in a weakening of the quality, or reduction in the virility, of our racial stock. In some of the nations today, infant mortality reduction, without concurrent birth control measures, has resulted in serious social and economic problems.

*Some exception may be taken to this statement, since the national health survey of 1959-60 showed a greater amount of illness, and particularly chronic illness, in the lowest economic groups that were studied. But as we have already noted, those in the lowest economic groups are not necessarily our poorest racial stock. There is good reason to believe that economic factors are responsible for the undue illness in these people. They may have great potential virility, which would emerge under favorable conditions. A good example of this fact is to be found in the Maritime Provinces of Canada. The most valuable export of Nova Scotia and New Brunswick to the United States has been the leadership and high intelligence of those who have emigrated to the United States, many of them coming from families of low economic status.

Reduction of the Birth Rate

A reduction of the birth rate has an advantage to the mother and to the family, if the infant mortality rate is reduced correspondingly.

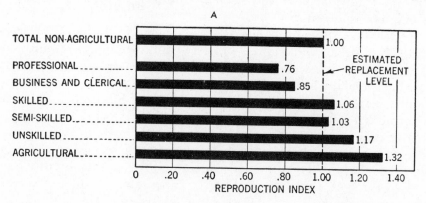

A. Estimated new reproduction rates per generation of broad occupational classes. (Adapted from Lorimer and Osborn, *Dynamics of Population.*)

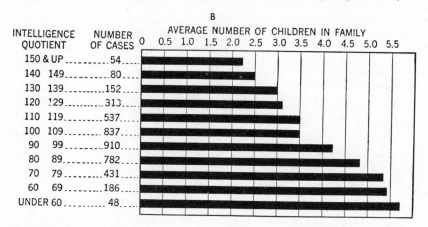

B. Distribution of families by size in relation to intelligence quotients of children. School and clinical data for 4,330 cases collected by Lentz. (From Lorimer and Osborn, *Dynamics of Population.*)

Figure 3. Relationship of occuaption and intelligence to the reproduction rate.

It is highly advantageous to the mother, in that she enjoys a marked reduction in the risks and the discomforts of pregnancy. If the infant death rate is low and the reduction in birth rate is intelligently accomplished, the average mother may have the risk of three children only, instead of eight, and the vital balance of the nation will be maintained. Furthermore, a proper spacing of children is most advantageous to the mother, for it will result in improvement of her health, and be equally advantageous to the baby. Eastman(3) has found that more healthy and stronger children are secured if proper spacing is employed.

Reduction of the birth rate is of advantage to the family, particularly in an urban civilization, and especially where the resources of the family are inflexible. On the whole, a smaller family results in a higher standard of living, better nutrition for each member of the family, better medical care, better education for each child, and better health status to all, with a resultant increase in the life expectancy of each member. Thus a reduction in the birth rate results in a lower morbidity and lower mortality rate for the whole community, and particularly in a continuous reduction of the infant mortality rate.

Nevertheless, the reduction of the birth rate, advantageous as it may seem, contains the elements of social disaster. The rate may fall so low that replacement does not occur, and the nation will rapidly decline in strength and virility. Still more insidious is the danger of the *selectivity* of the lower birth rate.

As we have noted, the advantages of a lower birth rate have accrued to the more intelligent and more wealthy families of the United States. The families of the poor, the ignorant, those who comprise the lowest economic and social levels, have not benefited by a lower birth rate. A herdsman would be considered highly incompetent if he replaced his flocks continually from his very poorest stock, but that is exactly what we may be doing in the nation at this particular moment. Is there any remedy for this situation?

Birth Control. How has the reduction of the birth rate been secured? Certainly not through reduction in fertility of the women of childbearing age. There is every reason to believe that the average woman of childbearing age in the United States is even more fertile, potentially, than in 1800. There is less sterility due to pelvic infections, better nutrition of these mothers, and better medical understanding of obstetrical problems.

The reduction in the birth rate has been secured by various methods of contraception.

Contraception. Dublin has stated:

The perfection of methods of contraception, and the spread of this knowledge over the whole civilized world are of the same order of importance as the extraordinary advances that have been made in saving human life. Together these two changes constitute, I believe, the most significant events of the last century(2).

The description of the simplest techniques of contraception are found in early literature, notably the Bible. Many natural methods have been utilized by mankind for centuries. Recently more scientific techniques have been developed. Each method has its advantages and disadvantages. It is not the function of this text to describe in detail the various techniques that may be employed in prevention of conception.* This subject belongs more properly to the fields of obstetrics and gynecology, and to prenatal care. It is our function to emphasize the responsibility of the state in this matter, and also to point out the special function of the physician in a community-wide program of family planning.

Responsibility of the State in Birth Control. In recapitulation, we wish to point out that:

1. Society has the obligation to reduce the death, morbidity, and infant mortality rates in every available effective way.

2. Reduction in infant mortality rates and, in general, death rates may result in eventual social disaster unless birth rates are reduced correspondingly.

3. This economic law has been applied in the United States, and disaster has been avoided by a lowering of the birth rate to such a degree that from about 1933 to 1940 the vital balance was reduced below the point of population maintenance. This curve was then reversed and by 1950 a net reproductive rate of greater than 1.0 had been re-established.

4. Much more important than numerical population maintenance is the improvement of existing national character and strength. Here we are in a precarious position: a change is required in the present selectivity of the birth rate, so that replacements of the population may not come from our poorest stock.

Does this not necessitate laws which permit dissemination of instruction by society to all social levels of people concerning the principles of planned parenthood and the techniques of contraception? The information which is now available to the wealthy and more favored economic groups should be made available to those who have low social standards and large families. Wise statesmanship would indicate removal of restrictions for dissemination of knowledge of contraception so that every family would have the opportunity for proper spacing of children and for adequate family planning.

*An excellent monograph on this subject is published by the Planned Parenthood Federation of America.

As a corollary also, sound statesmanship would require enactment of laws which would prevent conception in mothers in that very small element of society in which the progeny would, in all probability, become a social and economic burden to society.

Widespread practice of birth control would probably bring about a decrease in the birth rate in the lower income groups where, at the present time, contraceptive information is not within the reach of every married woman. But once the bearing of children became a voluntary and selective matter, then steps should be taken by society to aid parents to have "wanted" children. Modern society has the obligation to remove the obstacles that lie in the way of childbearing so that each family may be assured the economic security necessary for the children desired. The elimination of the present economic penalties that accrue when there are three or more children in each family may be secured by greater, and graded, tax exemptions for dependents, by provision for adequate housing for families, by adequate low-cost prenatal, maternal, and postnatal care, and by other suitable measures. The experience of Sweden in this social field is most encouraging. There, the program to encourage parenthood has been made a part of the national plan of social welfare. Government-sponsored clinics for planned parenthood have resulted not in a lower birth rate, but in a higher and more selective rate.

The Physician's Responsibility in Dissemination of Information Concerning Contraception. The practicing physician has a three-fold obligation in this field:

1. When pregnancy may jeopardize seriously the life and health of the mother. Under such circumstances, the physician is under obligation to give instruction to the parents so that suitable contraceptive methods may be employed which will prevent further pregnancy.

2. To prevent the birth of defective children. In certain families, it is quite obvious to the physician that conditions are such that the progeny will, in all probability, be defective mentally or physically, and will become a burden to the family and to the community at large. Under these circumstances, the family physician is under obligation to give suitable contraceptive advice to the parents, in order to prevent further pregnancy.

3. To prevent induced abortions. The family physician can be of great assistance in prevention of loss of life and the enormous amount of illness and disability that is caused by induced abortions.

No accurate record is available of the number of illegal abortions that occur annually in the nation. A reasonable estimate is about 4 to 5 illegal abortions per 100 pregnancies of married white women. It is estimated also that 90 per cent of all abortions are performed upon married women.

Illegal abortions are not only highly antisocial, they are stupid, dangerous, and quite unnecessary. The mother resorts to desperate measures because she is overwhelmed by the thought that further childbearing will result in family disaster.

The family physician, who has the complete confidence of his patients, can be of great assistance in prevention of illegal abortions. Often he can persuade the family that the pregnancy should be continued, or if abortion is medically indicated, he can make proper provision for the procedure. He can also be of aid to the mother, through proper instruction in contraceptive techniques, to prevent conception of future "unwanted" children.

Family Planning. Physicians are frequently asked for contraceptive advice by parents who believe that economic necessity requires that their family should be limited in order that every child of the family might have the maximum opportunity for health, happiness, and social advancement. This is a very delicate and difficult subject with religious and ethical implications that are not the province of this text to discuss.

The authors are under obligation, however, to express their own opinion, which is as follows:

We believe that every physician should consider it his obligation to aid parents in family planning and in spacing of pregnancy so that the greatest advantages may accrue to the health and happiness of the mother and the vigor and strength of each child. He should consider the economic status of the family and the nutritional requirements of the children, as well as the probable costs of the necessities of life and the probable inherent resources of the family. In so far as possible, he should help the family to plan its future so that each member will enjoy the greatest possible mental and physical benefit and the maximum opportunity for survival.

It is realized that this is a highly controversial subject and that instruction in contraceptive techniques by physicians is forbidden by law in certain states, except when pregnancy may endanger the life and health of the mother.

Every physician must be a law-abiding citizen, of course, and must conform to the legal restrictions in regard to these matters that apply

in his community. But if he has strong convictions upon these subjects, it is also his duty to express them and to aid in modification of
legal restrictions which he believes are not to the best interests of
the community.

Planned Parenthood Federation of America. This voluntary organization is administered along the same general lines as the other
nation-wide voluntary health associations, such as the National
Tuberculosis Association and the American Heart Association. It has
state and local chapters, and has had a far-reaching influence. Its
primary purpose is the education of the leaders of social, economic,
and political life so that our lawmakers may be enabled to promote
legislation concerning birth control.

The major functions of the Federation are educational, and
through its local chapters it reaches a great many people. As in the
developmental stages of the National Tuberculosis Association, the
local chapters sometimes give a direct service on a demonstrative
basis, through sponsorship of contraceptive clinics.

The Federation has met with very strong opposition. For the most
part this opposition has not come from physicians or from the organized medical profession, as was the case in the early development of
clinic services (under voluntary health agency auspices) for tuberculosis, venereal diseases, and the like. The opposition in this instance has arisen largely from religious groups that believe contraception is immoral and contrary to divine ordinance.

State-wide Contraceptive Clinic Services. Certain states, notably
North Carolina(4) and South Carolina, initiated state-wide programs
for instruction of all mothers in proper contraceptive techniques.
Other states have followed the example of the Carolinas with similar
types of organization. As a rule, the clinics are organized under the
auspices of the local health officer and under the sponsorship of the
state health department. The service is free but is limited to mothers
from the lower economic levels of the community. These clinics
are organized on much the same basis as any other public health
center clinic, and have been utilized extensively by the people that
they are intended to serve.

Sterilization of the "Unfit"

The authors are not in accord with a program of compulsory
sterilization to be utilized by the community to improve the racial
stock. Who is to be chosen as the infallible judge to decide what
racial stock is defective, and who is to determine which person must
be sterilized?

It is true that there are certain disease syndromes that are transmitted from parent to child. In a few instances, these diseases may produce such a degree of crippling or such important mental or physical defects that all the children born in the family that possesses these inherited traits will inevitably become a burden to the family and to the community. Under these circumstances, it may be advisable for the physician to recommend to prospective parents that sterilization of one or the other parent is indicated.

In some instances, feeble-minded women have no restraint and become prolific mothers. They are incapable of applying contraceptive techniques, and in many instances restrictive measures are not feasible. In these instances it may be of advantage to the community to insist upon compulsory sterilization of these women for social and economic as well as public health reasons.

The eugenist insists that the population must not be perpetuated from inferior stocks, and that the mentally and physically unfit must be prevented from having children. But we have so little evidence, as yet, concerning the hereditary nature of disease. Psychosis and mentally defective conditions are frequently cited as ample reason for sterilization. As we point out in the chapter on mental hygiene, science has provided only limited evidence that mental disease is transmissible from parent to child, and even mental deficiency states, which have been widely assumed to be a transmissible characteristic, are not so considered by many psychiatrists.

But, for the sake of argument, let us agree that certain types of mental deficiency, at least, are inheritable. If so, the characteristic is recessive. A short calculation indicates that it would have very little social effect if one sterilized *all morons* in the country. All the siblings of the mentally defective person must be sterilized as well if the disease is to be curtailed, since the characteristic is recessive; thus all the siblings are potential carriers of the defective genes (see Chap. 23).

A statistician once calculated that if mental defectiveness were hereditary, and if every mentally defective child in the nation were sterilized, and if this procedure were followed continuously over a long period of time, it would require at least five hundred years before the least diminution in the number of defectives in the population would become manifest. This calculation was based on the assumption that the condition is a recessively inherited characteristic and that every child with mental deficiency would be diagnosed and sterilized before puberty.

The first state sterilization law was enacted in Indiana in 1907.

California, Washington, and Connecticut followed suit in 1909. On January 1, 1960, 61,540 sterilizations(5) had been performed under mandate or sanction of state laws in 30 states.

The cause for performance of the operation was:

Insanity	50 per cent
Feeble-mindedness	48 per cent
Other causes	2 per cent

About 50 per cent of the subjects were women. California led all other states with over 20,000 sterilizations; five other states, Kansas, Georgia, North Carolina, Michigan, and Virginia, had more than 3,000 operations, whereas in 21 states the law is practically a dead letter, with fewer than 1,000 sterilizations in each state since enactment legislation.

Some states have laws that compel sterilization of certain types of the "habitual" criminal. If one were certain that criminality is a hereditary characteristic and is not due in part, at least, to impingement of social, economic, and environmental factors, we might feel more fully justified in advocating this procedure.

A prolonged period of genetic research, together with a study of the influence of heredity upon incidence of disease, is required before eugenic sterilization can be applied with intelligence and with real benefit to the state. There is no reason to believe that it will ever be an important preventive measure in our social and economic life.

POPULATION PROJECTION IN THE UNITED STATES

Prophecy is dangerous and often returns to confound the prophet, particularly if matters under consideration relate to social or economic change. Nevertheless, it is interesting and perhaps worth while to speculate on the changes in population composition, under the assumption that existing trends will be continued.

Probable Growth of the Total
Population in the United States
(in millions)

1900	76
1960	177
1980	260 (estimated)
2000	350 (estimated)

Birth Rate

During the "Great Depression" years, the birth rate declined to 18. A gradual increase then occurred. The peak birth rate was reached in the postwar year of 1947, with 26.6 births per 1,000 population. By 1960 the birth rate had more or less stabilized at 24 to 25. The trend has been away from large families of 7 to 8 children and also away from one-child families. The mean in fertile parents has centered around 2.8 children per family. Marriages tend to occur earlier.

Average Age at First Marriage
(years)

1890	Men — 28	Women — 22
1960	Men — 23	Women — 20

Parents have children earlier than their fathers did and space them more regularly. Most mothers have completed their childbearing tasks by the age of 30 years.

College graduates marry at a much earlier age than did their parents. They have more children earlier, and these more closely spaced.

A study(6) of attitudes concerning family planning indicates that the great majority of all families queried accepts the concept of family planning and tries to regulate the number and timing of births in relation to family needs and resources. Among fecund couples, 83 per cent practice contraception, and 7 per cent more plan to do so after having the children they want. The number of children wanted was a mean of 2.8 per family.(7)

Life Expectancy

The United States Census Bureau projection of life expectancy at birth is as follows:

	Males *(years)*	*Females* *(years)*
1955	66.7	72.9
1980	69.8	76.0

	Persons over 65 Years	*Per Cent of Population*
1900	3,080,498	4.1
1960	15,641,000	8.7
1975	21,872,000 (est.)	9.7 (est.)

Age expectancy at 65 years of age will gradually increase.

Age Expectancy at 65 Years

	1960 (years)	1975 (years)
White males	12.7	16.6
White females	15.4	19.6

Mortality Projections

Tarver(8) has made some interesting mortality projections to 1970.

1. Reduction in the death rate, 1955 to 1970, will be greater in infancy and early childhood than in adult and advanced ages.

2. At middle age and over, females will experience greater reduction in mortality than males. This will increase the number of widows and extend the duration of widowhood.

3. Diminished mortality will increase the chances of infants living to successive decades. This will augment the number reaching productive ages. By 1970 over 70,000 white males out of each cohort of 100,000 born can expect to attain 65 years of age. The gradual extension of life expectancy will thus increase the number of persons 65 years and over, enlarging the number of those receiving Social Security benefits. It also will lengthen the period that workers will spend in retirement.

Dependency Ratio

There will be not only more old people in 1980 but more young people as well. The "dependency ratio" is calculated as the number under 20 years and over 64 years per 100 persons in working ages 20 to 64.* This ratio reached a low point of 70.4 in 1940, but it has gradually risen and will be well above 100 by 1980 (see Fig. 4).

This would mean that every person in the production age group must support not only himself but at least one other nonproductive person.

Natural Increase Rate

One striking change has occurred in the natural increase rate in the United States. Formerly the balance of births over deaths was controlled largely by the death rate. Natural increase is now controlled by the birth rate. The birth rate tends to follow fluctuations in national economic and social changes and may be modified readily. Since the death rate is stabilized, population control on a nation-

---

*Most persons in the marginal ages under 20 and over 64 resent their classification as totally dependent since most of them are producing at least as much as they consume.

wide basis is attained by control of the birth rate. Control has proved to be a feasible procedure. This was apparent in Japan during the past decade. The authorities decided that the population was expanding too rapidly. Birth control measures were instituted. Success was due to the following factors:

1. High priority was given to family planning.
2. Most of the population are urban dwellers.
3. There is a high degree of literacy.
4. Widespread educational measures were employed.
5. Clinic service and medical advice were made readily available.

The results were as follows:

Birth Rate Per 1,000 Population
1947 — 34.3
1958 — 18.0

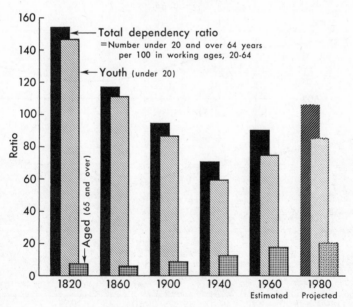

Figure 4. Rising dependency ratio. The dependency ratio represents the relationship of the dependent population (under 20 and over 64 years of age) to the economically active population (between 20 and 64 years). In 1820, there were 153 dependents to every 100 in the economically productive group. This ratio declined steadily until 1940 when there were only 70.4 dependents to 100 in the working ages. The ratio is now rising again and it will continue to rise in the next generation. (Population Reference Bureau: *Population Bull.*, Washington, D.C., 1960, *XVI*:99.)

Age Composition of the Population of the United States in 1980

The Population Reference Bureau(9) has estimated that the age composition of the United States in 1980 will be as follows:

	Per Cent of Population
Persons under 20	41.5
Productive age group	49.0
Old age — 65 years and over	9.5

The greatest proportional increase will be in age groups over 65 years, and the greatest decrease will be in the ages 40 to 64 (see Fig. 5).

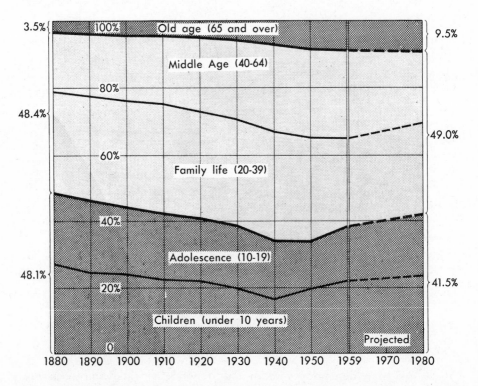

Figure 5. Century's change in age distribution. In 1880, 48 per cent of the population was under 20 years of age and somewhat more than 3 per cent was over 64. The proportion of youth declined until 1940, and it has increased steadily since then. Paradoxically, the United States population will grow both younger and older in the next 20 years. (Population Reference Bureau: *Population Bull.*, Washington, D.C., 1960, XVI:97.)

Conclusion

The changes in composition of our population during the next 25 years will have a strong influence upon our community planning for health protection and promotion. It will influence our thinking concerning facilities and personnel that must be provided to meet the needs of the coming generation.

Every physician and every health officer should be aware of the trends in population changes as well as their social and economic implications. He should plan his career to meet the changing needs of those people whom he will serve.

REFERENCES

1. WHELPTON, P. K.: *J. Am. Statist. A.*, 1936, **31**:468.

2. DUBLIN, L. I.: *Bull. New York Acad. Med.*, 1943, **19**:563.

3. EASTMAN, N. J.: *Am. J. Obst. & Gynec.*, 1944, **47**:445.

4. NORTON, ROY: *Am. J. Pub. Health*, 1939, **29**:256.

5. Human Betterment Association of America, 105 West 55th St., New York, N.Y., personal communication.

6. Population Reference Bureau: *Population Bull.*, Washington, D.C., 1959, **XV**(3):41.

7. Population Reference Bureau: *Population Bull.*, Washington, D.C., 1960, **XVI**(4):74.

8. TARVER, J. D.: *Milbank Memorial Fund Quarterly*, 1959, **XXXVII**:132-142.

9. Population Reference Bureau: *Population Bull.*, Washington, D.C., 1960, **XVI**(5):97.

3. STATISTICS IN PUBLIC HEALTH AND MEDICAL RESEARCH

Irwin D. J. Bross, Ph. D.
Roswell Park Memorial Institute for Cancer Research

The average young physician approaches statistics with apprehension and distrust. He hoped, when he became a student of medicine, that he could put his square roots and algebraic formulas behind him. All the tables and charts represent, to him, dull and uninteresting compilations of dry facts that bear little relationship to his medical activities and have no application to his future life.

It is only when the student begins to read the current medical literature that his interest is aroused. He soon realizes that at least half of the articles that are published in the journals must draw their conclusions from experiments that have to be interpreted on a statistical basis. His curiosity is aroused as to the validity of scientific conclusions that are founded on statistical tables, and suddenly the tables, graphs, and charts have real importance and become living things, full of expression and meaning.

Statistical techniques are of importance in the analysis of clinical and laboratory data. They also have an essential place in the field of public health. Vital data are the beacons of those who guide the public health activities of the states and the nation. Without a continuous and adequate compilation and interpretation of vital facts, all public health work would be carried out blindly and ineffectively.

The many different applications of statistical methods in modern medicine call for a wide variety of statistical principles and techniques. The procedures used in vital statistics differ from those commonly employed in laboratory studies, and clinical trials emphasize still other techniques. In a specialized area such as pharmacology, a large number of statistical tools (which go under the heading of "bioassay") have been developed for the experimental situations peculiar to the area. Hence this chapter will not attempt any comprehensive coverage of the title topic. Only a bare minimum of what a practicing physician needs to know about statistics will be presented here. Those doctors who go on in a specialized area of public health or medical research will need to acquire a working knowledge of the statistical methods of their specialty from some other source.

The first part will give some pointers on the sources and use of vital statistics. The second part will discuss some of the common procedures used in the presentation of statistical data. The third part will briefly consider some of the problems and pitfalls in the interpretation of statistical material.

SOURCE AND USE OF VITAL STATISTICS

Vital statistics is a measurement of achievement in human happiness and human welfare. A statistical statement that the infant death rate of the United States has dropped from 60 to 26 within a period of 25 years is tremendously vitalized when we realize what it means to the nation. If a person interprets these facts imaginatively, it brings a picture of thousands upon thousands of babies living in happy homes, of toddlers underfoot, of children thronging to school or playing with their friends. All of these children, if born under the conditions of only a generation ago, would have suffered illness and pain, and despite the travail of their birth, the sadness during their illness, the economic waste to the community by their loss, all would have died before they had reached their first birthday.

Vital statistics has been called poetically "the bookkeeping of humanity." As in all bookkeeping, the value of the data is minimal unless the facts that are collected are accurate and complete. The responsibility for accuracy and completeness is the direct function and duty of the family physician. It is one of the important community responsibilities which the physician assumes when he enters the practice of medicine. He must be the primary source of accurate and complete recording of the vital data of his community.

Registration and Collection of Vital Data

The collecting, recording, and interpretation of vital statistics are a function of government. The special responsibility of the physician in this field is the *registration* of vital data under governmental direction.

Only in recent years has collection of vital data been considered a governmental function in the United States. A great part of our national statistics was in chaotic state since local governments, and states as well, did not require registration of all births and deaths.

The federal government assumed leadership and formed a National Registration Area. The requirements for admission to this area by each state were:

1. A satisfactory state vital statistics law to set up the adequate machinery for collection of essential vital data.

2. Ninety per cent completeness in reporting of births and deaths.

Standardized forms for reporting deaths, births, stillbirths, and marriages were recommended. After a long and laborious trial period, all the states in the Union were finally admitted in 1933 to the National Birth Registration Area and also to the National Death Registration Area.

Vital Statistics Services

1. The Census. This is a complete enumeration of the population. It not only represents actual numbering of people, but it also considers such matters as age distribution, sex, race, geographic distribution, occupation, housing, and to some degree at least, income.

Bureau of the Census of the federal government takes a nation-wide census every tenth year. The estimate of the population of any area during an intercensal period may be obtained with a fair degree of accuracy. Various methods of estimate are used:

Arithmetic Method. The average annual increase or decrease of a community is determined between the last two successive censuses. This average annual increase (or decrease) since the last census is added (or subtracted) for the number of years since the last census.

For example: One wishes to estimate the population of a city in 1965. The 1960 census, as of July 1, 1960, gave a population of 50,000. The population of July 1, 1950, was 42,500. The average annual increase of the city between the census of 1950 and 1960 was 750. Thus, the estimated population for July 1, 1965, would be 50,000 + (5 × 750) = 53,750.

Geometric Method. This method postulates that the population is increased according to the *average rate* for the 10 intercensal years instead of the *average increase.* The geometric method is the method of compound interest. The mathematical formula is $P_n = P_c (1 + r)^n$.

P_n is the population to be estimated at n years. P_c is the last population census, and r is the rate of increase.

Supplementary Method. The National Office of Vital Statistics utilizes a method which takes into account the increase of reported births over deaths, together with all information that is available concerning migration of population. This method is of little value to the various states or local communities, since no accurate record is kept in the United States of the migration of people from one state or city to another.

Graphic Method. A local government may make a fairly satisfactory estimate of its population by the graphic method:

A curve is made of the growth of population through past decades, and this trend line is extended through to the period for which the estimate is desired.

Considering the gross errors due to population migration and the like, one method is about as good as another.

2. Registration. Registration is obtained by developing a machinery for the recording of individual certificates of vital facts. The most important data are births, stillbirths, marriages, and deaths. Records of morbidity, particularly for important communicable diseases, are also obtained with more or less accuracy in most states. A standard method of registration and collection of individual certificates has been devised by the National Office of Vital Statistics.

Governments are interested in the records of births and deaths, since they form the basis of the most interesting and valuable kind of bookkeeping: that of human population. One of the most dramatic of all stories is the result of the application of generations of research in medicine and public health now reflected in the gradually increasing span of human life and the reduction and disappearance of deaths from causes which until recently were accepted as inevitable. This achievement cannot be measured nor future campaigns planned without the guide provided by vital statistics.

There are three main points in each record of birth and of death. They are: (a) the individual concerned, (b) the event, and (c) the attending circumstances. In a birth certificate, the name and identification of the person and of his parents are of paramount importance, as are the date and place of occurrence, since these establish the identity, age, and citizenship of the individual. Additional questions are usually asked as to length of labor, complications, and so forth. When analyzed, these questions can give answers to many questions asked by the health officer who is interested in maternal and child hygiene.

The death certificate also identifies the individual and establishes the fact of his death, together with the time and place. These are facts comparatively easy to secure. In addition, the certificate asks for the "cause of death." Originally, this was a purely legal question, and the physician merely certified that the death was due to "natural causes" without suspicion of foul play. Gradually, however, it became obvious that the death certificate could furnish valuable – sometimes the only – information as to the presence and prevalence of various kinds of disease.

In view of the special interest of the health officer in many phases of vital-statistics reporting, it is not surprising that registration of births, deaths, and stillbirths is a function of the health department in every state but one, and in many foreign countries. Some health departments also register marriages and divorces.

The machinery of registration includes local registrars, to whom the original reports are given by the physicians (births) or undertakers (deaths). The local registrar must check the certificate for completeness and accuracy. His main job, however, is to see that every birth and death in his jurisdiction is recorded. For this reason it is necessary to select as registrars people with wide acquaintance in their community, for example, a postmaster in a small town, who is very apt to know everything that goes on. Originally, registration districts were very small. With increasing urbanization, however, districts have been consolidated so there is often only one local registrar for a city or even a county. This is generally the health officer or one of his deputies.

Certificates are usually mailed to state headquarters each month. In rural counties with well-organized health departments, however, it is becoming customary to appoint the health officer as a deputy registrar. The local registrars then send him the certificates immediately. This gives the health officer immediate information which is sometimes invaluable; it also gives him an opportunity to complete certificates or to have them corrected before they are sent to the state.

The state registrar is usually the state health officer or a deputy. When the certificates are received at state headquarters, they are checked again, coded and indexed, bound in permanent form, and filed in vaults, available whenever a copy is needed. The information is usually transferred to punch cards, which can be used in machines to analyze and tabulate the results.

Birth Certificates

Definition of a Live Birth. A child showing any evidence of life (action of heart, breathing, or movement of voluntary muscle) after complete birth should be registered as a live birth. Birth is considered complete when the child is altogether (head, trunk, and limbs) outside the body of the mother, even if the cord is uncut and the placenta still attached. The standard certificate of birth is filed with the local registrar within 10 days after the birth of the baby. The person responsible for filing the birth certificate is the person who is responsible for the delivery of the baby: usually a physician, sometimes a midwife. If the baby is born in the public wards of a hospital, the hospital superintendent is legally responsible for the filing of the certificate.

A copy of a standard certificate is illustrated in Figure 6. The writing must be legible and in black ink; no erasures or corrections are permitted. If no name for the baby has been selected, the certificate is filed without a given name, and a supplementary certificate with the chosen name must be filed within a year.

Some states require additional confidential information, which is written on the back of the certificate. It relates to the results of the mother's Wassermann test, the complications of pregnancy, congenital malformations, and birth injury, etc. None of this information would appear on a transcript of the certificate.

The major purpose of the birth certificate is to give legal proof of the status of an individual as a citizen. It is utilized to prove parentage, for purposes of inheritance, for obtaining passports, establishing the right to vote and to hold public office, to enter school, to engage in industry, and in many other important matters.

The various reasons why a birth certificate may be of great value to any individual are presented in detail in the *Physicians' Handbook on Birth and Death Registration*(1).

Stillbirths

Stillbirths are recorded on a special standard stillbirth certificate. The official United States Office of Vital Statistics' definition of stillbirth is: "A fetus showing no evidence of life after complete birth (no action of heart, breathing, or movement of voluntary muscle), if the 20th week of gestation has been reached."

The physician who is responsible for the care of the mother at the time of the stillbirth has the responsibility for filing the stillbirth certificate with the local registrar.

Death Certificates

A standard certificate of death is illustrated in Figure 7. It must be filed with the local registrar before a permit for interment can be secured. Usually a three-day limit is provided.

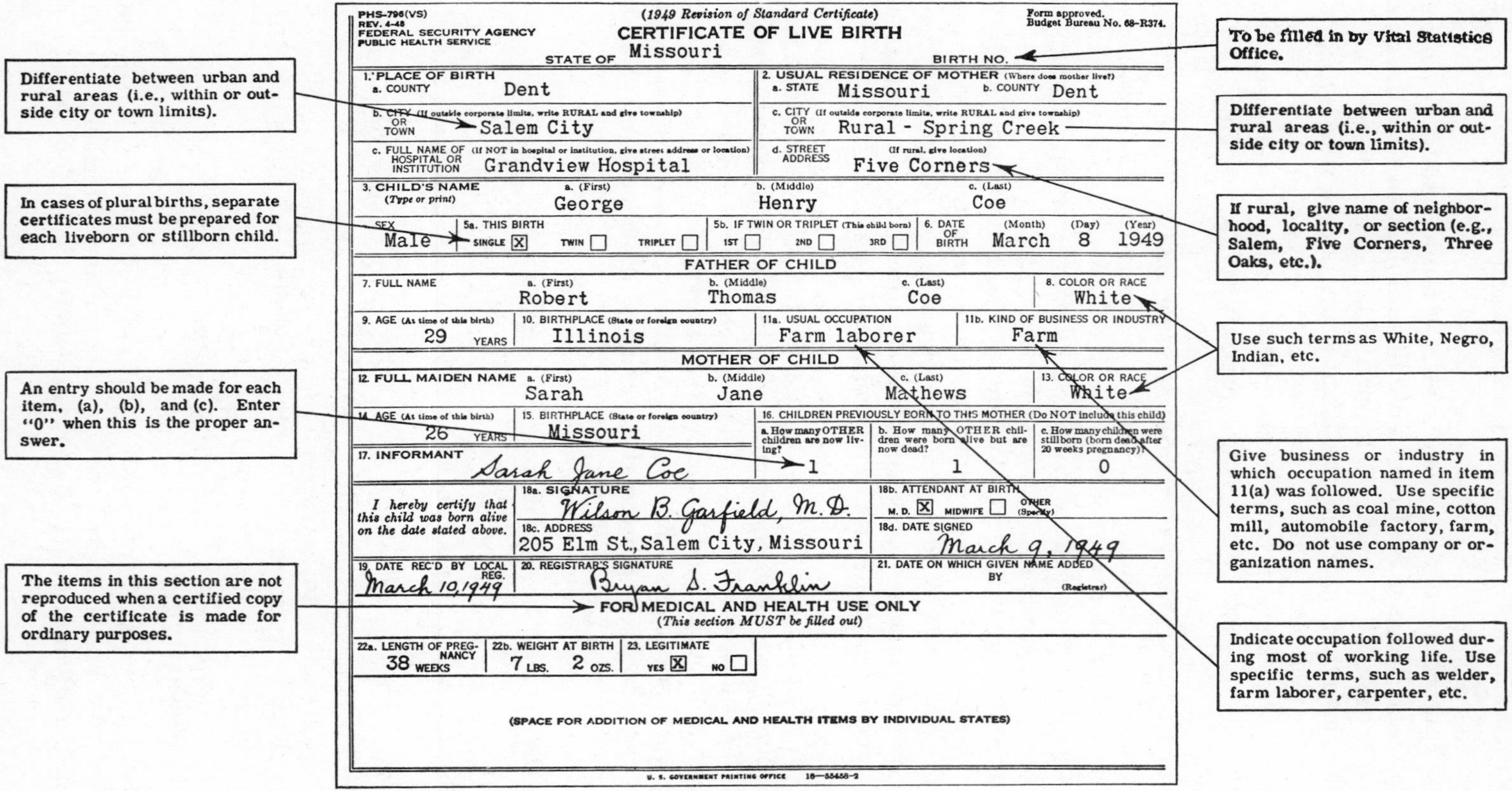
PHS-796(VS)
REV. 4-48
FEDERAL SECURITY AGENCY
PUBLIC HEALTH SERVICE

(*1949 Revision of Standard Certificate*)

CERTIFICATE OF LIVE BIRTH

Form approved.
Budget Bureau No. 68-R374.

STATE OF Missouri — BIRTH NO.

1. PLACE OF BIRTH
a. COUNTY Dent
b. CITY OR TOWN (If outside corporate limits, write RURAL and give township) Salem City
c. FULL NAME OF HOSPITAL OR INSTITUTION (If NOT in hospital or institution, give street address or location) Grandview Hospital

2. USUAL RESIDENCE OF MOTHER (Where does mother live?)
a. STATE Missouri — b. COUNTY Dent
c. CITY OR TOWN (If outside corporate limits, write RURAL and give township) Rural - Spring Creek
d. STREET ADDRESS (If rural, give location) Five Corners

3. CHILD'S NAME (*Type or print*) a. (First) George — b. (Middle) Henry — c. (Last) Coe

4. SEX Male — 5a. THIS BIRTH SINGLE [X] TWIN [ ] TRIPLET [ ] — 5b. IF TWIN OR TRIPLET (This child born) 1ST [ ] 2ND [ ] 3RD [ ] — 6. DATE OF BIRTH (Month) March (Day) 8 (Year) 1949

FATHER OF CHILD

7. FULL NAME a. (First) Robert — b. (Middle) Thomas — c. (Last) Coe — 8. COLOR OR RACE White

9. AGE (At time of this birth) 29 YEARS — 10. BIRTHPLACE (State or foreign country) Illinois — 11a. USUAL OCCUPATION Farm laborer — 11b. KIND OF BUSINESS OR INDUSTRY Farm

MOTHER OF CHILD

12. FULL MAIDEN NAME a. (First) Sarah — b. (Middle) Jane — c. (Last) Mathews — 13. COLOR OR RACE White

14. AGE (At time of this birth) 26 YEARS — 15. BIRTHPLACE (State or foreign country) Missouri

16. CHILDREN PREVIOUSLY BORN TO THIS MOTHER (Do NOT include this child)
a. How many OTHER children are now living? 1 — b. How many OTHER children were born alive but are now dead? 1 — c. How many children were stillborn (born dead after 20 weeks pregnancy)? 0

17. INFORMANT Sarah Jane Coe

I hereby certify that this child was born alive on the date stated above.
18a. SIGNATURE Wilson B. Garfield, M.D.
18b. ATTENDANT AT BIRTH M. D. [X] MIDWIFE [ ] OTHER (Specify)
18c. ADDRESS 205 Elm St., Salem City, Missouri
18d. DATE SIGNED March 9, 1949

19. DATE REC'D BY LOCAL REG. March 10, 1949 — 20. REGISTRAR'S SIGNATURE Bryan S. Franklin — 21. DATE ON WHICH GIVEN NAME ADDED BY (Registrar)

FOR MEDICAL AND HEALTH USE ONLY
(*This section MUST be filled out*)

22a. LENGTH OF PREGNANCY 38 WEEKS — 22b. WEIGHT AT BIRTH 7 LBS. 2 OZS. — 23. LEGITIMATE YES [X] NO [ ]

(SPACE FOR ADDITION OF MEDICAL AND HEALTH ITEMS BY INDIVIDUAL STATES)

U. S. GOVERNMENT PRINTING OFFICE 16—55458-2

Figure 6. The standard certificate of live birth. This is a permanent document. Type or use permanent black ink. Do not use ball-type pen.

The filing of the death certificate is the responsibility of the person who has charge of the interment of the body. The certificate has two parts: the social data and the medical data. The physician is responsible for the *medical certification,* which relates primarily to the time of death and cause of death.

The proper terminology for causes of death has been determined by a series of international conferences which has resulted in an "International List of Diseases, Injuries and Causes of Death" with suitable code. See the *Physicians' Handbook on Birth and Death Registration*(1), also the World Health Organization's *International Classification of Diseases*(2).

Every physician who attends a person in a fatal illness must determine: (a) the immediate cause of death, and (b) the underlying cause of death.

The interpretation and codification of the cause of death are the responsibility of the state department of vital statistics. The responsibility of the physician in attendance is to give a concise and exact statement of the cause of death. It is recommended that the approved terms listed in the *Standard Nomenclature of Diseases* be used(3).

All vague terms should be avoided. "Fracture from a fall" or "fracture from an automobile accident" is an incomplete statement. An exact statement would be: "Fracture of the base of the skull. Deceased was struck by a truck while crossing the street." "Cancer" is an unsatisfactory term. One must give the type and location of the lesion: for example, "carcinoma of the stomach" is more exact. Most states have prepared lists of undesirable terms of causes of death, illustrating common mistakes and pitfalls in medical certification of death. Each physician should familiarize himself with the list that is provided by his state department of vital statistics.

In certain instances, the physician is not responsible for certification of the cause of death even though he attended the patient in his last illness. In most states, for example, deaths due to violence must be certified by the coroner or by the medical examiner. If the patient has not been seen by his physician within the past ten days, then that physician cannot certify the cause of death in some states. Futhermore, if a physician who never saw the patient before is called in an emergency and finds the patient has expired or is dying, he would not certify the cause of death but would place this responsibility on the patient's family physician or on the medical examiner.

Death certificates are of incalculable value to both local and state health departments, in measuring achievement and in planning future programs for health protection. They also have an immense social value, because they enable the community to make farseeing studies of a changing population.

Details of the specific uses of death certificates have been compiled by the *Physicians' Handbook on Death and Birth Registration* as follows.

Uses of Death Certificates

Bereaved families often find themselves in urgent need of a legally recorded statement of the facts of death. The death certificate is the primary source of such information. Death certificates serve as the source of mortality statistics, which are of utmost importance to medical, health, and welfare organizations. The data are used for determining the importance of specific diseases as causes of death, for measuring the need for medical, health, and hospital services, and for evaluating progress in the prevention and control of diseases.

Following are some of the specific uses of death certificates:

1. Establishing the fact and date of death for such purposes as:
    a. Claiming life insurance carried by the decedent.
    b. Claiming pensions.
    c. Settling estates.
2. Providing certain facts about the deceased, such as:
    a. Circumstances of death, and its cause.
    b. Date or place of interment.
    c. Evidence as to age, sex, and race.
    d. Genealogical information.
3. Providing data for public health uses, such as:
    a. Determining the incidence of specific causes of death.
    b. Planning the control of communicable diseases.
    c. Investigating the nature and place of occurrence of fatal accidents.
    d. Establishing the need for health programs.
    e. Measuring the effectiveness of health services.

In addition to the uses cited above, death certificates or data derived from them are used by local, state, and national organizations, both governmental and private, for such purposes as ascertaining the best geographic distribution of their services, for program planning, and for clearing their files of the names of deceased persons.

Each certificate is checked by the local registrar, and in most instances it is then forwarded to a deputy registrar. Essential data are abstracted, and the local certificates are forwarded monthly to the

THE FUNERAL DIRECTOR IS TO COMPLETE ITEMS 1-3, 5-17, 24, 25.

To be filled in by Vital Statistics Office.

Differentiate between urban and rural areas (i.e., within or outside city or town limits).

Use such terms as White, Negro, Indian, etc.

Complete both 10(a) and 10(b) for all persons 14 years and over, even though disabled, retired, unemployed, or institutionalized.

In 10(a) give occupation followed during most of working life. Use specific terms, such as welder, farm laborer, carpenter, etc.

In 10(b) give business or industry in which occupation named in 10(a) was followed. Use specific terms, such as coal mine, cotton mill, automobile factory, farm, etc. Do not use company or organization names.

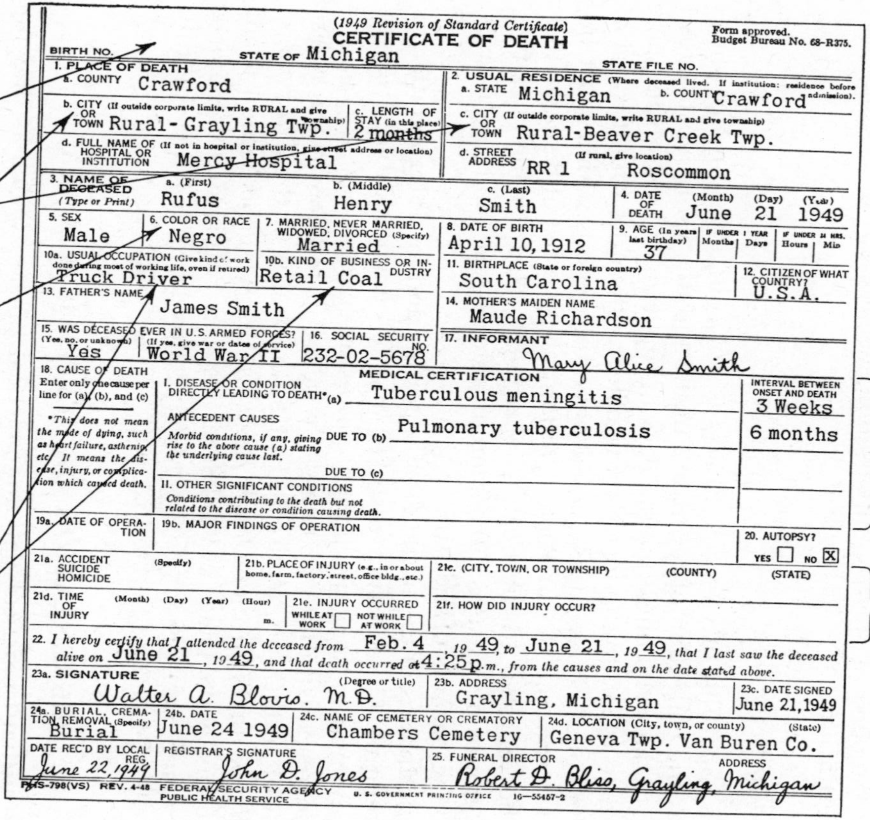

(1949 *Revision of Standard Certificate*)
CERTIFICATE OF DEATH
Form approved. Budget Bureau No. 68-R375.
BIRTH NO. STATE OF Michigan STATE FILE NO.
1. PLACE OF DEATH a. COUNTY Crawford
b. CITY OR TOWN (If outside corporate limits, write RURAL and give township) Rural-Grayling Twp.
c. LENGTH OF STAY (in this place) 2 months
d. FULL NAME OF HOSPITAL OR INSTITUTION (If not in hospital or institution, give street address or location) Mercy Hospital
2. USUAL RESIDENCE (Where deceased lived. If institution: residence before admission). a. STATE Michigan b. COUNTY Crawford
c. CITY OR TOWN (If outside corporate limits, write RURAL and give township) Rural-Beaver Creek Twp.
d. STREET ADDRESS (If rural, give location) RR 1 Roscommon
3. NAME OF DECEASED (Type or Print) a. (First) Rufus b. (Middle) Henry c. (Last) Smith
4. DATE OF DEATH (Month) June (Day) 21 (Year) 1949
5. SEX Male
6. COLOR OR RACE Negro
7. MARRIED, NEVER MARRIED, WIDOWED, DIVORCED (Specify) Married
8. DATE OF BIRTH April 10, 1912
9. AGE (In years last birthday) 37 | IF UNDER 1 YEAR Months Days | IF UNDER 24 HRS. Hours Min
10a. USUAL OCCUPATION (Give kind of work done during most of working life, even if retired) Truck Driver
10b. KIND OF BUSINESS OR INDUSTRY Retail Coal
11. BIRTHPLACE (State or foreign country) South Carolina
12. CITIZEN OF WHAT COUNTRY? U.S.A.
13. FATHER'S NAME James Smith
14. MOTHER'S MAIDEN NAME Maude Richardson
15. WAS DECEASED EVER IN U.S. ARMED FORCES? (Yes, no, or unknown) Yes (If yes, give war or dates of service) World War II
16. SOCIAL SECURITY NO. 232-02-5678
17. INFORMANT Mary Alice Smith
18. CAUSE OF DEATH Enter only one cause per line for (a), (b), and (c)
MEDICAL CERTIFICATION
I. DISEASE OR CONDITION DIRECTLY LEADING TO DEATH* (a) Tuberculous meningitis — INTERVAL BETWEEN ONSET AND DEATH 3 Weeks
ANTECEDENT CAUSES *Morbid conditions, if any, giving rise to the above cause (a) stating the underlying cause last.* DUE TO (b) Pulmonary tuberculosis — 6 months
DUE TO (c)
**This does not mean the mode of dying, such as heart failure, asthenia, etc. It means the disease, injury, or complication which caused death.*
II. OTHER SIGNIFICANT CONDITIONS *Conditions contributing to the death but not related to the disease or condition causing death.*
19a. DATE OF OPERATION 19b. MAJOR FINDINGS OF OPERATION 20. AUTOPSY? YES ☐ NO ☒
21a. ACCIDENT SUICIDE HOMICIDE (Specify) 21b. PLACE OF INJURY (e.g., in or about home, farm, factory, street, office bldg., etc.) 21c. (CITY, TOWN, OR TOWNSHIP) (COUNTY) (STATE)
21d. TIME OF INJURY (Month) (Day) (Year) (Hour) m. 21e. INJURY OCCURRED WHILE AT WORK ☐ NOT WHILE AT WORK ☐ 21f. HOW DID INJURY OCCUR?
22. *I hereby certify that I attended the deceased from* Feb. 4, 1949, *to* June 21, 1949, *that I last saw the deceased alive on* June 21, 1949, *and that death occurred at* 4:25 p.*m., from the causes and on the date stated above.*
23a. SIGNATURE (Degree or title) Walter A. Blovis. M.D. 23b. ADDRESS Grayling, Michigan 23c. DATE SIGNED June 21, 1949
24a. BURIAL, CREMATION, REMOVAL (Specify) Burial 24b. DATE June 24 1949 24c. NAME OF CEMETERY OR CREMATORY Chambers Cemetery 24d. LOCATION (City, town, or county) (State) Geneva Twp. Van Buren Co.
DATE REC'D BY LOCAL REG. June 22, 1949 REGISTRAR'S SIGNATURE John D. Jones 25. FUNERAL DIRECTOR ADDRESS Robert D. Bliss, Grayling, Michigan
FHS-798(VS) REV. 4-48 FEDERAL SECURITY AGENCY PUBLIC HEALTH SERVICE U. S. GOVERNMENT PRINTING OFFICE 16—55457-2

THE PHYSICIAN, MEDICAL EXAMINER, OR CORONER IS TO COMPLETE ITEMS 4, 18-23.

(See pp. 4-14 for further discussion of what should be entered here.)

In part I, give the sequence of events that led to death, specifying last the underlying cause which initiated the train of events. Do not report symptoms or mode of dying.

In part II, report other important diseases or conditions, if any, that contributed to the death but were not related to the causes given in part I above.

Complete items 21(a) - 21(f) if death was due to violence or external causes.

Figure 7. The standard certificate of death. This is a permanent document. Type or use permanent black ink. Do not use ball-type pen.

state department of vital statistics. The responsibility for the compilation, analysis, and interpretation of vital statistics rests with the state registrar of vital statistics. These certificates are deposited in fireproof vaults in the state archives.

Summaries of the statistical data are forwarded by each state to the United States Office of Vital Statistics for nation-wide interpretation. The local registrars are appointed officially by the state registrar and receive a small compensation, usually 25 to 50 cents for each certificate.

Morbidity Reporting

The reporting of cases of illness is not conducted on the same basis as the collection of records of births and deaths. In most states, the physician who encounters a case of reportable disease sends an immediate report to the local health officer. Often the report is made by telephone with a supplementary written report, which must be signed by the physician. Each state formulates a list of diseases that must be reported to the health department. This list includes two major groups of diseases: (a) communicable diseases and (b) diseases due to the hazards of industry.

Descriptions of the methods of reporting and the interpretation of data relating to industrial diseases and to communicable diseases will be found in their appropriate places in this text.

The responsibilities of every physician in relation to the registration of births and deaths are set forth clearly in the *Physicians' Handbook on Birth and Death Registration*, which is issued to all physicians by the Office of Vital Statistics, U.S. Public Health Service. Each practicing physician should have this handbook in a readily accessible place and be familiar with its contents.

PRESENTATION OF STATISTICAL DATA

To utilize statistical data for practical purposes such as drawing conclusions, making recommendations, or taking action to prevent or to treat a disease, it is first necessary to put the original data in a form that is intelligible, meaningful, and usable.

Tabulation of Data

The collection, tabulation, and correlation of vital data, or of clinical and laboratory observations, constitute at best a slow and laborious process. When a large series of data or case records—more than 500 units—is to be studied, the information should be coded, placed on a standard punch card, and analyzed by a standard automatic tabulating machine.

A clinical or laboratory study of 100 to 500 units may be tabulated effectively on the Gregg type of simplified punch card. This is a 4-by-6-in. stiff card with some 62 holes in the margin. Each item to be assembled is assigned a hole on the card; if the item is positive, this hole is given a special punch. The cards are assembled, and a knitting needle is passed through the hole that will give the desired information. If the punched cards are then shaken out, all positive cards are released.

Tabular information should always be simply presented and clearly summarized. Many splendid scientific papers are rendered uninteresting and lose much of their effectiveness because the data are presented in too great detail, without suitable analysis and without proper summarization.

Graphical Presentation

Certain more or less traditional methods have been devised to present statistical data in a simple and graphic form. All of these methods have distinct limitations. The most direct method of presentation of data is in simple summary tables, but most readers are unwilling to go to the trouble of studying tables in detail.

The usual order in reading an article in a medical journal is to read (a) the title, (b) the author's name and his affiliation, (c) the conclusion, and glance at (d) the graphic presentation. Tables are always read as a last resort—an evidence of great interest. Thus the author is driven to present his pertinent data in a graphic manner.

The graph is a device used frequently for the graphic presentation of vital statistics as well as clinical and laboratory data. It has many limitations: it gives an incomplete impression, for it cannot tell the whole story; it must be used properly or it will distort the data and give a false picture. The graph must be correct in form as well as in detail; it must be legible and clear, telling its whole message at a glance. Tables must be studied slowly and carefully, for they require analysis and interpretation. A graph should drive home the point to be presented at once; thus it must be so constructed that it calls for no analysis or special interpretation.

There are a few simple rules that should be followed in presenting a good graph:

1. The graph must be simple and legible.

2. Not more than three, preferably only two, elements should be compared in a single graph. For example, in a line graph, there should never be more than four trend lines.

3. The graph should be a simple summary of tabulated data. The tables should be available for those who wish to analyze the data in greater detail.

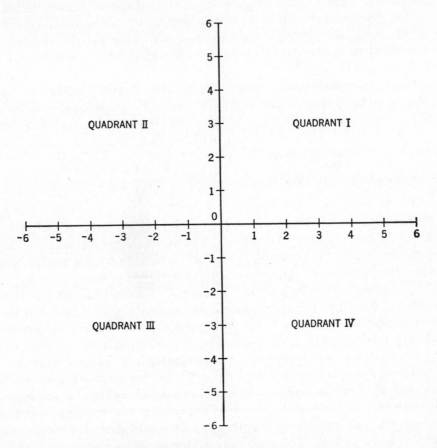

Figure 8. The basic form of the graph.

Some Principles in Graphing

The principle of the graph is the plotting of related data on two axes, which are formed by the intersection of a horizontal with a perpendicular line. The horizontal line is called the abscissa, and the perpendicular line the ordinate. This gives four quadrants (see Fig. 8).

Quadrant I, the positive quadrant, is the most frequently used in presenting medical data. Zero for all quadrants is at the intersection of the two lines.

The Line Graph

In the simplest graphs, two variables are plotted as a series of points, and a line is drawn connecting them. This is called the line graph. Conventionally, the passage of time is plotted on the abscissa, traveling from left to right. Frequency, or intensity, is plotted on the ordinate, beginning with zero.

The best illustration of a traditional line graph is the temperature and pulse chart of the hospitalized patient. A hospital chart of a patient's temperature illustrates the chief characteristics, the essential values, and the intrinsic weakness of the line graph.

The most common mistake in a line graph is that the baseline does not indicate *zero*. Unless zero is indicated on the graph, the presentation obviously is misleading.

Illustrations of simple line graphs comparing two sets of data are presented in Figures 1 and 2 in Chapter 2.

Shading and crosshatching may be utilized in bringing out the contrast of comparisons of values in the line graph.

Histogram

A histogram is a columnar diagram which has a purpose similar to the line graph, but under some circumstances it gives a more accurate picture of the facts. It is presented as a series of perpendicular rectangles and is used effectively in presenting cumulative frequency distribution. An example of a histogram is given in Figure 9.

The data in this histogram might be presented as a line graph by drawing a line through the top of each rectangle, and the presentation as a line graph would be a valid one but not as informative as the histogram. Combined cumulative frequencies may be presented in a histogram with effect.

Bar Diagram

The bar diagram contains no element of time. It is used chiefly to compare incidence of like phenomena at any given period of time. For example, a comparison of the death rate from pulmonary tuberculosis in ten large cities in the United States during the year 1960 would be represented traditionally by a series of horizontal rectangles. Volume

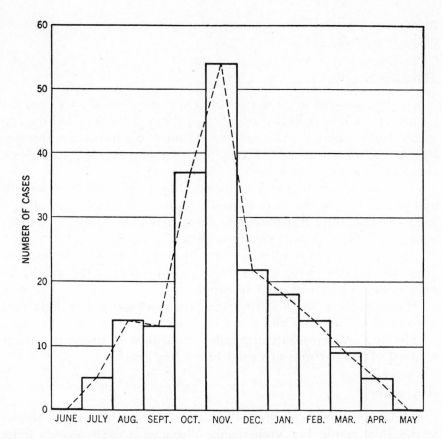

Figure 9. Chart illustrating the use of the histogram. Monthly incidence of cases of primary atypical "virus" pneumonia occurring in a student health service.

is indicated on the abscissa. Usually the rectangle of greatest length is placed at the top of the chart with graduations in series to the bottom.

Special Graphic Devices

Spot maps and shaded maps are frequently utilized in the interpertation of epidemiologic data. They have a special and definite place in graphic presentation.

Percentage distribution of variables is often presented graphically as a "pie diagram": a circle representing the whole is divided into component parts, each section representing one of the variables. Usually shading is employed to emphasize the important elements.

The pie diagram does not give a true picture and is not good graphics, but it is a useful device in health education.

The "pine-tree graph" is a special device used in comparing a series of paired events. It utilizes quadrants I and II. For example, age distribution of males and females in a given population may be presented as a series of left and right bar diagrams, or rectangles (see Fig. 10).

The "three-dimensional graph" has a special place in the presentation of vital data. It is a combination of a series of flat graphs superimposed upon one another, giving the conception of depth and perspective.

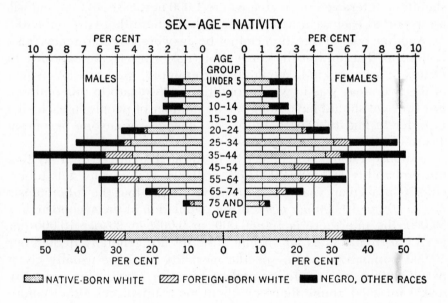

Figure 10. Pine-tree graph. *(Kips Bay-Yorkville*, 1940, edited by Earl L. Koos. The Department of Public Health and Preventive Medicine, Cornell University Medical College, New York, 1942.)

Rates and Ratios

As an alternative to graphs, a numerical mode of presentation is used by many authors. There are as many kinds of graphs as there are different kinds of tabulations and numerical summary statistics. No one method is "best" for all study situations, although there is usually a "method of choice" in a given situation. The choice of an appropriate summary statistic is by no means obvious, and the medical literature is full of examples of poor choices leading to obscurity, confusion, and misleading conclusions.

Rates and ratios are the most frequently encountered summary statistics in the medical literature, and these indices have often been badly used. There is nothing terribly complicated about these simple indices. A little background, experience, and common sense will obviate many mistakes.

All mathematics originally started with counting. We still count events in vital statistics and usually call the count a "frequency." There is something to be learned from frequencies. If, for example, we are planning the location of a new tuberculosis sanatorium, we should be interested in an area where 1,000 new cases of tuberculosis are reported each year as against another where there are only 100.

Another type of question cannot be answered by frequency. This is the sort that implies the concept of "risk," that is, the exposure to factors of a given kind. We might, for example, want to know which of the two areas was in worse condition with regard to tuberculosis. For this, we should have to know the number of people in each area in order to find the "probability" or "chance" of anyone becoming a case of tuberculosis in a year.

Suppose 1,000,000 people live in the first area. We then say that the probability is 1,000/1,000,000, or 0.001, that anyone gets tuberculosis in a given year. More usually, we say that the tuberculosis *rate* is 10 per 10,000 *per year*. If the population of the second area is 50,000, the rate there is 100/50,000, or 0.002, or 20 per 10,000 per year. (Morbidity rates for specific diseases are generally quoted per 10,000 population, while specific mortality rates are usually given per 100,000, and "crude" mortality rates per 1,000. This generally makes for good, round figures without too many places either before or after the decimal.)

It will be noted that the frequency and the rate furnish different types of information and answer different questions. The first area furnishes the most cases of tuberculosis and will fill the larger sanatorium. It may be, however, that tne second area needs sanatorium care more than the first. It might be a better place to expend our efforts in control of tuberculosis.

It will also be noted that the rate is per year. In general, rates involve the idea of time: a year for general phenomena, but sometimes longer or shorter periods for events that move slower or faster.

Similar to a rate, but not involving time, is a quotient sometimes called a rate but, more accurately, a *ratio*. Such is the "case-fatality ratio" in which we divide events (deaths) by events (cases of the disease) without regard to the length of time involved. It is generally accepted, for instance, that the case fatality in typhoid fever is 0.1, or 10 per 100.

The following questions now arise:

1. Would you expect every sample of ten typhoid cases to show just one death? Even if the treatment were just the same?

2. What would happen to a case-fatality figure if only a small proportion of all cases were reported? May one infer that the published case fatality for measles in the average city is correct?

3. Would case fatality vary with the severity of the disease? What sort of measles case is most usually brought into a children's hospital? Is it possible that the hospital's measles case-fatality ratio does not represent the general condition for the community as a whole?

4. Should case fatality be based on: (a) cases hospitalized, (b) cases clinically diagnosable, (c) cases proved only by laboratory, or (d) all cases which could conceivably be the disease in question, during an epidemic? How may one secure a case-fatality estimate for, say, poliomyelitis?

One thing to be remembered from this discussion is that rates and ratios are fractions and that fractions have numerators and denominators. If either varies, so does the fraction.

If one is going to compare two conditions by means of rates (or ratios), it is extremely important to make sure that the denominators are comparable. There is a fallacy called the "hidden classification," which is a very hard thing to avoid and sometimes even difficult to discern when it is present. For instance, one may find that the tuberculosis rate among policemen is 100 per 10,000, while in the general white population of the state it is only 50. The enumerator may have been careful to make the comparison with general white population, because most of the policemen are white. Perhaps one is comparing, as he should, the rates for white policemen with general white rates only.

The denominator for white policemen — that is, all white policemen — contains, however, a much heavier proportion of Irish than does the entire white population. If white policemen show higher tuberculosis rates than expected, is it due to their occupation or to the fact that they are Irish and may have a higher tuberculosis incidence? On the other hand, before deciding that Irish have more tuberculosis than other groups, one should be sure that it is not because so many of them are policemen and because, perhaps, policemen have more tuberculosis. In other words, there are at least two factors in the denominator which might be connected with variations in the tuberculosis rate: occupation and nationality. There may be others which must be carefully investigated, such as age and length of service on the force. If, for example, a given occupation leads to a disease, it may be that this occurs early in susceptible individuals and that employees of long standing will have a lower rate than do newcomers.

In order to compare two groups, one must try to have them comparable in everything but the one variable being measured. We do not expect an old and a young population to have the same death rate; we do not expect a white population and a colored population to produce a similar incidence of tuberculosis; an army camp will not have as many births per thousand population as will a suburban town. Yet we sometimes see weight laid, on comparison of two towns by means of crude death rates (total deaths per year per 1,000 population) in total disregard of the fact that these towns differ from each other in every respect that has been mentioned as well as in many others.

Some Commonly Used Ratios

Certain terms are commonly utilized in the expression of summaries of vital data for a given community or state. The terms that are recommended by the National Office of Vital Statistics are as follows:

1. Crude Birth Rate. The number of live births reported in the calendar year per 1,000 actual or estimated population at the middle of the year.

2. Crude Death Rate. The number of deaths reported in the calendar year per 1,000 actual or estimated population at the middle of the year.

3. Age-specific Birth Rate. The number of births to women of a certain age (e.g., 15 to 45 years) per 1,000 women of the same specified age groups of the whole population.

4. Age-specific Death Rate. The number of deaths in a specified age group (e.g., 25 to 35 years) per 1,000 population in the same specified age groups.

5. Standardized Death Rate. The number of deaths which would have occurred per 1,000 in some standard population (e.g., the population of England and Wales in 1901) if its age-specific death rates were the same as that of a given community. Method of computing:

$$\frac{\text{Sum of} \left(\begin{array}{c}\text{Standard population} \\ \text{in each age group}\end{array}\right) \times \left(\begin{array}{c}\text{Specific death rates in each} \\ \text{corresponding age group of} \\ \text{the given community}\end{array}\right)}{\text{Total standard population}} \times 1{,}000$$

Five age groups may be selected, namely, under 12 months, 1 to 19 years inclusive, 20 to 39 years inclusive, 40 to 59 years inclusive, and 60 years and over.

Various details of the methods of estimating rates by a standard population method will be found in A. B. Hill's *The Principles of Medical Statistics*(5).

6. Specific-cause-of-death Rate. The number of deaths from a specific disease (e.g., measles, pneumonia) per 100,000 population. Method of computing:

$$\frac{\text{Number of deaths from a specific disease}}{\text{Total population}} \times 100{,}000$$

7. Maternal-mortality Rate. The number of deaths ascribed to puerperal causes per 1,000 live births. (In some instances "total births" including stillbirths is used rather than "live births." However, on account of the great variation in stillbirth reporting, "live births" is the usual basis.) Method of computing:

$$\frac{\text{Number of maternal deaths}}{\text{Total number of live births}} \times 1{,}000$$

8. Infant-mortality Rate. The number of deaths of infants under 1 year of age during the calendar year per 1,000 live births during that same period. Method of computing:

$$\frac{\text{Number of infant deaths under 1 year}}{\text{Total number of live births}} \times 1{,}000$$

9. Neonatal-mortality Rate. The number of deaths of infants under 1 month of age per 1,000 live births. Method of computing.

$$\frac{\text{Number of infant deaths under 1 month}}{\text{The number of live births}} \times 1,000$$

10. Morbidity Rate. The number of reported cases of a given disease (e.g., tuberculosis, whooping cough) per 100,000 (10,000 or 1,000) population. Method of computing:

$$\frac{\text{Number of cases of a given disease}}{\text{Total population}} \times 100,000 \ (10,000 \text{ or } 1,000)$$

11. Case-fatality Rate. The number of deaths ascribed to a specified disease or condition per 100 (or 1,000) reported cases of the same disease or condition. Method of computing:

$$\frac{\text{Number of deaths from a specified disease or condition}}{\text{Reported cases of the specified disease or condition}} \times 100 \ (\text{or } 1,000)$$

Summary Statistics for Measurements

Three types of variables are used in medical studies. Sometimes the variables are described by verbal categories and at other times by numbers.

1. When there are only two verbal categories (dichotomous classification) such as lived-died or cured-not-cured, rates and ratios are ordinarily used to summarize the data.

2. When the study employs *metric* variables (i.e., numerical measurements such as physical measurements of length or weight), a different set of summary statistics is used. The arithmetic mean or average is the principal tool for summarizing metric data, but a number of auxilliary statistics are also used.

3. Between dichotomous classification and metric data is a wide "borderland" consisting of ordered verbal categories (e.g., minor, moderate, severe) and numerical indices that are not genuine metrics. A statistical technique called ridit analysis is often useful with borderland variables(6).

Some of the common summary devices for measurement variables are defined below.

1. Frequency distribution. A statistical table constructed from a series of observations, showing the number of observations in each

classification group. For example, a table showing the number of deaths occurring in each age group.

2. Arithmetic mean or average. The sum total of values recorded in a series of observations, divided by the number of observations.

3. Median. The center value in a series of observations, when the observations are ranged in order from highest to lowest.

4. Mode. The value which occurs most frequently in a series of observations.

5. Range. The distance between the lowest and highest values recorded in a series of observations.

6. Average deviation from the median (A.D.). The arithmetic mean of all the differences between each observation in a series and the median of the series, the differences being added without regard to their sign, i.e., whether an observation is above or below the median of the series.

7. Standard deviation (S.D.). The square root of the sum of the squares of the differences between the observations in a series and the mean of the series divided by the degrees of freedom.

8. Standard error (S.E.). A measure of the sampling error of a statistical quantity, such as the mean, standard deviation, percentage, which shows the variability of that quantity when repeated samples are drawn at random from the same universe of observations.

9. Probable error (P.E.). The probable error of a value is 0.6745 times its standard error.

Illustrations of the Use of These Terms. We have selected the incubation period, in days, of ten cases of malaria and ten cases of typhoid fever, which are taken from a large series.

The data are as follows: Ten cases of typhoid fever with known incubation periods of 5, 11, 32, 8, 6, 21, 15, 12, 14, and 16 days, respectively. Ten cases of malaria taken at random had the following incubation periods: 15, 12, 14, 10, 16, 15, 17, 14, 15, and 12 days each.

The data are tabulated in columns A and A_1 of Table 1.

The mean of each series, according to our definition, is the total divided by the number of observations. It is 14 days in each instance.

The median is the midpoint in each series. In Table 1, the median incubation period for typhoid fever is 13 days; for malaria it is 14 1/2 days.

The deviation from the median is determined in Table 1 in columns B and B_1. In the typhoid fever series it is 13 days $\pm$ A.D. 5.6, and in malaria, 14.5 days $\pm$ A.D. 1.6.

The range in the typhoid fever series is between 5 and 32 days, or 27 days; in malaria it lies between 10 and 17 days, or 7 days. The mode is not selected in a small series such as we are considering. It is only of import in a much larger series of data. In the malaria series, it is 15, e.g., the number that is observed most frequently in the series.

TABLE 1

Incubation Periods of Ten Cases of Malaria and Typhoid Fever

Typhoid Fever		Malaria	
A	B	A_1	B_1
Days	Median deviation	Days	Median deviation
5	− 8.0	10	−4.5
6	− 7.0	12	−2.5
8	− 5.0	12	−2.5
11	− 2.0	14	−0.5
12	− 1.0	14	−0.5
(13 median)		(14.5 median)	
14	+ 1.0	15	+0.5
15	+ 2.0	15	+0.5
16	+ 3.0	15	+0.5
21	+ 8.0	16	+1.5
32	+19.0	17	+2.5
Total 140	56.0	140	16.0
Mean 14		14	
A.D. from the median	5.6		1.6

Standard Deviation from the Mean. The standard deviation about the mean, or average, is a measure of dispersion. In any series it is the square root of the sum of the squares of each deviation from the mean divided by the degrees of freedom. For individual series the degrees of freedom will be one less than the number of observations.

The steps in the determination of the standard deviation are:

1. Determine the mean, or average.
2. Determine the deviation of each number in the series from the mean.
3. Square these deviations.
4. Total the column of the squares of the deviations.

5. Divide by the number of observations minus one.

6. Take the square root of this number.

The result is the standard deviation. A computational shortcut is available(7).

In Table 2, the standard deviation of the series of incubation periods of typhoid fever and malaria has been determined by proceeding step by step as we have just described.

Thus, the standard deviation in this series is 8.0 days for typhoid fever, and 2.2 days for malaria.

TABLE 2

Determination of Standard Deviation

(INCUBATION PERIODS OF TYPHOID FEVER AND MALARIA IN DAYS)

	Typhoid Fever				*Malaria*	
Days	A *Deviation* *from mean*	A_1 *Square of* *deviation*		*Days*	B *Deviation* *from mean*	B_1 *Square of* *deviation*
5	− 9	81		10	−4	16
6	− 8	64		12	−2	4
8	− 6	36		12	−2	4
11	− 3	9		14	−0	0
12	− 2	4		14	−0	0
14	− 0	0		15	+1	1
15	+ 1	1		15	+1	1
16	+ 2	4		15	+1	1
21	+ 7	49		16	+2	4
32	+18	324		17	+3	9
Total 140		572		140		40
Mean 14				14		

Sum of squares
  divided by the
  degrees of freedom(9)
		63.56				4.44

Square root of this quantity		8.0				±2.2

The standard deviation and the standard error are conceptually similar. It is customary, however, to use the term standard deviation when referring to the original observations (as in the above example) and to use the term standard error when referring to calculated quantities such as averages. Ordinarily the standard error of a mean is estimated from the standard deviation of the observations by dividing by the square root of the number of observations going into the mean. For example, the standard error of the average incubation period for typhoid fever would be $8.0/ \sqrt{10} = 2.5$. When observations are *independent*, the precision of an average is greater than that of an individual observation, and hence the standard error of the mean is less than the standard deviation of an individual observation.

For reasons to be explained later, standard deviations and standard errors are often multiplied by a factor of about 2 and reported in this way: Mean ± 2 (standard error). Unfortunately, the plus-or-minus symbol, $\pm$, is used in other ways so when this notation is used in a scientific paper the reader must sometimes guess which convention the author is using.

INTERPRETATION OF STATISTICS

Scientific Inference

The medical literature is riddled with examples of incorrect, misleading, and pointless applications of statistical methods. This unhappy state of affairs is often blamed on the statistical methods—the arithmethic is too extensive, the mathematical formulas are too abstruse, the principles are too complex. However, more often than not the root of the trouble goes much deeper: The investigators simply do not understand the process of scientific inference—the procedure for going from data to scientific conclusions. Since statistical methods are merely tools that are useful in scientific inference, they cannot be effectively used without an understanding of the procedure for drawing scientific conclusions.

The basic rule for statistical inference is the Galilean rule: A theory must fit the facts. Although the rule is easy to state, it is hard to put into practice. There are three phases in the application of the Galilean rule. First, there is the task of putting the theory in a testable form—in a form which permits definite and unambiguous predictions of the observations. Second, there is the task of collecting data adequate in quality and quantity relevant to the theory under test. Finally, there is the task of testing the agreement between theory and fact in some systematic and explicit fashion.

At first sight the testing phase might seem simple—either the theoretic predictions agree with the observations or they do not. However, in any scientific study the data itself shows variability. This ubiquitous phenomenon of variability goes by several names (e.g., sampling variation, experimental error, biological variability).

However whatever name is used, the investigator faces the basic problem of every scientific study: In a large series of observations, the reports show differences and inconsistencies. Consequently, the investigator can neither reject nor accept a theory in any *absolute* sense. He therefore must learn to think in terms of probabilities or odds. He can reject a theory as unlikely, or he can show that the theory accords reasonably well with the facts. There are no certainties or absolute truths in science.

The procedures employed in scientific inference are very different from those used in making inferences in formal logic or mathematics. This point is sometimes confused, because both logic and mathematics are used in the theoretic phase of scientific inference. For example, if a theory employs several postulates (i.e., statements assumed to be true), the implications can be explored by formal logic. However, formal logic is inadequate in the face of variation and probabilities. Hence as soon as data are introduced, the tools of statistical inference are necessary.

There is one peculiar feature of scientific inference that leads to many misunderstandings, although the basic concept is simple. Scientific inference has a negative or "inverted" structure. Instead of proving directly that a given hypothesis is likely, the investigator shows that other explanations or theories are unlikely. Since there are always numerous choices, this process of elimination in a scientific argument tends to be long and tedious. Because the argument has many steps, there is a risk of leaving gaps or loopholes. Hence it is important to proceed carefully and systematically, with a clear idea of both the task and the obstacles. It is the failure to appreciate this process — not the difficulties with statistical methods — that brings disappointment to many medical investigators.

Steps in a Scientific Argument

The following study of lung cancer in women(8) is used to illustrate the steps of a scientific argument. The working hypothesis was: Cigarette smoking increases the risk of epidermoid lung cancer in women. The data were obtained by interviews and mailed questionnaires; 196 women with histologically confirmed lung cancer and 1,304 women with cancers or benign tumors at sites other than the respiratory or upper alimentary tract participated in the survey. A further comparison of smoking habits could be made with a nationwide sample survey conducted by the United States Bureau of the Census.

TABLE 3

Distribution According to Amount Smoked and Histologic Type

COMPARISON OF OBSERVED AND EXPECTED NUMBER

Smoking Status (No. of cigarettes per day)	Epidermoid Carcinomas		Adenocarcinomas		Anaplastic Carcinomas		Unclassified Carcinomas	
	Observed	Expected*	Observed	Expected*	Observed	Expected*	Observed	Expected*
Nonsmoker	16	30	29	32	5	10	9	7
Smoker	25	11	12	9	9	4	0	2
1 to 9	3	4	4	3	2	2	0	1
10 to 20	10	6	7	5	3	2	0	1
21	12	1	1	1	4	0	0	0

*On basis of smoking habits of controls of comparable ages.

A portion of the data (the distribution by amount smoked and histo-logic type for the lung cancer patients) is shown in Table 3.

If the working hypothesis were correct, the epidermoid series should show a large excess of cigarette smokers, especially in the pack-a-day (20 per day) and higher consumption categories. Inspection of Table 3 shows a striking difference between the epidermoid and adenocarcinoma series. The epidermoid series also shows a marked departure from the "expected" numbers, which were obtained from the 1,304 controls by a procedure that will be explained later.

Mere inspection does not entitle us to jump to the conclusion that the working hypothesis is correct. To reach that conclusion it is first necessary to rule out all other hypotheses that might possibly account for the result. The first step is to detail those hypotheses. The possible explanations fall into four broad categories:

I.   The results are due to sampling variation alone (i.e., the kind of differences that will occur even when two samples are drawn from the same population).

II. The results are due to artifacts or biases, i.e., the measuring instrument (here a questionnaire), or the method of obtaining the sample, or to other procedures used in the collection and processing of the data.

III.   The results are due to "accepted" factors, e.g., such factors as age and sex in epidemiologic studies (for which extensive evidence of relationships already exists).

IV.   The results are due to "proposed" factors without, i.e., factors that have been suggested in the literature but without extensive evidence.

To build a scientific demonstration for the working hypothesis, a process of elimination is applied to the above counterhypotheses. In other words, we eliminate those hypotheses which are highly unlikely in view of the basic data and the precautions taken in collecting the data. In so doing, we are employing the principle of scientific simplicity (Occam's Razor), i.e., we do not propose a new hypothesis if a simpler explanation is at hand. Each step presents a challenge, and an appropriate procedure (often statistical) is needed to meet this challenge. Clearly the process of scientific inference is more than simply jumping to conclusions!

The following summary from Wynder *et al.*(8) illustrates the process of elimination utilized in the lung cancer study.

I. The statistical methods (significance tests) used here indicate that it is extremely unlikely that the differences between the smoking habits of the women in the series of cases of epidermoid lung cancer and those of the women in the comparison series [Table 4] are due to sampling variation alone. On the other hand it is not unlikely that the differences between the adenocarcinoma series and the control series and between the control series and the national sample are due to sampling variation alone.

II. A statistical examination of the basic data suggests that it is unlikely that there are sizable biases or artifacts (slight biases could not account for the markedly different smoking habits found in the epidermoid series):

a. It is likely that there are sizable biases in the measuring instrument because two different instruments (an interview and a mailed questionnaire) were used, but the results were very similar in both cases.

b. It is unlikely that there were sizable biases in the histologic classifications because an independent review by expert pathologists gave similar classifications.

c. It is unlikely that there were sizable biases in the selection of the epidermoid series because such a bias should also have appeared in the adenocarcinoma series. The adenocarcinoma series provides an especially good control series because the two types of cancer can be distinguished only by a microscopical examination of lung tissue. This is a unique feature of this study.

d. It is unlikely that there were sizable biases in the selection of the comparison series. The similarity of the adenocarcinoma series, the control series and the national sample affords a striking validation of the sample—a degree of validation that is rarely possible in epidemiologic studies.

III. Statistical analysis of the data reveals that it is highly unlikely that the results are due to age. Sex is not a variable since all the subjects in the primary series are women. As a precaution several different analyses have been run adjusting for age only, age and education and so forth. All these different analyses lead to the same conclusion.

IV. A strong effort was made to include in the interviews all the factors that have been suggested as bearing on the etiology of cancer, such as occupational exposure, air pollution (residence) and previous medical history. No demonstrable difference was found between the series for these factors. This does not mean that these factors play no part, because with relatively short series it is only possible to detect very strong environmental factors. However, it does mean that it is highly unlikely that the results are due to these factors alone or to correlations between these factors and smoking.

As a result of this process of elimination, we are left with the hypothesis that cigarette smoking substantially increases the risk of epidermoid lung cancer in women. In accordance with scientific principles, we are entitled to assert this hypothesis as a "posit" (as the most probable hypothesis on the basis of our evidence). This is all that can be demonstrated in any field of science, including the physical sciences. We note that we are unable to reject the hypothesis that cigarette smoking does not increase the risk of adenocarcinoma of the lung in women.

Hypotheses Based on Sampling Variation

The first step of a scientific inference is the elimination of hypotheses based on sampling variation. The statistical techniques currently employed for this purpose are called *significance tests* or *test of hypotheses*. The rationale for these statistical methods employs the characteristic "inverted" or negative argument. The general approach is as follows:

1. A testable hypothesis is set up which involves only sampling variation (or experimental error). This hypothesis is often called a null hypothesis, because it postulates that there are no real relationships.
2. On the basis of the null hypothesis, the value of a statistic is predicted in a probability sense. In other words, a theoretical statement is derived of the form: If the null hypothesis is true, then most of the time the observed value should fall in a specified range (e.g., between zero and 3.86).
3. The statistic is then calculated from the sample.
4. If the statistic falls outside of the specified range, then the null hypothesis is rejected.

In practice the investigator usually does not have to take the theoretical step himself, because this has already been carried through in the standard statistical tables. He has only to locate the proper "critical number" (e.g., 3.86) in the table and to compare his calculated statistic with this number. A variety of significance tests are now available. These include the chi-square test, the student *t*-test and *F*-test, the sign test, and many others.

In using significance tests, the investigator should be aware that he is controlling—not eliminating—his risk of reaching an erroneous conclusion. In medical research the 5 per cent (or 1 per cent) probability level is generally used. This means that there is only 1 chance in 20 (or in 100) that the null hypothesis will be erroneously rejected (i.e., rejected if it is true). Thus the risk of a "false positive" conclusion (also called type I error) is controlled if the investigator uses significance tests in analyzing his data. There is also a risk of a "false negative" conclusion (type II error). In other words, there is a chance that a real effect will not be distinguishable from the effects of sampling variation. The second risk can be quite large if the number of observations is small. For this reason it is incorrect to argue from a nonsignificant statistical test that there are no real effects in the data. We can only say that no real effects were demonstrable.

To illustrate the use of significance tests, the chi-square test will be applied to the lung cancer data. For this test we first make a 2 x 2 contingency table from the original data, then border the 2 x 2 table with row and column totals:

Series	Nonsmokers	Smokers	Totals
Epidermoid carcinoma	$a = 16$	$b = 25$	$T_e = 41$
Adenocarcinoma	$c = 29$	$d = 12$	$T_a = 41$
Total	$T_s = 45$	$T_n = 37$	$T = 82$

We then apply the chi-square test (with Yates' correction) by using the formula below.

$$\text{Chi-square} = X^2 = \frac{\left(\mid ad-bc \mid - \frac{T}{2} \right)^2 T}{T_s T_n T_e T_a} = \frac{(\mid 16 \times 12 - 29 \times 25 \mid - 41)^2 \times 82}{(45 \times 37)(41 \times 41)}$$

The vertical bars in the above formula are "absolute signs" and tell us to disregard the sign of the quantity between the bars:

$$X^2 = \frac{(\uparrow 533 \uparrow - 41)^2 \, 82}{(1{,}665)(1{,}681)} = 7.09$$

The calculated value exceeds the critical number for the 5 per cent level (3.84) and also the 1 per cent level (6.64) that is found in the chi-square table for one degree of freedom and corresponding probability levels. Therefore we reject the null hypothesis that sampling variation alone can account for the difference. Note that the statistically significant result does not give any license to jump at once to the desired conclusion – many more steps are needed. We might also note that since any data constitute a sample, it is always possible to frame a counterhypothesis based on sampling variation.

The chi-square test used above does not take account of the amount smoked. However, there are other significance tests which make better use of the data(9). The choice of statistical method is not always obvious, and in some studies it is necessary to construct a test to meet specific requirements.

Most standard statistical tests are variants of one basic rule – the two-sigma rule. If μ and σ are the *true* mean and standard deviation of a population and if y is an observation drawn at random from the population, then the two-sigma rule tells us that about 95 per cent of the time the value of y will lie between $\mu - 2\sigma$ and $\mu + 2\sigma$. Although this rule is often considered a property of one kind of population (the normal distribution), it holds for most populations encountered in actual research. Because of the two-sigma rule, the range between the arithmetic mean -2 standard deviations and the arithmetic mean $+2$ standard deviations will include roughly 95 per cent of a population.

Hypotheses Based on Artifacts

Although significance tests control the risk of being misled by random fluctuations of sampling variation, they do not necessarily provide protection against consistent or systematic effects that arise from the way in which the data were collected or processed (i.e., artifacts). The main safeguard against artifacts is good design. If the investigator can show that he has taken design precautions which eliminate or control a given artifact, then critical counterhypothesis based on this artifact can be ruled out.

An example of a device to control a potentially serious artifact is the "blind" or "double blind technique" that is widely used in clinical trials of new drugs. In a double blind trial, neither the patient nor the doctor doing the evaluation knows which of the agents under test has been given. The practical procedure is to compound the agents so that they look and taste alike and to assign them code numbers. Hence if either the patient or the doctor happens to have strong opinions about the agents under test, those opinions will not influence the reports of response. At the end of the study, the code is broken and an analysis is made.

In the lung cancer study, the interviews were blinded in the sense that the histologic type was not known to the interviewers. Hence even if interviewers had wanted to obtain results in line with the increased-risk hypothesis, they would not have been able to influence the result.

When a potential artifact cannot be conveniently controlled by a design device, it may be possible to insert a protocol step which will at least provide a warning of impending trouble. For example, in the lung cancer study the histologic classification was a potential source of difficulties since it depended on the judgment of pathologists. As a precaution the available slides were independently reviewed by two experts (without knowledge of previous histologic classification or smoking history). In 4 of the 41 cases, the new diagnosis disagreed with the previous one, but changing the status of these patients did not result in any essential change in the findings.

When a serious artifact appears, it is sometimes possible to make statistical adjustments to try to compensate for the effect. However, an analytic approach is the most difficult and least satisfactory way to deal with artifacts. When the hypothesis which the investigator is trying to establish involves a factor subject to *direct* control, such as therapy, an important design device for dealing with artifacts (and also extraneous real factors) is *randomization*. In controlled clinical trials, the allocation of treatments to the patients (or the sequence of treatments) is made with the help of a random number table (which is similar in principle to drawing numbers out of a hat). Since the allocation is determined by a mechanical procedure, it is not dependent on personal opinions or predilections. While randomization is the method of choice in experimentation, it cannot be used when the study factor is not subject to the investigator's control.

Hypotheses Based on "Accepted" Factors

Occam's Razor advises us "not to multiply entities without necessity." In other words, if the data can be explained by well-known factors there is little reason to introduce new factors. When we turn to alternative hypotheses based on substantive factors, background or contextual knowledge of the field of the study plays a key role in the process of drawing conclusions.

In an epidemiologic study, such as the lung cancer example, there are certain "accepted" factors—age and sex, for instance—which would have to be ruled out before any new factor could be advanced. Since this lung cancer study is confined to females, the results cannot be explained in terms of sex differences. However, age effects would have to be ruled out.

The relationship between age and smoking habits in women can be seen from Table 4 for the 1,304 controls. Without going into details, it can be seen that the younger women tend to smoke more than the older women so that smoking habits are related to age. Moreover the epidermoid lung series tends to be younger (median age 56) than the adenocarcinoma series (median age 62). Consequently, we must consider a counterhypothesis that the difference between the two lung cancer series might be explained by the factor of age alone.

TABLE 4

Distribution of Control Patients According to Age and Amount Smoked

Age (Years)	Number of Patients	Patients Smoking Zero Cigarettes Daily (Per cent)	Patients Smoking 1 to 9 Cigarettes Daily (Per cent)	Patients Smoking 10 to 20 Cigarettes Daily (Per cent)	Patients Smoking 21 + Cigarettes Daily (Per cent)
30-39	225	51	17	26	6
40-49	429	55	13	28	5
50-59	354	72	8	18	2
60-69	219	85	6	7	1
70+	77	90	7	4	0

The procedure for testing whether the hypothesis that the age factor (or age and sampling variation) can account for the smoking habits found in the epidermoid and adenocarcinoma lung cancer series is the "method of expectations." The approach is similar to that employed for sampling variation alone:

1. A testable hypothesis is set up. Here we can frame the hypothesis that, in a given age group, a lung cancer patient and a patient from the comparison series (1,304 cases) would have the same chance of falling into a specified smoking category.

2. On the basis of this hypothesis, we can predict the expected number of cases in each smoking category. For each lung cancer patient, we write down the proportions in the line of Table 4 for this age category. We then add the numbers to get the expected values for a given smoking category that are shown in Table 3.

3. We then compare the observed and expected numbers, making due allowance for sampling variation. If there are marked differences between the observed and expected numbers, the hypothesis would be rejected.

The refined significance test for expectancies is somewhat complicated, but a useful approximate test (where the control series is much larger than the study series) is quite simple. First, take the categories where departures from the hypothesis under test ought to show most strongly—here the 21-per-day category or a combination of the 10-to-20-per-day and 21-per-day categories. Then calculate:

$$\frac{(\text{Observed-expected})^2}{\text{Expected}}$$

and see if the calculated value exceeds 3.86. Combining the two highest smoking categories here we get:

$$\text{Epidermoid:} \qquad \frac{(22-7)^2}{7} = \frac{15^2}{7} = 32.1$$

$$\text{Adenocarcinoma:} \qquad \frac{(8-6)^2}{6} = \frac{2^2}{6} = 0.7$$

We are able to reject the age hypothesis for the epidermoid series but not the adenocarcinoma series.

The method of expectations outlined above is only one of a number of analytic devices used to control or "standardize" the "accepted" factors in a study. When large numbers of observations are available, as in vital statistics, two or more "accepted" factors may be controlled simultaneously, as in "age-sex standardized rates" or in rates adjusted for age, sex, and socioeconomic status. An alternative approach is to try to balance out the extraneous factors by a *post-hoc* pairing or matching of series. For example, it would have been possible to take a case from one of the lung cancer series and to pair that case with a patient from a large control series, who was in the same age group, had similar education, and was similar in other factors that we might want to balance out. Instead of a pairing or case-for-case matching, a control series might be constructed similar to a lung cancer series in average age and education. One advantage of over-all matching rather than case-for-case matching is that the control series would not be whittled down to the size of the study series, but the disadvantage is that the matching would not be as close.

When an "accepted" factor has a strong influence on the response variable under study, the "raw" results of a study might be quite misleading. In studies of therapeutic results, the disease severity is often a strong factor. For example, in cancer the stage of the disease (as determined by the size and spread of the tumor) strongly influences survival. Usually surgery is attempted only in the earlier stages of the disease, since once the cancer has metastasized (spread through the body) removal of the original tumor cannot halt the disease. Consequently a comparison of "raw" survival rates for surgically treated cases with corresponding rates for untreated cases is likely to be deceptive.

For forward-going studies such as controlled clinical trials, there are design devices for dealing with "accepted" factors that do the job in a simple, straightforward fashion that gives clear-cut conclusions. These devices are based on the balancing principle, but the balancing is done in advance instead of *post hoc*. A simple example is the use of a patient as his own control. In analgesic testing studies, the patient is given a series of test agents, and the responses can be compared within the same patient. Thus all stable patient factors (e.g., age, sex, severity) are automatically balanced out. The time sequence of administration can be balanced out by using designs of the Latin square family plus randomization. When an "accepted" factor is balanced out in advance by a Latin square(7), or other design, the task of ruling out the "accepted" factors is greatly eased.

Hypotheses Involving "Proposed" Factors

It would be unrealistic to require the proponent of a scientific hypothesis to rule out all possible hypotheses involving new or vaguely specified factors. With a bit of ingenuity it is always possible to imagine some new factor which might have led to the observed results. Many of these factors—such as "stress"—have no generally accepted measure and hence are untestable at present. So it is necessary to draw a line somewhere and to restrict consideration to *tenable* hypotheses. A tenable hypothesis is one which is testable and which meets the usual requirements for tenability in the subject matter field of the study. In epidemiology, for example, the minimal requirement for tenability is that the hypothesis be in reasonable agreement with the incidence pattern for the disease. For example the hypothesis should be consistent with the time changes in age-sex specific rates from vital statistics, with age distributions, sex ratios, and with other characteristics of the disease and related diseases.

The following remarks from the lung cancer paper of Wynder *et al.*(8) illustrate how the tenability of a "proposed" hypothesis can be developed.

In addition to the data of this study there is the evidence from vital statistics as well as previous data on lung cancer; therefore, the posit can be tested against the other data. This has been done and it has been found that the posit is consistent with the following:
The United States Vital Statistics on the death rate from lung cancer in males and females over the past decades. In particular both the lower death rate among females and the slower rise in this death rate can be explained by this posit. According to our posit the rate should not rise very much in the next decade (a twofold increase is unlikely even though the younger women are smoking more heavily than the older women).

The change in the sex ratio in lung cancer in the preceding decades.

The relative frequency of adenocarcinoma and epidermoid lung cancer in males and females, as well as the changes in this relative frequency over the past decades in the two groups.

Previous studies of the relation between smoking and lung cancer in males.

The posit not only is consistent with the body of data known to us but also resolves some of the apparent paradoxes concerning lung-cancer rates in women. We therefore assert the posit that cigarette smoking increases the risk of epidermoid lung cancer in women.

The tedious task of ruling out tenable counterhypotheses based on new factors can be greatly simplified if the study situation permits the use of randomization. The effect of randomization is to balance out extraneous factors in a long-run sense (i.e., if the series is large enough). Note that this balancing out occurs even though the investigator is unaware of an important extraneous factor. Thus randomization is the investigator's shield against the "slings and arrows of outrageous fortune."

Scientific Conclusions

If the investigator has carried through the exhaustive argument outlined here and has eliminated the rivals of the original working hypothesis, can he now assert that he has proved his hypothesis? Yes, provided that he is circumspect about his claims. There are two reasons why no dogmatic claims can be made. First, the counterhypotheses have not been ruled out in any absolute sense but only in the probability sense that they are unlikely. Hence the investigator's thesis can be asserted only in a probability sense—as a *posit*. In other words, the hypothesis is asserted as a "best bet"—as a sensible guide to action (but not an infallible one). The second limitation is that no scientific result is final—the whole matter can be reopened at any time if new evidence comes to light.

Perhaps this modest claim seems inadequate recompense for the lengthy task of scientific inference, but there is no royal road to scientific knowledge! When medical scientists try to short-cut the careful, tedious process of scientific inference, their work is likely to result in one of the futile and disruptive controversies that so often stalemate medical progress for years or decades. Here the longest way saves time.

The process of scientific inference is a kind of self-discipline that keeps a medical scientist from being carried away by his own ideas and opinions. Statistical methods are useful tools for carrying through the process in a systematic and explicit way. Before accepting the various statements and assertions that appear in the medical literature, it is wise to test the argument in the paper by the process of scientific inference.

REFERENCES

1. *Physicians' Handbook on Birth and Death Registration.* Office of Vital Statistics, U.S. Public Health Service, Government Printing Office, Washington, D.C.

2. *International Classification of Diseases.* World Health Organization, Geneva, Switzerland, 1959.

3. JORDAN, E. P.: *Standard Nomenclature of Disease and Standard Nomenclature of Operations.* American Medical Association, Chicago, 1942.

4. ARKIN, H., and COLTON, R. R.: *Graphs: How to Make and Use Them.* Harper & Bros., New York, 1936.

5. HILL, A. B.: *The Principles of Medical Statistics.* The Lancet, Ltd., London, 1950.

6. BROSS, I.: *Biometrics,* 1936, **14**(1):18-38.

7. SNEDECOR, G. W.: *Statistical Methods Applied to Experiments in Agriculture and Biology.* Iowa State College Press, Ames, Iowa, 1956.

8. WYNDER, E. L., BROSS, I., CORNFIELD, J., and O'DONNELL, W.: *New England J. Med.,* 1956, **255**:1111-1121.

9. BROSS, I.: *Federation Proc.,* 1954, **13**(3):815-819.

4. EPIDEMIOLOGY

Epidemiology has been defined as "the science which considers infectious diseases—their courses, propagation, and prevention."(1) This definition considers the field of epidemiology in its narrowest sense. Dr. W. H. Welch once called epidemiology "a study of the natural history of disease."

A more comprehensive and modern conception of epidemiology was expressed by W. H. Frost(2):

It is the science which considers the occurrence, distribution, and types of diseases of mankind, in distinct epochs of time, at varying points on the earth's surface; and secondly, will render an account of the relations of these diseases to inherent characteristics of the individual, and to the external conditions surrounding him and determining his manner of life.

Under this definition there is an epidemiology of diabetes and cancer as well as an epidemiology of smallpox. The term is most frequently applied in its narrow sense, but potentially it includes the study of all the diseases of mankind.

Epidemiology is a complex science. The epidemiologist requires long, arduous training and extensive field experience before he is competent to handle all the types of problems that he may be called upon to solve. These problems cannot be considered in detail in this text. We can only point out certain features of epidemiology as a science, particularly as they are related to the practice of medicine.

The Basic Factors in an Epidemiologic Study

1. **Etiology—Direct Causative Agent.** This agent can be a virus, a bacterium, a chemical substance, or a physical agent. It might be unknown, as in cancer or atherosclerosis. Even though the exact nature of the etiologic factor is not understood, the epidemiologist can undertake valuable studies and reach valid conclusions. He usually assumes, however, that the etiologic factor is a definite

74

entity with uniform and predictable characteristics. Examples of this principle in epidemiologic studies are the early work on the prevention of smallpox with cowpox vaccine by Jenner, and Snow's studies which correlated the occurrence of cholera with the drinking of water from certain sources. These studies produced important and life-saving procedures long before the etiologic agents were known.

However, the possibility of *multiple etiology* must be kept in mind—particularly with respect to chronic and nonparasitic diseases. Even in the case of infectious diseases, simultaneous or concordant infections may occur in the same population (or even in the same individual) to produce disease which by clinical or epidemiologic criteria seems to be of single etiology. The characteristic incidence curve of influenza in a semiclosed population is shown in Figure 11; yet careful study of this outbreak revealed that simultaneous infection with two immunologically distinct forms of influenza virus (A and B) was occurring in that children's institution. Simultaneous summertime outbreaks of enterovirus infection have long

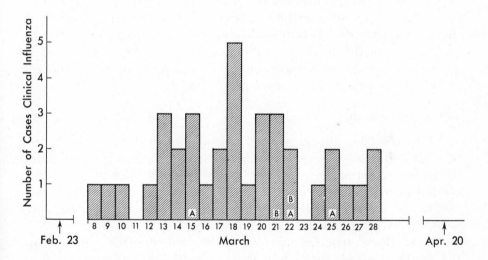

Figure 11. Chronology of an epidemic. An apparently homogeneous institutional epidemic of influenza resulting from simultaneous outbreaks of influenza A and B. The letters *A* and *B* represent virus types isolated on the days indicated. Serologic studies demonstrated that of the 115 children under observation, 25 were infected with influenza A virus, 11 with influenza B virus, and 10 with both viruses. (Kilbourne, E. D., Anderson, H. C., and Horsfall, F. L., Jr.: *J. Immunol.*, 1951, 67:547.)

confounded the epidemiology of poliomyelitis, and there is a suspicion that severe paralysis sometimes results from the synergistic
effects of two enteroviruses.

Nevertheless, it is generally true that in acute epidemics, a single
causative factor should be assumed and sought.

The Host

The susceptibility or resistance of the host is an important variable
that is often puzzling to the epidemiologist because individual resistance to a causative agent of disease is so difficult to measure. Inherent genetic factors may play a much more important role than we
have suspected in host resistance and susceptibility (see Chap. 21).

Host susceptibility may be determined or influenced by age or
sex as well as by genetic endowment. With infectious diseases, the
increased resistance associated with age is usually the result of
earlier childhood contact with the infectious agents. If such specific
immunity is not engendered in childhood, then contact with the
parasite at an older age can lead to disease more severe than in the
younger patient. In other words, increasing age of the host can be
accompanied by either greater or lesser resistance to a given disease
than is characteristic of childhood—depending on his past experience.

The sex of the host may influence susceptibility directly, as in
sex-linked hereditary diseases (p. 287), or indirectly by influencing
occupational exposure to infections or toxic agents.

The Environment

Ordinarily one speaks of the environment as the climatic factors
to which the host is exposed: temperature, humidity, barometric
pressure, radiation, etc. Other environmental factors intimately
related to individual living (the host's "microclimate") include such
factors as socioeconomic conditions, food, sanitation, living and
working environment, poverty, and illiteracy (see Fig. 14).

These three major factors—the seed, soil, and the climate—are
the basic concepts with which the epidemiologist must deal in
developing the field of epidemiology.

The Interrelation of Etiologic Agent, Host, and Environment

The incidence and severity of disease are a function of the interrelationship of host and etiologic agent as each or both together are
influenced by environment.

These relationships can be simply expressed as:

Disease (incidence or severity) =

$$\frac{\dfrac{\text{Host or population susceptibility}}{\text{Environment}} \times \dfrac{(\text{Etiologic agent} \times n)}{\text{Environment}}}{\text{Environment}}$$

where n = the numbers or quantity of the etiologic agent.

Thus, the environment can affect the etiologic agent in such a way that the agent is either increased or reduced in concentration (n) or even eliminated. The environment might so alter the host that he has greater or less susceptibility to contact with or invasion by the agent; or possibly after contact with the agent, the development of disease could be modified by environmental influences upon the infected or affected host.

Investigation of an Epidemic

Usually the epidemiologist is called upon to study an outbreak of disease because practicing physicians have noted an undue prevalence of the specific infection in their community. The study of the outbreak is based upon an analysis of all cases of the disease.

Case Records. Every epidemiologic study requires an accurate and complete record for each case. The case record is, in fact, the very heart of epidemiologic investigation. Each case record is studied by the epidemiologist in relation to all other cases that have occurred at about the same time and in the same geographic area.

Practicing physicians furnish most of the initial data upon which these records are based. Thus the clinician is responsible for the early and accurate diagnosis of reportable diseases and for prompt reporting of all cases of these diseases that may be encountered in his practice. The physician might see only one segment of the epidemic. He might see only a single case and not consider it of sufficient import to warrant an immediate report. But this case is an integral part of the epidemic and could be the key to the solution of the source of infection.

A comprehensive study of the status of morbidity reporting in the United States by Deuschle and his associates(3) has disclosed that two thirds of state health officers are dissatisfied with the accuracy of such reporting by physicians. Nevertheless, both state and local health officers felt that even inadequate data could provide a guide to public health programming.

Diagnosis. In the face of a pending epidemic, diagnosis must be accurate and rapid. The epidemiologist who is called in to investigate a situation first sees a sufficient number of cases of illness to be certain that the tentative diagnosis suggested is correct and that all the cases of illness in the area are due to the same cause.

Once the diagnosis is made, he must pause and consider the following points:

1. The characteristic epidemic curve of the disease.
2. The extreme limits of the incubation period of the infection.
3. The degree of communicability of this particular infection.
4. The effect of secondary factors upon susceptibility to this type of infection. Among other factors that must be considered are: age, race, sex, and distribution of the persons involved, as well as community housing, nutrition, climatic factors, seasonal factors, and other characteristics of environment that may affect this type of illness.
5. The various possible sources of infection in the disease.
6. The most common methods of transmission of the infection.
7. The most effective methods of control.

With this information in mind, the epidemiologist then secures as many case records as possible in a short space of time, fits each of the reported cases into its proper relationship with all others, and then quickly he constructs the natural history of the epidemic.

Normal Prevalence

How does the epidemiologist determine that an epidemic is pending? This is usually determined on the basis of any deviation from normal prevalence. Case reports of all reportable diseases have been secured by the epidemiologist from practicing physicians in all communities, over a considerable period of time, within the state or other jurisdiction. As these accumulate, the epidemiologist is able to determine the prevalence and the true sequence of the cases and to delineate the geographic distribution and seasonal prevalence of each type of illness. This accumulation of past experience in each community develops a *normal prevalence curve* for any given disease in any given area at any given season of the year. Slight deviation from normal prevalence immediately indicates that the situation may be hazardous and that an epidemic may be pending.

The word "epidemic" is a very loose term. Any unusual prevalence of an infectious disease in a community, as indicated by deviation from a normal prevalence curve, may be termed an epidemic. Thus two cases of rabies or Rocky Mountain spotted fever, occurring in a small New England town, might well be considered as an epidemic for that community and warrant an immediate epidemiologic investigation.

Epidemic Characteristics of Disease

Every infectious disease possesses its own characteristic epidemiologic pattern which distinguishes it from other conditions. Some of the elements which may be assembled to make up the whole picture are:

1. The clinical nature of the disease.
2. Incubation period of the disease. (For the most part, incubation periods are contained within narrow limits.)
3. The various means by which a disease may spread.
4. The speed of penetration of a disease into the community.
5. The rapidity of disappearance of a disease from a community.

Practically all infectious diseases have a characteristic "epidemic curve," with a fairly constant period of invasion, an upswing, a peak, a downswing of the curve, and finally a period of disappearance which may be prolonged and, in fact, may never reach the baseline. The upswing of the curve to the peak is almost always more rapid than the downswing, after the peak has been passed.

A striking illustration of these characteristics is the epidemic curve of influenza (see Chap. 13). In this disease the incubation period in the individual is very short (24 to 48 hours); susceptibility of the various members of the community is relatively high; the mode of transmission is usually by direct contact, and thus the penetration through the community is rapid. In an urban area, the epidemic is "two weeks up and three weeks down!" This expression simply means that following a short invasion period of about a week, the curve of incidence rises sharply and almost in a straight line for 14 days. The peak is reached at the end of the second week, and the curve then begins to fall sharply and symmetrically. The downswing lasts about 21 days (see Fig. 24). The epidemic is now practically over. This phenomenon is so constant that the officials in any city who have charge of medical and hospital facilities, and who are faced with an impending influenza epidemic, can make their preparations and plan for the day-to-day requirements of the emergency upon the basis of this characteristic prevalence curve. They know not only how many

hospital beds must be available for tomorrow and for Thursday of
next week but can even make a fair estimate of the number of additional coffins to be prepared and the number of graves to be dug for
people in the community who are, at the moment, perfectly well.

Purpose of an Epidemiologic Study

The epidemiologic investigation of any outbreak of a disease has
great value in that it enhances our knowledge of the natural history

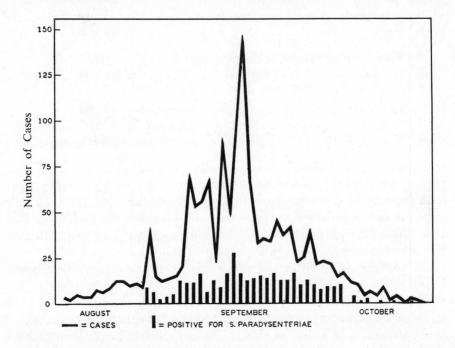

**Figure 12. Epidemic curve of bacillary dysentery. An epidemic curve of
fly-borne bacillary dysentery in North Africa.**

of that disease. But such a study has also more immediate and practical import. Primarily, epidemiologic studies are undertaken to
prevent further spread of the immediate hazardous situation. When
an outbreak is reported, the investigator must act at once—often on
the basis of very meager information. Once the diagnosis of the
etiology of the outbreak has been determined by clinical diagnosis
and laboratory aids, he must find the source (or sources) of infection
in that particular outbreak. This requires comprehensive information
concerning all possible modes of transmission of the type of infection

under scrutiny. The epidemiologist cannot assume, for example, that the epidemic of typhoid fever is water-borne, as it may well be, but he must fit every possible method of transmission of the disease into the epidemiologic characteristics of the outbreak. Then he must determine by a suitable analytical process of elimination the most probable source of infection in that instance.

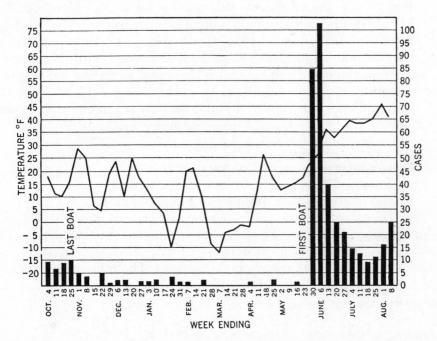

Figure 13. **Epidemic of acute respiratory infections. Spitsbergen. Acute respiratory infections, Longyear City, Spitsbèrgen, by weeks, 1930-1931, with a curve showing mean weekly minimum temperature.** (Paul, J. H., and Freese, H. L.: *Am. J. Hyg.*, 1933, *17*:517.)

The Epidemic Curve

Figure 12 illustrates many of the points under discussion. It is an illustration of an epidemic of bacillary dysentery that occurred in a large military bivouac(4). The diagram shows that the cause of the epidemic was *Shigella paradysenteriae*. Additional information in the graph is as follows:

Number of cases reported: 1,577.
Population at risk: not given (for military reasons).
Geographic limitations: a single bivouac.

Character of incidence curve: two weeks' invasion, four weeks' upswing, sharp peak, five weeks' downswing, rapid disappearance.

Seasonal prevalence: late summer.

Causal factors: flies infected in improperly operated "straddle-trench" latrines. *Shigella paradysenteriae* were actually isolated from the flies collected in the mess area and from the latrines as well as from 90 per cent of patients that were examined bacteriologically.

Figure 13 illustrates an epidemic of acute respiratory disease that occurred in Spitsbergen in 1931, in a highly susceptible population of 500 coal miners(5). The village had no contact with the outside world from October 25 to May 23. Ships came in during the summer from Norway to take out the coal.

The outbreak was due to a single source of infection; the exact moment of initial exposure of the community was known.

The curve gives the following data:

1. The incubation period of the disease.
2. The rapidity of its penetration in the village.
3. The degree of susceptibility of the population.
4. The short duration of immunity of a few individuals (e.g., repeat infection during the last week in August), and the disappearance of the infectious agent because of lack of susceptible material. The graph suggests that carriers do not exist. The influence of season and the lack of influence of low temperature upon infection also are shown.

Tracing of Contacts

In order to prevent further spread of an epidemic, the epidemiologist must trace those *contacts* who have been exposed to infection and who, if susceptible, may be in the incubation period of the disease. Here again a knowledge of the natural history of the disease is required. In an epidemic of syphilis, for example, only the most intimate personal contacts of the initial case need be traced, whereas in a smallpox outbreak, even a most casual contact of a susceptible person with a case of the disease in its early stages will result in infection.*

Another important activity of the epidemiologist is to search for the *missed* cases of the disease: the mild cases and the silent carriers.

---

*An epidemic of smallpox was studied in which one person, in the initial stages of the disease, attended a Christmas dance in a large hall. Every nonimmune person who attended the dance developed smallpox within a period of 14 days.

These individuals may not even have been seen by a physician, but they are an integral and important part of the epidemic picture and are often a very important source of transmission of further infection. For example, the case of faucial diphtheria is not a great community menace. The disease is spread by the mild missed case of nasal diphtheria.

In any outbreak, if the source of infection is determined and the contacts traced, then prompt action can be taken to prevent further spread of infection, and the epidemic will be brought under control.

The various methods that may be employed by the epidemiologist in the control of communicable disease have already been discussed. He is given authority by law to eliminate probable sources of infection, to isolate actual cases of disease, and to quarantine susceptible contacts during the incubation period of their infection.

Basic Epidemiology

Thus far we have discussed the functions and activities of an epidemiologist who is actually in the field and who has been investigating and analyzing a specific outbreak of infection. It is fascinating work, and the solution of a complex and intricate epidemic situation, with resultant control of a dangerous outbreak, is a most satisfying experience.

A more important though less spectacular aspect of the science we have termed *basic* epidemiology. It represents that phase of the subject that considers "the occurrence, distribution, and type of diseases of mankind, in distinct epochs of time, and at various points on the earth's surface." The chief elements of this science are time and painstaking effort. Results are not secured by an individual working alone but by the long-continued accumulation and compilation of data from day to day by workers in many parts of the land. Studies of disease prevalence must be made on a large scale under widely varying environmental conditions. All the various factors that could play a part in the incidence of the condition and its distribution through the mass of people must be properly evaluated.

Epidemiology of Noninfectious Illnesses

Since epidemiology is by definition "a study of the natural history of disease"(1), every disease entity can be studied from the epidemiologic point of view.

An excellent example is the study of morbidity and mortality caused by accidents.

The approach to the problem is analogous to studies of infectious disease, and the principles involved and procedures employed are closely related to the epidemiologic methodology of infectious disease studies (see Chap. 26).

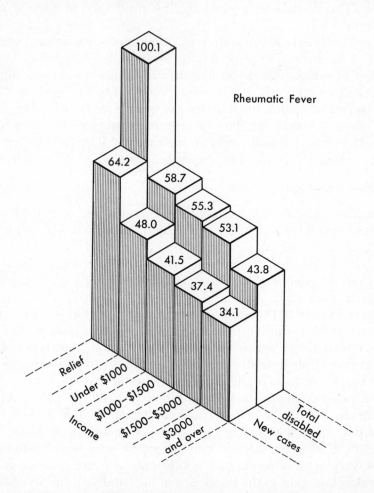

Figure 14. Effect of poverty on development of rheumatic fever. Incidence of rheumatic fever and prevalence of disability per 100,000 in children, 5 to 19 years of age, in canvassed white families of different income levels – 84 cities and towns in 19 states during the 1930's. (Data from Collins: 1947, *Pub. Health Rep.*, Supp. No. 198. From Paul, J. R.: *Clinical Epidemiology*, University of Chicago Press, 1958.)

Epidemiology of Chronic Illness

A great amount of valuable information concerning various types of chronic illness has been accumulated in recent years through epidemiologic studies of chronic illnesses and the disabilities resulting from these conditions.

Certain difficulties are encountered since the basic etiology of most chronic diseases is not known. Cancer is not a disease entity but has a very wide spectrum. The term "cardiac disease" encompasses a wide variety of clinical conditions. In most instances the etiology is not well understood. Arthritis is a symptom of a variety of chronic illnesses, and the same is true of hypertension. Even diabetes, which is a fairly clear-cut entity, does not have the concise epidemiologic features of an infectious disease.

Furthermore, the epidemiologic study of chronic disease cannot be carried out over a short space of time but must be continuous, beginning with factors that might influence the incidence of the disease in childhood and be carried through adolescence, early adult life, and into old age. A chronic disease that might not become clinically manifest until 60 years could have had its onset at 20 years. Multiple environmental factors could have played a part in production of eventual manifestations of chronic disease and disability (Fig. 14).

It is conceivable that this epidemiologic approach to studies of chronic disease could give clues to the clinician concerning the etiology of certain disease entities. Furthermore, epidemiologic evidence can be of great value in providing information for community planning of adequate facilities for medical care and the rehabilitation of those suffering from chronic disease.

In subsequent chapters we discuss the importance of epidemiologic information in relation to various types of chronic illness — with special reference to cardiac disease, cancer, arthritis, diabetes, and other chronic debilitating afflictions.

Epidemiology as a Research Method for the Identification of Etiologic Factors

Careful epidemiologic studies, because they entail the definition of the natural history of a disease as well as its geographical distribution, can provide valuable clues to etiology. A notable example is the relationship of lung cancer and cigarette smoking — a relationship which was established by classical epidemiologic methods. The disease was known to have its highest incidence in elderly males. Males smoke more than females. The incubation of cancer might be long. There are carcinogens in tobacco tar. Smoking might carry the carcinogens to the site at which cancer develops. Therefore, an etiologic relationship was suggested. It was then established by Wynder and his associates(6) that the incidence of lung cancer was proportional to the number of cigarettes smoked and was not obviously related to other factors.

Yet even this situation is not clear-cut. The protests of some workers that air pollution and not smoking is of critical importance in the genesis of lung cancer may be assuaged by the studies of Stocks and Campbell(7). Their work illustrates the possible synergism of the two effects — if urban residence can be equated with air pollution (see Fig.15).

Clinical Epidemiology

The clinician considers the individual affected with an illness. The unit of his study is one person or, at most, a family. The unit of study of the epidemiologist is the community. Each individual case of illness in the area under consideration is a *symptom*; it is a fractional part of the complete picture that must be assembled. This epidemiologic point of view which gives consideration to the community as the unit of investigation is a very difficult concept for most physicians to grasp, but it is one of the most fundamental features of a successful approach to the study of epidemiology.

As J. R. Paul(8) has so clearly indicated, every alert clinician is a potential epidemiologist. The cultivation of the science of epidemiology is not limited to the public health worker in the field nor to the laboratory worker with his experimental animals and scientific equipment.

Every case of illness is an epidemiologic problem. The basis of all sound work in this science is the accurate observation and recording of host factors. A compilation of these data and a study of environmental variables affecting the individual patients may readily lead to better understanding of unknown etiological factors in production of illness — as indicated earlier in this chapter.

Conversely, it is also true that the intelligent practice of medicine and the optimal evaluation of the individual patient demand that the patient's disease be considered in the context of disease in the community. Only when this is done can encephalitis in an infant be related to the mild "fever blister" of the mother, and the presumptive diagnosis of herpes simplex encephalitis be entertained. As indicated

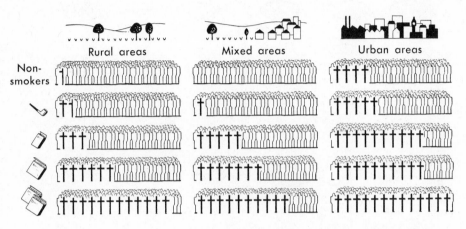

Figure 15. The relation of lung cancer to smoking and to residence in urban areas. Synergism of two postulated causes of lung cancer. Merseyside and North Wales. 1952-1954. Males. Ages 45-74, incl. Each cross represents 30 deaths per 100,000 men. (An attempt at health education of the public.) (Stocks, P., and Campbell, J. M.: *Brit. Med., J.*, 1955, 2:933; and *News Chronicle*, April 26, 1956. From Morris, J. N.: *Uses of Epidemiology*, 1957, E. And S. Livingston, Ltd., Edinburgh and London.)

in Figure 16, the full spectrum of disease (e.g., herpes simplex) is not discernible by the individual practitioner in the individual patient. The pediatrician attending a premature infant is impressed with the lethal potential of the virus in his patient with viremia or encephalitis; the internist or dermatologist considers the virus as a nuisance—a mere annoying cause of "cold sores" or "fever blisters." Neither view is wholly correct nor wholly incorrect. Only through an understanding of epidemiologic principles and of the divergent responses conditioned by age and specific immunity, can the whole range of disease be revealed and divergent views be reconciled.

Experimental Epidemiology

Thirty years ago W. C. C. Topley(9) developed the concept that epidemiology could be studied under laboratory conditions in which variable factors relating to the etiologic agent, the host, and the environment could be brought under a reasonable degree of control.

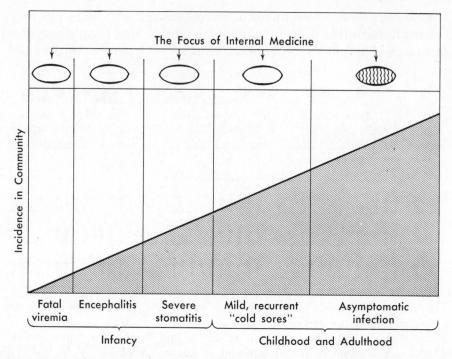

The Focus of Internal Medicine

Incidence in Community

| Fatal viremia | Encephalitis | Severe stomatitis | Mild, recurrent "cold sores" | Asymptomatic infection |

Infancy   Childhood and Adulthood

Figure 16. The spectrum of disease associated with herpes simplex virus infection—the restricted view provided by study of the single case.

He then attempted to hold certain variables constant and to modify one or perhaps several other variables. These studies were carried out, for the most part, on colonies of mice. His results were most illuminating. L. T. Webster(10), and later Howard Schneider(11), at the Rockefeller Institute, New York, carried these studies further under carefully controlled conditions with large colonies of mice. Using mouse typhoid as a prototype, they demonstrated the importance of genetic variation in both host and parasite as well as showing the importance of host nutritional status in the epidemiology of disease. Experiments of this kind make it possible to study the effects of predetermined, precisely measured quantities of the etiologic agent upon hosts of uniform age, sex, genetic constitution, and immunologic experience. When these factors are controlled, the role of subtler influences on disease can then be studied.

If, for example, mice are infected first with avirulent influenza virus, then three weeks later with a virulent strain, the "live virus vaccine" given initially will protect them completely from pneumonia

TABLE 5

Effect of Cortisone on Acquired Specific Active Immunity to Influenza: Challenge of Mice Previously Inoculated with Avirulent Virus*

	Day 1	Day 14		Day 21		
Group	Initial Inoculation	Challenge Inoculum	Cortisone (mg)	d / t †	Pneumonia (per cent) ‡	Virus in Lungs
1	Saline	Virulent virus	0	4 / 6	72	—
2	Saline	Virulent virus	5	4 / 5	80	—
3	Avirulent virus	Virulent virus	0	0 / 6	0	0
4	Avirulent virus	Virulent virus	5	0 / 6	10	+
5	Avirulent virus	Virulent virus	5 mg × 3 §	0 / 6	33	+
6	Avirulent virus	Saline	0	0 / 6	3	0

* From data of E. D. Kilbourne (12).
† Number of dead mice / total in group.
‡ Per cent of lung volume.
§ On days 13, 14, and 15; this dose does not depress antibody concentrations.

and death (Table 5). If, however, in the same experiment, similar mice, similarly immunized, are physiologically modified by the injection of cortisone, their resistance is so affected that pneumonic lesions develop (group 5) and virus persists in their lungs.

A problem of contemporary interest which is being studied epidemiologically in mice is the possible synergistic effect of respiratory viruses and air pollutants in the causation of pulmonary cancer.

REFERENCES

1. STALLYBRASS, C. O.: *Principles of Epidemiology and the Process of Infection.* Macmillan, London, 1931.

2. *Papers of W. H. Frost*, K. F. Maxcy, ed. The Commonwealth Fund, New York, 1941.

3. DEUSCHLE, K. W.; STRAUS, R.; and ENROTH, R. M.: *The Status of Morbidity Reporting: National and State (Kentucky).* Unpublished data.

4. KUHNS, D. M., and ANDERSON, T. G.: *Am. J. Pub. Health,* 1944, **34**:750.

5. PAUL, T. H., and FREESE, H. L.: *Am. J. Hyg.,* 1933, **17**:517.

6. WYNDER, E. L.; BROSS, I.; CORNFIELD, J.; and O'DONNELL, W.: *New England J. Med.,* 1956, **255**:1111-1121.

7. STOCKS, P., and CAMPBELL, J. M.: *Brit. Med. J.,* 1955, **2**:923.

8. PAUL, J. R.: *Clin. Epidemiology.* University of Chicago Press, Chicago, Ill., 1958.

9. TOPLEY, W. C. C.: *Proc. Roy. Soc., London,* series B, 1941-42, **130**:337.

10. WEBSTER, L. T.: *Medicine,* 1946, **25**:77.

11. SCHNEIDER, H.: *J. Exp. Med.,* 1948, **87**:103.

12. KILBOURNE, E. D.: *Proc. Soc. Exp. Biol. and Med.,* 1956, **90**:685.

SPECIAL REFERENCES

To the reader interested in the field of epidemiology, the following books are suggested as an introduction to the subject:

CHAPIN, CHARLES: *The Principles of Epidemiology.* The Commonwealth Fund, New York, 1934.

GREENWOOD, MAJOR: *Epidemic and Crowd Diseases.* Williams & Norgate, Ltd., London, 1933.

MORRIS, J. N.: *Uses of Epidemiology.* E. & S. Livingstone, Ltd.; Edinburgh and London, 1957.

SIMMONS, J. S. *et al.*: *Global Epidemiology.* J. B. Lippincott Co., Philadelphia, 1944.

SMITH, GEDDES: *Plague on Us.* The Commonwealth Fund, New York, 1941.

AND THE PARA

with

Book One

PUBLIC HEALTH
SITISM OF MAN

a note on newer hazards

In the underdeveloped areas . . . release of the resources of the countries from the tangled undergrowth of mass disease is a prerequisite of development. Just as the Panama Canal could not be constructed until Gorgas had mastered yellow fever, so the technical resources of these countries cannot be effectively exploited until the conditions of better health have been created. . . . Somehow governments will have to finance the capital requirements of health.

United Nations (1952) *Preliminary Report on the World Social Situation with Special Reference to Standards of Living*, New York

When man completes his first brief journey and emerges from the birth canal into this vale of tears he is immediately beset with a host of microparasites with which he will live in a state of armed neutrality for the rest of his days. If he is unluckier than most, he may emerge already deafened, blinded, or crippled by the ravages of intrauterine infection, or he may quickly succumb to an ambush of pathogens within the canal itself. Toward the end of his life, as his strength ebbs and his defenses fail, his final illness, no matter how initiated, will be attended by recrudescence of earlier infections or fresh attacks from without.

The microorganisms which may invade the human host vary enormously in size and biologic activity and include metazoan (multicellular) organisms as well as protozoa, bacteria, rickettsia, and viruses. The inequities of circumstance dictate an unequal distribution of these parasites among the world's population with the ironic result that economic "have-nots" have more than their share of parasites. Thus, the lives of whole populations are governed as much by the tertian tides of malarial plasmodia within them as by the diurnal tides of the ocean without. The incredible toll of such infestations cannot be measured in terms of mortality or even manifest morbidity in those who have never known true well-being. It is a basic problem of public health that the inverse ratio of man's economic and parasitic possessions is a self-perpetuating one. Much of the added burden of infectious disease in so-called "underdeveloped areas" is a corollary of a rural, crowded, impoverished existence in which the laws of economic survival require intimate contact among men in which they share one another's filth and the proximity of animals and their excreta. When man is thus forced to share the habitats of animals, he shares also their parasites and diseases. Or it may be that lesser beings will share their parasites with him — as does the malarial mosquito. Chronically debilitated by these parasites, the impoverished population finds it difficult to develop the simple but expensive machinery of environmental sanitation to which the Western countries owe their relative freedom from all but the obligate parasites of man himself.

Yet in those countries with higher living standards, the problems of human parasitism are far from solved, and new problems have followed in the wake of sanitation, artificial immunization, and new antimicrobial drugs. Thus, the restriction in infantile fecal-oral contact resulting from modern sanitation has almost eliminated typhoid fever in some countries, but in those same countries "infantile" paralysis, now postponed from infancy, has become a disease of older children and adults.

It is the purpose of the discussions which follow to consider the parasitic or infectious diseases of man not as clinical entities but as complex natural phenomena influenced by both host and environment. It is the province of clinical medicine to define and study disease in the individual patient, and the province of medical microbiology to classify and study the microorganisms which cause disease. It is a major point and purpose of public health to study and then influence the interrelatedness of host, parasite, and environment. The discussions and classifications of disease in this book are unconventional by clinical and microbiologic standards, but they derive from the ecology and transmissibility of infectious diseases and provide a logical basis for public health practice. Infections such as malaria and typhus will not receive detailed consideration in these pages. Important as these infections are to large numbers of the world's population, they are, in a scientific sense, diseases of the past because their ultimate control awaits only the general application of well-established principles of sanitation. They are basically economic rather than medical problems.

The complicated life cycles of the larger parasites are well presented in standard parasitology texts and will be considered here only in summary fashion as they relate to important problems of human disease.

A major emphasis of this book will be upon the communicable diseases directly transmissible from man to man. These are the diseases such as influenza which are relatively unaffected by the practice of environmental sanitation, and hence emerge as problems of the mid-twentieth century in the United States. They are predictably the incipient problems of the near future for those areas which have not yet experienced industrial revolution.

SECTION I

Infectious Hazards of the Environment

The infections with which environmental sanitation has been traditionally concerned are those in which the parasite either can or must exist for a time outside the human host. Such infections include:

1. The zoonoses or infections primarily of animals.
2. Infections primarily human but with an arthropod vector (filariasis).
3. Human infections (typhoid) caused by agents which may survive without multiplication in soil or water.

To these may be added certain clostridia and staphylococci which induce the formation of toxins in food, thus contaminating the environment of man. Despite the diversity of these agents and the diseases they cause, it is useful to consider them together as threats of man's environment.

5. INFECTIONS PRIMARILY OF ANIMALS THAT ARE TRANSMISSIBLE TO MAN

In the case of certain infections, man is an accidental victim or "innocent bystander" who is attacked by a parasite that is a primary or usual pathogen in lower animals. In diseases of this sort the existence of man is not necessary for the continued survival of the parasite, and in most instances further transmission of the parasite directly from man to man does not occur. Infections which primarily involve animals are caused by a wide variety of microbial species and may be transmitted from animal to man in many ways. The more important infections of this type are considered in Table 6 (pp. 100-101) and in the discussion below.

Trichinosis

The antiquity of this problem is illustrated by the ancient religious dietary proscriptions of pork. Raw pork may contain viable encysted larvae of the nematode *Trichinella spiralis*. When ingested, the larvae are liberated by digestion and attach to the mucosa of the upper portion of the small intestine. After developing to sexual maturity in approximately two days, the adult worms copulate. Subsequently, following development and hatching of the ova within the female's uterus, living larvae are gradually ejected over a six-week period into the host's intestinal lymphatics. Striated muscle is invaded by the larvae via the systemic circulation. In the muscles, necrosis and inflammation occur about the coiled (spiraled) encysted larvae, followed by eventual calcification within a year. In the absence of human cannibalism, the infestation then reaches a "dead end" in man.

The perpetuation of the cycle in swine involves essentially the ingestion of raw pork in uncooked garbage, or less frequently the consumption by the swine of trichina-infected rats.

Estimates of the frequency of human infection (based on autopsy

[*Text continued on p. 102.*]

99

TABLE 6

Animal Infections of Public Health Importance Transmissible to Man

MAN AN ACCIDENTAL HOST

Infection	Agent	Principal Hosts	Principal Methods of Transmission
Nemathelminthic			
Trichinosis	*Trichinella spiralis*	Swine, rat	Ingestion
Echinococcosis	*Echinococcus granulosus* (larva)	Dog (adult worm) Sheep, swine, cattle (larva)	Ingestion
Bacterial			
Anthrax	*Bacillus anthracis*	Herbivorous animals	Direct contact
Brucellosis	*Brucella abortus* *Brucella melitensis* *Brucella suis*	Cattle, swine, goats, horses Goats, sheep, cattle, swine Swine, cattle, horses	Contact, ingestion, inoculation, air-borne
Leptospirosis	*Leptospira icterohaemorrhagiae* (Many others)	Rodents, swine, cats, dogs, horses, poultry, calves	Direct contact(?)
Plague (bubonic)	*Pasteurella pestis*	Wild rodents	Insect (flea) bite
Salmonellosis (food poisoning)	*Salmonella typhimurium,* *S. choleraesuis, S. oranienburg*	Rodents, fowl, swine	Ingestion
Tetanus	*Clostridium tetani*	Horses, cattle	Inoculation or contact with animal feces
Tularemia	*Pasteurella tularensis*	Wild rodents	Contact, arthropod bites, ingestion
Tuberculosis (bovine)	*Mycobacterium tuberculosis*	Cattle	Ingestion, air-borne

100

Rickettsial			
Q fever	*Rickettsia burnetii*	Cattle, sheep, goats	Contact, air-borne ingestion
Spotted fevers			
Rocky Mountain spotted fever	*Rickettsia rickettsii*	?	Tick bite
Rickettsialpox	*Rickettsia akari*	Mouse	Mite bite
Typhus fever (murine)	*Rickettsia mooseri*	Mouse	Flea bite
Viral			
Psittacosis	Psittacosis (ornithosis) virus	Birds, including domestic fowl	Air-borne
Arbor viruses (group A)			
Western equine encephalitis	Western equine encephalitis virus	Birds	Mosquito bite
Eastern equine encephalitis *(group B)*	Eastern equine encephalitis virus		
St. Louis encephalitis	St. Louis encephalitis virus	Fowl, birds	Mosquito bite
Japanese B encephalitis	Japanese B encephalitis virus	Birds, heron (?)	Mosquito bite
Russian tick-borne encephalitis	Russian tick-borne encephalitis virus	Sheep, goats (?)	Tick bite, ingestion in milk
Yellow fever (jungle type)	Yellow fever virus	Monkey	Mosquito bite
Rabies	Rabies virus	Dog	Dog bite

data) vary widely, but in North America the incidence approaches 16 per cent.

Echinococcosis

The larval forms of the tapeworm *Echinococcus granulosus* encyst in the viscera of man to produce hydatid disease if he ingests material contaminated with tapeworm eggs from the feces of dogs in which the adult worm is parasitic in the small intestine. This tapeworm and the human disease are widely distributed throughout the world, particularly in sheep-raising countries. The disease is perpetuated by intimate contact between dogs and sheep and dogs and man. The canine infection is acquired from ingesting the viscera of infected sheep. Reduction in the intimacy of contact of dogs and humans, especially children, and efforts to prevent canine infection can reduce the incidence of the disease.

Anthrax

This virulent disease of ruminant animals can be transmitted to man through his direct contact with infected animals on farms or in slaughterhouses or, less directly, through animal products which carry the hardy viable spores of *Bacillus anthracis*. A notable example of indirect contagion occurred with the spread of anthrax through shaving brushes made from pig bristles. Less commonly, the infection can be acquired by ingestion of infected meat or by inhalation (wool sorters' disease).

Anthrax is perpetuated through the prolonged persistence of spores of the bacillus in soil used for pasturage. As originally shown by Pasteur, the bacilli may remain infectious in such contaminated soil for as long as twelve years. At least one outbreak of the disease in animals in the United States resulted from the importation of contaminated bone meal from overseas.

It is possible that saprophytic multiplication of *B. anthracis* occurs in soil, although the persistence of viable spores is adequate explanation for the epidemiology of this infection.

Brucellosis

Three species of the bacterial genus *Brucella* can be transmitted to man from various animals, producing both infection and disease. The species name indicates the animal which is the primary reservoir of infection as in the case of *Brucella melitensis,* which most often infects goats, and *Brucella suis,* which chiefly infects swine. *Brucella abortus* is identified with infectious abortion or Bang's disease in cattle. A newly identified species is *Brucella ovis,* which induces genital disease and abortion in sheep; it has thus far been recognized mainly in Australia and New Zealand. The *Brucella* species have broad pathogenic potential, however, so that *Brucella melitensis* can infect swine, and *Brucella suis* can infect cattle. The three common *Brucella* species can infect man and produce disease. Infection with *Brucella abortus* results in less severe disease than that induced by *Brucella suis* or *Br. melitensis.*

Although the small coccobacillus of brucellosis can survive for months in animal carcasses, it has no spore phase, which permits predictable extra-animal survival, as do *Bacillus anthracis* and the *Clostridia.* Thus, the chain of transmission depends on infection transmitted from animal to animal by direct or indirect contact. Transmission from animal to man commonly occurred by ingestion of milk prior to the widespread use of pasteurization. At present, brucellosis is principally an occupational disease of those in contact with ruminant domestic animals or their products. A higher attack rate in men than in women is apparently related to the greater exposure of men to sources of infection.

Leptospirosis

A wide variety of clinical syndromes is now recognized to be associated with leptospiral infection. In addition to Weil's disease, lymphocytic meningitis, arthritis, iridocyclitis, and grippe have been identified as manifestations of human leptospiral infection. Of the more than twenty strains associated with human infection, the most common in North America are *Leptospira icterohaemorrhagiae, L. canicola, L. pomona, L. autumnalis, and L. grippotyphosa.*

Leptospirosis is primarily an asymptomatic infection of rodents. It is incidentally transmitted to man or domestic animals through contamination of food or the environment with rodent urine containing spirochetes. The *Leptospirae* survive only briefly outside the living host, but the density and frequency of contamination of small bodies of water, rice paddies, or damp soil can lead to human infection without direct rodent-human contact. At special risk are those with occupations requiring exposure to rodent-infested areas, such as mines, sewers, abattoirs, rice fields, and farms. The infected flesh or urine of domestic animals slaughtered for food is also a source of infection for man by contact.

The exact mode of infection of man is disputed, but it is generally presumed to be through direct invasion of the abraded skin. Certain cases are probably acquired by ingestion or inhalation of *Leptospirae*.

Plague

Plague is essentially an endemic and epidemic infection of rats and other rodents, which can be transmitted to man by rodent fleas. The resulting disease in man is bubonic, i.e., characterized by necrotic lymph node swellings known as buboes. If in the course of a severe bubonic infection, the lungs are invaded by *Pasteurella pestis*, the disease becomes pneumonic. The pneumonic form is associated with a higher fatality rate and can spread directly from man to man with great rapidity.

The perpetuation of plague in the rodent population results from constant endemic infection in wild (rural) rodents which have developed immunity following epizootics and from exposure to recurrent epizootics in urban rats. Man is constantly threatened by these rodent reservoirs of infection. It is an ancient observation that epidemics in man are preceded or attended by epidemics in rats. When human infection becomes highly prevalent and sanitation is very poor, plague can be spread from man to man by the flea. Usually, however, the relatively low concentration of *P. pestis* in human blood as compared with that in the rat is prohibitive to this method of dissemination.

Salmonellosis

Salmonella typhosa and three other *Salmonella* species (*S. paratyphi, S. schottmülleri* and *S. hirschfeldii*) are primarily human pathogens and cause the clinical syndrome of typhoid fever (enteric fever). There is little evidence that these species infect animals or are maintained in nonhuman mammalian hosts. However, it is apparent that an increasing number of other *Salmonella* species infect animals principally, and man secondarily. Such species include *S. typhimurium* of rodents, *S. choleraesuis* of swine and cattle, and *S. oranienberg* of chickens. The human disease resulting soon after ingestion of these organisms is usually a brief, acute gastroenteritis, in contrast to the primary intestinal involvement and protracted febrile course of typhoid or paratyphoid. Severe infections can occur, however, and be associated with septicemia and its pyogenic sequelae.

The gastroenteritis induced by the "nontyphoid" *Salmonella* results from the ingestion of contaminated food and is one of several types of microbial "food poisoning."

Tetanus

The inclusion of tetanus in the present category of animal infections transmissible to man is an editorial convenience. Although the reservoir of *Clostridium tetani* is definitively in the intestines of horses and cattle and in soil fertilized with animal manure, infection in the sense of tissue invasion is not necessary for the perpetuation of the parasite. However, the virtual absence of the *Clostridium* from uncultivated virgin soil emphasizes the importance of proximity to animals and their excreta in the cause of human infection. Occasionally the human intestine may harbor the pathogen.

Clostridium tetani has little capacity to invade viable tissue or to extend its invasion from the wound site into which it is introduced. Its capacity to induce disease is related to the formation of a highly potent exotoxin which migrates to the central nervous system via peripheral nerves. The failure of toxin to enter the blood may explain the puzzling failure of the disease to evoke immunity following an attack.

Tularemia

Pasteurella tularensis is notable as a pathogen because it has been transmitted to man by every known method, including direct contact, inhalation, ingestion, and the bites of arthropods. However, the principal factor in the human epidemiology of this endemic "plague" of wild rodents is direct contact with infected animals (especially rabbits) during their butchering or preparation for the table. In contrast to plague, human-to-human transmission has not been reported even from cases of tularemic pneumonia.

Bovine and Avian Tuberculosis

Mycobacterium tuberculosis has the ability to infect many animal species, but only bovine and avian infections are of epidemiologic importance to man. These infections are chiefly caused by the variants *bovis* and *avium*. Although these variants differ slightly in biochemical and pathogenic properties from the human type of bacillus, they cause similar disease in man. Infection of man with the avian type is very rare, but infection with the bovine type accounts for much human tuberculosis in all but a few countries such as the United States. Such infection may be air borne but usually results from ingestion of contaminated milk or inadequately cooked meat. The differing clinical and pathologic nature of human infection with bovine and human types of M. *tuberculosis* probably reflects the differing routes of infection rather than important pathogenic differences in the parasites.

Q Fever

Rickettsia burnetii (Coxiella burnetii) is widely distributed in nature, in arthropods, cattle, sheep, and smaller animals in many parts of the world. Much information has been gathered concerning the epidemiology of this rickettsial infection, yet the mode of transmission to man is not completely clear. In animals, the infection is probably perpetuated by biting arthropods, notably ticks, much as tularemia is perpetuated in wild rodents.

Infection of man appears to be derived chiefly from contact with infected cattle or sheep. In many cases such contact is quite indirect, the infection occurring from inhalation of dust, wool, or aerosols of contaminated placental and amniotic fluid during "lambing" or calving" of infected animals. Some human infection is acquired by the ingestion of contaminated milk but, as with brucellosis, the disease in the United States is chiefly an occupational hazard of workers exposed to domestic animals or their products.

The Spotted Fevers

A variety of similar diseases characterized by prostration, high fever, and petechial rash is induced by infection with *Rickettsia* transmitted from wild animals to man by the bite of hard-shelled ticks. These diseases include Rocky Mountain spotted fever (caused by *Rickettsia rickettsii*) encountered throughout the United States, boutonneuse fever of the Mediterranean, South African tick-bite fever, and the rickettsioses of North Queensland, Australia, Kenya, Africa, and India. Minor immunologic differences distinguish the *Rickettsia* that cause this group of infections. Common to all these infectious agents is their endemic parasitism of small animals, such as the field mouse, and their capacity to survive in (and indeed propagate within) a number of ticks, chiefly *Dermacentor variabilis* and *Dermacentor andersoni* in the United States. Transovarian congenital transmission from tick to tick implicates the arthropod itself as a potential reservoir as well as a vector of infection.

Murine Typhus

Primarily a mild rodent infection of *Rickettsia mooseri*, this less severe form of typhus is spread from the infected rat to man by the bite of the rat flea *(Xenopsylla cheopis)*. When man-to-man transmission occurs, it is effected by the human louse, as with epidemic typhus.

Psittacosis

Birds of many species are endemically infected with the virus of psittacosis. Either ill or inapparently infected birds (parrots, parakeets, pigeons, domestic fowl) excrete the virus in their feces and nasal discharges. Inhalation of virus from such dry materials may induce pneumonia in man. Man-to-man transmission of infection via the sputum has been reported but is uncommon. The ubiquity of avian infection in other than psittacine birds has led to adoption of the term "ornithosis" as a name for the infection of nonpsittacine birds(1).

The Arbor Virus Infections

In recent years it has been discovered that many aberrant and seemingly unrelated viral infections of man and animals possess certain common biologic features. This has led to their classification as "arthropod-borne" or "arbor" viruses. Each of the nearly fifty viruses in this group has (a) the capacity to multiply in an arthropod vector and (b) the capacity to infect and multiply in vertebrate hosts with the production of viremia. In addition, many of the viruses within this large category have been found to be antigenically related to one another.

The studies of Casals and Reeves (2) have established two major antigenic groups (A and B), a small group (C), and a fourth unclassified group. The fourth group includes such viruses as those of Colorado tick fever and sandfly fever, which are antigenically unrelated to each other or to other arbor viruses.

This new method of classification admittedly overlooks viral characteristics other than antigenic relatedness, so that the agents of such epidemiologically and clinically different infections as St. Louis encephalitis and yellow fever are classified together as group B viruses. However, this classification has proved worth-while in evaluating antibody studies in human and animal populations; it constitutes the best method yet proposed for understanding this complex group of viruses. The infections with certain of these viruses, which are described briefly below, represent the more important diseases of this group in which man is not the necessary vertebrate host for the perpetuation of the infection. Thus, these may be considered infections transmissible from animal to man.

Eastern and Western Equine Encephalitis. These two infections are caused by different viruses, and as the names imply, the geographic distribution of the infections in the United States also differs. Eastern equine encephalitis is a disease of greater severity with a higher fatality rate (60 per cent). However, the epidemiology of the two infections is so similar that they may be considered together. Both "equine" diseases are misnamed because the horse is neither the primary host nor is he important in the spread of the infection to man. Although the presence of encephalitis in horses may signal the presence of virus in the area, the horse, like man, is a "dead end" in the infection chain after he has acquired his infection from the mosquito vector. These infections are primarily endemic in wild birds in swamp and woodland areas. Aviophilic mosquitoes maintain the infection in birds that often show no evidence of disease. If horses or men are incidentally bitten, they can acquire the infection; this infection need not result in encephalitis but can be clinically inapparent.

St. Louis Encephalitis. As with the equine encephalitides, the name of this disease is misleading except for its historic implications. The infection is sporadically present throughout much of the United States, but was originally recognized in the region of St. Louis, Missouri. The primary reservoir of infection is probably in birds and perhaps in domestic fowl. The mosquito vector seems to vary in different localities. Evidence is even stronger than with eastern and western equine encephalitis that most human infections are asymptomatic.

Japanese B Encephalitis. This infection, which is present in most of eastern Asia, is also characterized by a high rate of nonencephalitic or inapparent infections, although the clinical manifestations in man can be very severe. As with the other encephalitis viruses, wild birds, including the heron, are suspected of harboring this virus endemically. Various mosquitoes are capable of transmitting the infection. Local differences in epidemiology may be explained on the basis of a differing natural history of these vectors.

The Russian Tick-borne Complex. Olitsky and Clarke(3) believe that four widely differing infections transmitted by ticks of the family

Ixodidae are caused by different strains of the same virus. The infections are:

1. Louping ill, a disease of sheep and occasionally of shepherds in the British Isles.
2. Russian spring-summer encephalitis.
3. Central European tick-borne virus encephalitis.
4. Kyasanur forest disease in India.

Epidemics of these infections are directly related to the seasonal activities of the tick vectors. In contrast to mosquitoes, which are exclusively vectoral, the tick may be both vector and reservoir, and it can remain infectious for a long period and transmit the infection to its offspring. Many small animals as well as domestic sheep and goats have been found to be infected with these virus strains, but their role in the whole epidemiologic pattern is not clear.

Yellow Fever (Jungle Type). Only when effective methods for the curtailment of classical urban yellow fever were developed did the epidemiologic entity of jungle yellow fever emerge into view. The urban type of yellow fever and the mosquito vector *Aëdes aegypti* were imported into the Americas from Africa with the slaves. The classical experiments of Walter Reed established the role of the *Aëdes* mosquito in man-to-man transmission of this disease. Sanitation directed against the urban-dwelling *Aëdes* eliminated the disease in many areas. However, persistent endemic and occasionally epidemic foci were noted in rural or jungle areas demonstrably free of aedes mosquitoes or pre-existing infection in man. It has since been shown that in these jungle areas monkeys or small marsupials were infected with the virus. Forest mosquitoes which perpetuated the monkey disease cycle infected men who penetrated into the jungle to clear land for coffee planting. Women and children outside the jungle were not secondarily infected because the usual urban vector, *Aëdes*, was not present in the area. These fascinating studies thus clarify what had been a strange epidemiologic puzzle—the almost exclusive occurrence of jungle yellow fever in adult males, and the absence of secondary epidemic spread in their villages unless *Aëdes* species are present (see Fig. 17).

Rabies. Two differing epidemiologic patterns of rabies have been described by Johnson(4), depending on the occurrence of the disease in urban or rural areas. The more familiar urban disease is dependent upon the domestic dog for its perpetuation. Dogs with the encephalitic form of rabies spread the causative virus in their saliva by

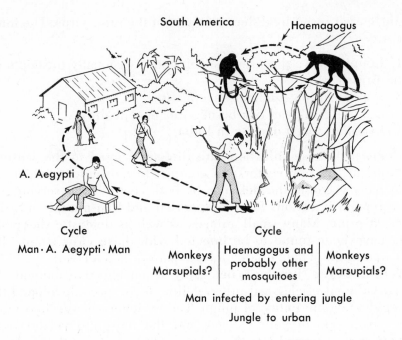

Figure 17. Man goes into jungle, becomes infected, returns home and, if *A. Aegypti* are present, may initiate the urban or man-mosquito-man cycle. (*The Status of World Health*, U.S. Government Printing Office, 1959. Adapted from Karl F. Meyer, 1955.)

biting dogs, men, and other animals. The infection is usually not transmitted further except by newly infected dogs.

In rural and sylvan areas, rabies appears to be maintained not primarily in dogs but in other canine species (including wolves, foxes, coyotes, and jackals) as well as the mongoose, ermine, and other members of the weasel family. All mammalian and most avian species are susceptible to rabies infection, although the disease is chiefly manifest in carnivores. Any such infected animal is theoretically capable of spreading the virus to man. However, the victims (chiefly cattle) of paralytic rabies transmitted by the vampire bat do not become vicious or bite.

Not only the vampire bat but noncarniverous bats as well have recently been found to be carriers of rabies virus. Several human fatalities have been traced to attacks by nonvampire species. Infection of the vampire may be unique in that it may be unassociated with disease, apparently involving only the salivary glands of this species.

The major source of rural rabies varies from time to time and country to country (wolves in Iran, foxes in the eastern United States, skunks in the western United States, wild dogs and jackals in India). The failure of rabies to establish itself in isolated canines, as in Alaska and parts of Africa, has suggested that presently unrecognized reservoirs of virus (e.g., smaller animals) might be necessary for the perpetuation of the sylvan disease.

REFERENCES

1. *Control of Communicable Diseases in Man*, 8th ed. Am. Public Health Ass., New York, 1955.
2. CASALS, J., and REEVES, W. C.: *Viral and Rickettsial Infections of Man*, 3rd ed., p. 269. T. M. RIVERS and F. L. HORSFALL, JR., eds. Lippincott, Philadelphia, 1959.
3. OLITSKY, P. K., and CLARKE, D. H.: *op. cit.*, p. 305.
4. JOHNSON, H. N.: *op. cit.*, p. 405.

6. INFECTIONS PRIMARILY OF MAN IN WHICH THE INFECTIVE AGENT HAS A REQUISITE PERIOD OF EXTRA-HUMAN RESIDENCE BEFORE TRANSMISSION

Certain microorganisms, although they are primarily pathogenic to man, are not spread directly from man to man but have a requisite stage of existence in man's external environment. This can be a passive stage in water or soil as with the agents of amebiasis or coccidioidomycosis (Table 7), or it may be part of a complicated cycle involving intermediate animal hosts, as with schistosomiasis or tapeworm infestation. Infection from these environmental reservoirs may be initiated through direct transcutaneous inoculation of parasites by biting insects, overt invasion by free-swimming cercariae, or passive inhalation of mycotic spores.

Schistosomiasis

Three species of blood fluke with an incredibly complicated life cycle induce the disease complex known as schistosomiasis or bilharziasis. *Schistosoma mansoni* and *S. japonicum* reside in intestinal venules and cause so-called intestinal schistosomiasis, whereas *S. haematobium* induces urinary vesicle schistosomiasis by invasion of vesical and pelvic venous plexuses. The paired adult worms release eggs into the visceral venules; these eggs pass into the intestinal and bladder lumina, and thence are voided into fresh water. There, hatching of the eggs releases swimming miracidia, which penetrate certain species of snail. In the snail, development into a free-swimming cercarial form occurs. The cercaria invade the human host through cutaneous or mucous membrane capillaries whence they eventually reach the portal circulation after passing through the right heart and pulmonary circuit. Acute and chronic disease accompanies host inflammatory reaction to the transvisceral migration of ova.

112

In the case of *S. japonicum*, mammals other than man can be reservoirs of infection.

Tapeworm Infections

Intestinal infections of man are induced by many species of tapeworm but are caused principally by beef, pork, or fish tapeworms (*Taenia saginata*, *T. solium*, and *Diphyllobothrium latum*). When inadequately cooked beef or pork is eaten by man, the encysted larval form (cysticerus) of the tapeworm attaches by a head or scolex to the intestinal wall. There it matures and grows by the segmental addition of potentially independent units called proglottids. Attached worms can reach 10 to 20 feet in length. Eggs liberated into the bowel and shed in human feces in areas where the animals feed constitute the source of infection of swine or cattle. In these food animals, the eggs hatch, releasing embryo worms which invade and encyst within the muscles. Here they comprise a potential source of human infection. If man ingests the eggs, he too may be the victim of visceral and somatic cestodiasis from the encysting larva (cystocerus). Although the development cycle of the fish tapeworm is more complex (it involves a first larval stage in a water flea), the infection is similarly transmitted to man by fish which contain a larval stage. The source of infection of fish is the eggs shed from the human intestinal tract.

Whipworm Infection

Infection of man with the roundworm *Trichuris trichuria* usually does not have serious consequences. It is widely prevalent in tropical and semitropical regions of the world. The whiplike male and female parasites live in the cecum and colon of man. Infection with this exclusively human parasite is acquired by ingestion of ova which have embryonated in warm moist soil contaminated by human feces.

Ascariasis

This very common infestation results from the ingestion of the ova of *Ascaris lumbricoides* which have undergone embryonation to the effective larval stage in the soil. Ingested eggs containing the larvae hatch in the small intestine. The larvae then reach the lungs via the mesenteric veins, liver, vena cava, and right heart. They penetrate to the alveoli, proceed up the airway to the pharynx, then descend to mature in the small intestine. Passage of eggs by the female worm

TABLE 7   **Infections Primarily of Man in Which the Infective Agent Has a Requisite Period of Extra-human Residence before Transmission**

Infection	Agent	Extra-human Phase	Intermediate Host or Vector	Transmission
Helminthic				
Schistosomiasis	*Schistosoma mansoni* *S. japonicum* *S. haematobium*	Water	Snail	Ingestion, skin penetration
Tapeworm	*Taenia saginata* *T. solium* *Diphyllobothrium latum*	Cattle Swine Fish	— — —	Ingestion Ingestion Ingestion
Whipworm	*Trichuris trichuria*	Soil	—	Ingestion
Ascariasis	*Ascaris lumbricoides*	Soil	—	Ingestion
Filariasis	*Wuchereria bancrofti* *W. malayi*	Mosquito	Mosquito	Skin penetration
Hookworm	*Ancylostoma duodenale* *Necator americanus*	Soil	—	Skin penetration
Protozoan				
Amebiasis	*Endamoeba histolytica*	Soil	(Fly)	Ingestion
Malaria°	*Plasmodium vivax* *P. malariae* *P. falciparum* *P. ovale*	Mosquito	Mosquito	Mosquito bite
Trypanosomiasis	*Trypanosoma gambiense* *T. rhodesiense* *T. cruzi*	Fly Fly Triatoma	Glossina (fly) Glossina Triatoma	Fly bite Fly bite Insect bite
Leishmaniasis	*Leishmania donovani* *L. tropica* *L. braziliensis*	Phlebotomus (fly)	Phlebotomus	Fly bite
Mycotic				
Coccidioidomycosis	*Coccidioides immitis*	Soil	—	Air-borne
Histoplasmosis	*Histoplasma capsulatum*	Soil	—	Air-borne
Bacterial				
Relapsing fever	*Borrelia recurrentis*	Arthropod ?Wild rodents	Louse, tick	Skin penetration
Rickettsial				
Typhus (epidemic)		Louse	Louse	Skin penetration
Viral				
Yellow fever (urban)	Yellow fever virus	Mosquito	Mosquito	Mosquito bite

°Actually, an infection primarily of the mosquito.

completes the cycle if the eggs reach soil appropriate for their matura-
tion.

Filariasis

Filariasis is an infection of the peripheral lymphatics of man with
the threadlike nematodes *Wuchereria bancrofti* or *W. malayi*. This
infection usually involves the lymphatics of the extremities or external genitalia. Chronic obstruction of lymphatic drainage may lead
to lymphedema and elephantiasis of the legs, arms, or the external
genitalia. The acute and earlier stages of infection may be asymptomatic in children. In adults, an allergic type of inflammatory
reaction may occur.

The bite of an insect (usually *Culex fatigans* or other mosquito)
initiates infection by inoculation of filariform larvae into the skin.
By one year after infection, the adult female worm has matured and
produced embryonic forms known as microfilaria, which migrate via
the blood to the viscera. In most types of filariasis, a nocturnal periodic increase in microfilaria in the peripheral blood is demonstrable.
Ingestion of human blood by insects results in transfer of the microfilaria, which then mature to an infective larval stage that may infect
man.

Hookworm

Hookworm infection follows penetration of human skin by the
soil-dwelling filariform larvae of *Ancylostoma duodenale* or *Necator
americanus*. These larvae reach the lungs via the blood stream, then
proceed up the bronchial tree, then down the enteric tract to the
jejunum. There development to the adult stage occurs. Eggs shed by
the adults may reach the soil via the feces. In the soil, rhabditiform
larvae emerge from the egg, later developing to the infective filariform
stage.

This widespread infection is climatically restricted because the
larvae cannot develop in the soil in areas where the mean monthly
temperature is cooler than 50° F.

Amebiasis

Amebiasis is a chronic infection of the colon of man with the
protozoan *Endamoeba histolytica*. The infection is most prevalent
in the tropics, but has a world-wide distribution. Although usually

mild, the disease is likely to recur in acute episodes. Infection is acquired by the ingestion of the cyst form of the parasite. In the cecum, trophozoites emerge from the cyst and thereafter invade the colonic mucosa. Cysts passed in human feces may contaminate the soil and its products and serve to propagate the infection. The most severe illnesses and outbreaks are usually the result of contamination of drinking water by sewage.

Malaria

Four species of human-specific plasmodium protozoan parasites cause the varied clinical types of malaria in man. *Plasmodium vivax* and the less common *P. ovale* have similar developmental cycles; they induce the mild but frequently relapsing tertian type of malaria, which typically is manifested by fever every other day. *Plasmodium malariae* causes the somewhat more severe quartan malaria with two-day intervals between febrile attacks. The most severe type of disease, which may be attended by the complications of blackwater fever (hemoglobinuria) or cerebral involvement, results from infection with *P. falciparum*. A relatively specific type-homologous immunity follows infection; however, this immunity appears to be specific for the locally encountered strains, suggesting antigenic strain differences within each plasmodium species.

The disease is perpetuated in human populations by the bites of several varieties of mosquitoes. The mosquito serves as more than a passive vector of the parasite because fertilization of the sexual forms (gametocytes) occurs within the mosquito's foregut. Following fertilization, the oocyte develops and then liberates sporozoites to the salivary glands. With the bite of the mosquito, the sporozoites are injected into the human host. After a latent period that varies with the plasmodial species, asexual forms appear in the erythrocytes of the infected host. Release of these merozoite forms from the ruptured red blood cell induces symptoms of the disease. Later, sexual forms are produced which, when ingested by the mosquito, insure the further transmission of the infection.

Trypanosomiasis

African sleeping sickness or trypanosomiasis results from the bite of the tsetse or *Glossina* fly, which inoculates *Trypanosoma gambiense* or *T. rhodesiense* resident in its salivary glands. It is in dispute whether animals other than man are important reservoirs of infection, although they serve to maintain the existence of the vector, *Glossina*, by supplying blood for its feedings. As in malaria, the protozoan parasite undergoes development in the insect vector. Unlike malaria, both sexes of the vector ingest human blood and can transmit the disease.

The distribution of trypanosomiasis is completely dependent upon the varying local prevalence of *Glossina* species, which thus far are restricted to Africa. *Trypanosoma gambiense* is sporadically distributed throughout tropical Africa, but *T. rhodesiense* is present only in East Africa.

American trypanosomiasis (Chagas' disease) differs importantly from the African infection in the following respects:

1. Many species of small animals (including cats and dogs, and in the southwest United States, the armadillo) are reservoirs of infection with *T. cruzi*, the etiologic agent.

2. Several species of nocturnal hematophagous insects of the family Reduviidae transmit the disease.

3. Chagas' disease is manifested initially by ocular or cutaneous lesions, then later by meningoencephalitis in the infant or carditis in the adult or older child. Except in Brazil and Argentina, however, the prognosis of most cases is good.

4. The intracellular location of *T. cruzi* has made therapy more of a problem in Chagas' disease than in the African type.

Leishmaniasis

Visceral leishmaniasis or kala-azar is caused by *Leishmania donovani*. This chronic infection of the reticuloendothelial system is widespread in China, Eastern India, Asia Minor, and parts of Africa adjacent to the Mediterranean. Some cases have been reported from South America.

As with the other protozoan infections, malaria and trypanosomiasis, a developmental stage of the parasite occurs in the insect vector, the *Phlebotomus* fly or sandfly in which flagellated leptomonad forms of leishmania are seen. These forms contrast with the nonflagellated, oval Leishman-Donovan bodies, which infect the vertebrate host.

The domestic dog is also subject to the infection and with the sandfly constitutes a reservoir of the disease in some areas.

Kala-azar, if untreated, is attended by a high mortality. It is most common in children.

Cutaneous leishmaniasis, which is of less importance than kala-azar, is caused by *L. tropica* in the Orient and by *L. braziliensis* in Central and South America, where it occasions high morbidity and sometimes mortality in jungle areas.

Coccidioidomycosis

This usually benign infection has been recognized mainly in the southwestern United States, where the causative fungus, *Coccidioides immitis* is present in the dry soil of desert areas. The infection is usually acquired by inhalation, resulting in acute pulmonary involvement characteristic of the primary infection. Pure cutaneous transmission is occasionally observed.

Histoplasmosis

The fungus *Histoplasma capsulatum* has a world-wide distribution, and consequently human disease associated with its inhalation is sporadically widespread. However, most recognized infections have occurred in the Mississippi and Ohio valleys of the United States. The epidemiology of the infection has not been definitively clarified, but the fungus has been recovered from soil and in the manure of pigeons, chickens, and bats. Epidemics have been related to inhalation of such material in dried form. Pulmonary calcifications following infection may simulate those resulting from tuberculosis and hence confound roentgenographic surveys.

Relapsing Fever

A number of species of spirochete (genus *Borrelia*) may cause the symptom and epidemiologic complex known as relapsing fever. The prototype *Borrelia recurrentis* is louse borne, but other species or strains of borrelia are carried by ticks. The tick-borne and louse-borne diseases do not differ clinically. The spirochete is transmitted to man through the skin, either as a result of the arthropod vector or through contamination of the skin with the crushed vector or its excretory products. Multiplication and persistence of borrelia occur in both the human body louse and the tick (genus *Ornithodorus*); transovarian transmission of the spirochete to its progeny occurs in the case of the tick.

As with typhus, the epidemic form of the disease is usually associated with lice; the endemic form follows tick transmission. The occurrence of the disease is related to the distribution of its arthropod vectors and to population upheavals, which favor the spread of the human body louse. Most cases have been reported from Southeast and Central Europe, China, and North Africa.

Epidemic Typhus

The ancient scourge of typhus, like relapsing fever, also follows disruption in man's environment, which expedites the transmission of its vector, the human body louse *(Pediculus humanus)*. The causative microorganism, *Rickettsia prowazeki,* is transmitted to man through the skin following its excretion in the feces of the louse. The louse is infective if it feeds on a victim of the infection in the early phase when rickettsiae are present in the peripheral blood. Lice do not carry the rickettsiae for long but die as the result of infection of the gut with the organism. It has been postulated that infected lice tend to leave promptly the source of the infection as the host is usually febrile. The louse in seeking a new host then spreads the disease before its own demise.

Yellow Fever (Urban)

In contrast to the sylvan or jungle-type yellow fever described earlier, no animal reservoir is needed for the perpetuation of the classical or urban type of the disease. Instead, the virus is spread from human to human by the bite of the town-dwelling *Aëdes aegypti.* Virus ingested by the mosquito coincident with viremia in its victim must remain in the arthropod for at least nine days before it is transmissible to man.

The infection has been endemic in Africa and the New World for centuries but has never appeared in the Far East.

7. INFECTIONS DIRECTLY TRANSMISSIBLE FROM MAN TO MAN IN WHICH THE INFECTIVE AGENT MAY PERSIST IN THE ENVIRONMENT

The infective agents of certain diseases, although they may be transmitted directly from man to man, may be capable of survival for long periods in the external environment. From this location they may threaten man through his water, his food, even through the air he breathes. This epidemiologically defined group of microorganisms is somewhat heterogeneous, but for the most part includes bacteria and viruses that cause primarily enteric infections. The infections so classified are listed in Table 8 and are considered briefly here with respect to their transmissibility.

Cholera

Although the *Vibrio comma* survives demonstrably for only a few days in infected human feces, extra-human survival is sufficiently protracted to allow the dissemination of the organism through contaminated water and food. Certain features of the epidemiology of the disease, including its seasonal incidence, remain puzzling. The possibility of an extra-human interepidemic reservoir has not been excluded.

Bacillary Dysentery

This "disease of the tropics" is in fact world-wide in distribution, although it is more common in tropical areas where poor sanitation and transport by flies contribute to its spread. Although the *Shigella* are not particularly hardy organisms, they can survive for several days in sea water; occasionally they induce epidemics through their survival in water and food. For the most part, however, infections result from direct human contact through the medium of fecal contamination of hands.

Typhoid Fever

In contrast to infections of man caused by other salmonella, typhoid fever is a specifically human infection which is transmitted directly from human to human via fecal-oral contact. Because only a few bacilli of *Salmonella typhosa* are required to initiate infection, contaminated water in which fecal contamination is highly diluted can serve as the vehicle of spread. Similarly, shellfish in contaminated water can harbor the bacilli and spread infection if eaten raw.

Typhoid carriers with chronic biliary tract infection can contaminate the food they handle and thus transmit the bacilli; milk serves as a vehicle of infection even after pasteurization if it is improperly handled in the bottling process.

Staphylococcal and Streptococcal Infections

Infections with certain strains of *Staphylococcus aureus* and of group A *Streptococcus pyogenes* are usually the result of direct human-to-human transmission of these bacteria, with entry into the upper respiratory tract. However, both of these "air-borne" organisms can cause cutaneous infections which are not necessarily associated with respiratory tract infection of the patient. "Surgical scarlet fever" following secondary infection of surgical wounds has long been recognized.

The increasingly important problem of intrahospital infections seems to be associated with increased numbers of staphylococci in the general environment as well as a "carrier state" for the organism in hospital personnel. Although the relative importance of human carriers and the environment per se must be decided by further study, the fact is that both the staphylococcus and streptococcus can survive in the air and dust and upon bedclothes and linens long enough to serve as sources of infection.

Tuberculosis

The situation with respect to human tuberculosis is similar to that described above for staphylococcus and streptococcus. The mycobacterium, however, can survive in dried sputum and in dust for even longer periods of time, serving as a potential source of infection. It is likely, however, that such environmental sources are

TABLE 8

Infections Directly Transmissible from Man to Man in Which the Infective Agent Persists or Multiplies in the External Environment

Infection	Infective Agent	Sites of Persistence	Transmission
Bacterial			
Cholera	*Vibrio comma*	Water, food	Ingestion
Dysentery (bacillary)	*Shigella*	Water, food	Ingestion
Typhoid fever	*Salmonella typhosa**	Water, food	Ingestion
Staphylococcal diseases	*Staphylococcus aureus**	Food, air,	
Streptococcal diseases	*Streptococcus pyogenes**	environment in	Inhalation,
Tuberculosis	*Mycobacterium tuberculosis*	proximity to man	contact
Viral			
Smallpox	Smallpox virus	Air, dust, environment in proximity to patient	Inhalation
Infectious hepatitis	Hepatitis virus A	Water, food	Ingestion
Coxsackie virus disease	Coxsackie viruses	Water	Ingestion
ECHO virus disease	ECHO viruses	Water	Ingestion
Poliomyelitis	Poliovirus	Water, food	Ingestion

* May multiply in the environment.

122

relatively unimportant in the spread of tuberculosis and that direct human contact is the usual mode of infection.

Smallpox

The virus of smallpox survives desiccation for weeks or months. This fact accounts for the effectiveness of the primitive immunization by variolation with smallpox scabs. Epidemiologic evidence indicates that some infections with the virus have followed exposure to objects handled by smallpox victims long before. But again, the importance of environmental reservoirs of the respiratory pathogen is probably as slight as with the bacterial agents of staphylococcal, streptococcal, and tuberculosis infections.

Virus Infections of the Intestinal Tract. Infectious Hepatitis, and the Enterovirus (Coxsackie, ECHO, and Poliovirus) Infections

Viruses that infect the human intestinal tract are singularly resistant to denaturation: they can survive for long periods in human feces, in sewage, and even in water chlorinated by the usual methods. No infections have been linked to water-borne epidemics from any but the hepatitis virus, but the low clinical attack rate of the infections may prevent recognition of cases from a common source. That most infections with these viruses are the result of direct human-to-human transfer seems unequivocal, although the relative importance of the respiratory and the enteric routes is still debated.

8. DISEASES CAUSED BY PREFORMED MICROBIAL PRODUCTS WITHOUT TRUE INFECTION OF THE DISEASED HOST

Certain microorganisms while in the external environment may multiply and produce poisons or toxins. If eaten by man, these microbial products can induce severe symptoms and even death. These disease states are not true infections, as they can be induced experimentally by the exotoxin *in the absence of the bacteria,* and because the microorganisms are incapable of invading and multiplying in the tissue of the host. These toxic diseases are to be distinguished from such infections as diphtheria and tetanus in which disease results from exotoxin, following and coinciding with invasion of the host tissues by microorganisms. Because the diseases caused by preformed microbial toxins are food-borne, they are often confused with acute food-borne infectious gastroenteritis caused by the Salmonellae.

Botulism

Botulism is a serious disease that fortunately is quite rare. It is reported more commonly in the United States in the Midwestern and Far Western states. The symptoms of the disease appear from 18 hours to 4 or 5 days after infected food has been eaten. Death results in one third to one half the cases.

The characteristics of the outbreaks are related to the ecology of the infecting organism. *Clostridium botulinum* is a spore-forming anaerobe. It is found in the intestines of many animals and is encountered freely in farm soils. It is not pathogenic to man or animals per se, but it grows freely in protein foods and produces a highly potent, soluble toxin. Even a few drops of fluid from a jar of infected home-cooked vegetables have caused death to man and to experimental animals.

The organism grows under anaerobic conditions, producing gas and a characteristic odor so that infected food has a "tainted" taste. The toxin has a special affinity for nerve tissues. Although five toxicogenic types are recognized, only two groups of organisms, A and B, are commonly encountered. Their toxins differ somewhat, so that type-specific antitoxin must be administered in order to save the patient's life. The toxin is killed by a temperature of 80° C, maintained for 20 minutes. Boiling destroys it almost at once. The organism itself is quite heat resistant: a temperature of 120° C maintained for 10 minutes is required to kill the spores.

Staphylococcal Food Poisoning

An unknown number of staphylococcal strains has the capacity to produce an enterotoxin (not to be confused with endotoxin) under appropriate culture conditions. Such conditions are provided by a wide variety of protein foods (notably those containing egg or milk products) and inadequate refrigeration. The widespread carriage of staphylococci in the nasal secretions and on the skin of healthy people makes contamination of food almost inevitable. If the protein food is not stored at refrigerator temperature, rapid multiplication of staphylococci can occur with concomitant production of enterotoxin (sometimes in less than six hours.) This preformed toxin is the agent of the acute and transiently devastating gastroenteritis that occurs in man within 3 to 12 hours of its ingestion.

The disease is obviously an intoxication and not a true infection. Symptoms are caused by the filtered toxin in the absence of the staphylococcus, and staphylococci capable of forming enterotoxin can be ingested without ill effect. These facts are reflected by the brevity of the incubation period, the course of the acute illness, and the absence of the fever and pyogenic sequelae that characterize staphylococcal invasion of tissues.

This form of food poisoning is by far the most frequent and contributes enormously to morbidity, if not to mortality. The difficulties in control of this disease, even in industrialized countries are related to:

1. The ubiquitous occurrence of *Staphylococcus aureus.*
2. The rapid rate of bacterial growth and toxin production in unrefrigerated foods.
3. The heat stability of the toxin, which can withstand boiling temperatures.
4. The absence of taint, odor, or other indication of food spoilage in toxin-containing foods.

The importance of the time element in *Staphylococcus aureus* toxin formation is well illustrated in the following epidemic:

Eighty-eight students and nine faculty members of P. H. Academy ate the same food. Within a period of three months, seven outbreaks, with a total of 242 illnesses, occurred. Each outbreak was explosive, all persons becoming ill within 30 minutes of one another and always about three hours after a meal.

Milk was incriminated as the source of the infection. The academy had its own dairy and did not pasteurize the milk. One of the cows had an infection of the udder, and *Staphylococcus aureus* was isolated from the lesion and from the pooled milk, and from the vomitus of the patients. The organisms were cultured in broth and 3 ml of the filtered broth, added to a glass of milk, was swallowed by students. Characteristic toxic symptoms developed in the volunteers.

The households of the farm manager and of the school principal drank the milk, but none of these persons became ill. This was easily explained on the basis that milk sent to these households was put into small containers and refrigerated immediately, so that the organisms, though present, did not grow and form toxin. The milk for the student body was placed in large containers and cooled slowly, affording ample opportunity—two or three hours—for growth of organisms and development of toxin.

The total disability produced by this brief and ultimately benign disease can be a serious threat if it involves key personnel participating in complicated or essential procedures. For this reason, members of the crews of commercial airlines are not permitted to eat at the same time. The wisdom of this regulation may be judged from the following description of an epidemic published in the *Morbidity and Mortality Weekly Report of the U.S. Public Health Service*(1):

A violent gastroenteritis was reported among 13 of 28 passengers arriving by air in Honolulu on January 16, 1961. The flight originated at Vancouver, B. C.; a stop was made at San Francisco but no food was taken aboard. About one and one-half hours out, 13 passengers became violently ill with nausea and vomiting. All who were ill reported eating breast of chicken Jeanette. Those who had not partaken of the chicken did not become ill. Items from lunch and dinner served prior to the outbreak were received for bacteriological examination. No organisms commonly associated with food poisoning were found in any of the specimens of foods submitted, except three portions of breast of chicken, which showed a coagulase-positive *Staphylococcus aureus* 187 in counts up to 11,000,000 per gram.

The pilots and other crew members who do not eat the food that is prepared for the passengers, did not become ill. It is worth noting that this precaution is designed to prevent a disastrous Staphylococcal food poisoning episode among crew members. As an additional precaution, the hours of eating for the pilot and co-pilot are staggered on trans-oceanic flights.

REFERENCE

1. *Morbidity and Mortality Weekly Report of the U.S. Public Health Service*, 1961, **10**(11):8.

SECTION II

The Control of Infectious Diseases Acquired from the External Environment (the traditional mission of public health and environmental sanitation)

In the preceding pages a number of infections of widely varying biological types has been discussed together with the problem of their transmissibility to man. These disparate infections have one common attribute: their agents threaten man from their residence in his general *biological* environment, which comprises the food he eats, the water he drinks, the air (and dust) he breathes, and the animals (vertebrate and invertebrate) with which he comes in contact. Literally, the environment also includes other people, but in terms of infectious disease "other people" constitute a very special environmental problem which is considered elsewhere in this book (Sections III and IV of Book One).

It is obvious that control of infections emanating from the environment can be accomplished by appropriate manipulation of this environment. This fact was recognized long before the germ theory of disease was postulated. The ancients drained the marshes to control malaria because they recognized the association of filth and disease, and they also established empirical dietary laws against the eating of certain foods.

This manipulation of the environment of man is essentially the science of *sanitation* as it now exists in public health practice. It has been pointed out elsewhere in this text that public health legislation did not originate within the medical profession but was dictated more by esthetic and olfactory considerations.*

*The recently revised sanitary code of New York City has at last relieved the Commissioner of Health of his obligation to look for dead horses in the street.

129

THE CHANGING ECOLOGY OF INFECTIONS

Details of public health practice with respect to sanitation will not be considered here, but the *rationale* of sanitation for infectious diseases is discussed in relation to the *ecology** and mode of transmission of infections. Before discussing the application of sanitation to the problems of environmentally-linked infections, it should be emphasized that unplanned changes in the environment may change radically the relation of host and parasite to the advantage or detriment of either. Thus, floods are notoriously associated with epidemics of enteric infections since sewage and drinking water are mixed by rising water. An unusually rainy summer in New Jersey in 1959 increased the mosquito population and could well have contributed thereby to a human epidemic caused by mosquito-borne eastern equine encephalitis virus.

The traditional human urge to "kill the vermin" resulted not only in the extermination of mice in a New York City apartment house but also in the appearance of a new disease, rickettsialpox, as parasitic mites left the cold bodies of their murine hosts to seek succor on the warm bodies of the human tenants of the buildings. This episode is, of course, no indictment of the killing of mice per se; if the mice had survived, they might have transmitted lymphocytic choriomeningitis virus instead. The lesson is the old one: the "balance of nature" even in a New York apartment house should be disturbed only with due appreciation of the consequences.

The Geographic Determination of Infections

There is little evidence that the races of man differ in their susceptibility to the acquisition of infection. Therefore, differences in the geographic distribution of infectious disease may be assumed to result from factors determining local prevalence of the infectious agent. Such varying prevalences are in the large sense geographically determined, but they will depend definitively upon climate, the presence of an appropriate vector or intermediate host, or upon regional peculiarities of habit which permit man to come in contact with the parasite.

Thus, the "geographic" restriction of African sleeping sickness (trypanosomiasis) to Africa reflects the apparent restriction of the vector Glossina fly to that continent, although perpetuation of the infection is also dependent on the prevalence of infected mammals.

*Ecology is the branch of biology which deals with the mutual relations among organisms and between them and their environment.

On the other hand, the spotty global distribution of coccidioido-mycosis and hookworm reflects primarily the occurrence of arid or damp climatic conditions, respectively. In the case of hookworm infection, however, the further requirements of poor sanitation (with respect to sewage disposal) and an unshod human foot are needed for the disease to occur.

Although it can be predicted that hookworm will never become a problem in Denver, Colorado, it cannot be said that yellow fever or malaria will never again threaten the continental United States. The insect vectors and susceptible population are present; only the intro-duction of human infection is required to complete the chain.

What factors, then, can be manipulated to prevent infections from the environment?

The essential jobs of current public health sanitation are:

1. Water purification.
2. Sewage disposal.
3. The control of food.

To a lesser extent public sanitation is concerned with insect and vermin control, housing, and other aspects of the socioeconomic environment. The newer and urgent tasks of control of air pollution and other twentieth century environmental hazards are considered in Section V of Book One.

9. THE CONTROL OF INFECTIONS CARRIED BY WATER

Because the most common and important water-borne infections derive from the human intestine, the problems of sewage disposal and water purification are interlinked. Inadequate methods of sewage disposal can compromise the safety of water treated by optimal methods.

In cities of the United States the average daily consumption of water per capita is about 150 gal. Most of this water is used in industry. Only about 50 gal per capita are required for total household purposes. Since it is not feasible to have one water supply for domestic use and another for industrial use and fire protection, it becomes necessary for the entire water supply to be treated and purified as though every drop were to be used for drinking purposes.

Every community, from the small village to the largest city, has a primary obligation to provide a water supply that is adequate for all nutritional, household, industrial, and fire-protection requirements. Large cities may find it necessary to go great distances, to tap large watersheds, to tunnel mountains, to drain rivers, to inundate towns, and to depopulate large areas in order to provide storage facilities for their water supplies. Extensive and intricate systems of transportation of water, purification plants, and distribution systems must be supplied. These are all problems in sanitary engineering. It is sufficient for the physician to know that a water supply must be provided to each of the individual homes in the community which is adequate, potable (i.e., free from taste, odor, and color), and free from pollution, and that will not produce disease.

The development of community water supplies in the United States in the first half of this century was phenomenal. In 1900, only 3,200 cities and towns had community water systems. In 1950, nearly 15,000 cities had public water supplies, which served well over 100,000,000 people. During this period the typhoid death rate dropped from 23 per 100,000 population to less than 0.5, and the death rate from diarrhea, enteritis, and dysentery for the U.S. Registration Area was cut to one tenth of the former rate.

The physician is primarily interested in the water supply because it may be an important factor in the transmission of disease. Waterborne infection practically always results from pollution of the water supply with human wastes, particularly with the urine and feces of

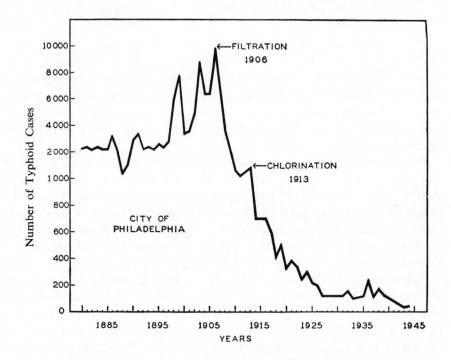

Figure 18. Reduction of typhoid fever in Philadelphia following treatment of the water supply. (Data supplied through the courtesy of Dr. Angelo M. Perri.)

persons with active intestinal diseases, or perhaps by the carriers of disease agents.

There are exceptions to this rule—notably anthrax, which is a disease of animals that has been transmitted to human beings through water. Tularemia also, another primary disease of animals, has been reported as being transmitted to human beings through infected water.

Water is used almost universally as a means of disposal of home and community wastes, especially the disposal of sewage. As areas become more densely inhabited, the problem of prevention of water-borne disease becomes more acute and difficult. During the developmental period of America, the great importance of water as a vehicle of infection was not fully recognized. Epidemic after epidemic of typhoid fever, cholera, and other intestinal infections occurred as a direct result of community-wide water pollution. The solution of these problems has been one of the great triumphs in sanitary engineering (see Fig. 18).

Water-borne Epidemics. In former years, widespread epidemics of disease due to pollution of community water supplies were of annual occurrence. These outbreaks have almost entirely ceased in municipalities, and also in institutions having a common water supply. This result has been brought about through the vigilance of state and municipal divisions of sanitary engineering and by the development of proper methods of water purification, together with the establishment of suitable procedures for constant checking of possible pollution. From time to time, the methods that have been worked out so carefully fail to function, and disaster results.

Water-borne outbreaks of disease are still all too common in small communities and in rural areas. In the seventeen years from 1920 to 1936, there were 412 reported water-borne epidemics of disease in the United States, affecting nearly 116,000 persons, and causing 955 deaths(1).

In recent years, the constant vigilance of municipal and state health authorities has continued the decline in community-wide water-borne epidemics. Temporary labor camps, summer trailer parks, and other places where groups of people utilize primitive sanitation are now our chief source of water-borne outbreaks of disease.

Sources of Water

Surface Water. Water for individual homes and for casual use, as on picnics and summer outings, is frequently derived from small, rapidly running streams. This water has an excellent taste, for it is cool, well aerated, and free from odor, but it is always potentially dangerous because it is so frequently open to pollution from human sources. No person should drink from a spring or mountain stream, no matter how inviting, unless he is sure that the entire watershed is free from human pollution. Infection may be carried for many miles in a mountain stream, and the aeration produced by the splashing over the rocks does not destroy infective agents. No home should utilize spring water, nor water from streams, nor even the water from shallow wells, unless the householder has complete control of the watershed and can be sure that there has been no opportunity for human pollution of the water supply.

Lakes and Rivers. Communities both small and large frequently find that the most convenient source of water is surface supplies, such as rivers, lakes, and reservoirs. This type of water supply has less dissolved matter than ground water and is not hard; usually it is free from taste and odor. It cannot be used with safety, however, unless careful plans are made for proper sanitary safeguards.

Ground Water. Ground water comes from driven wells. It is a very reliable and constant source of water, practically always free from pollution. The disadvantage of ground water is that these supplies often contain dissolved elements from the soil, which affect the taste of the water and are detrimental to its use in the household and for industrial purposes.

In soils with a limestone substratum, polluted surface waters sometimes filter rapidly through the rocky crevices and infect the ground water of driven wells. Many outbreaks of typhoid fever have occurred in zones of limestone formation, because it was not understood that surface pollution can penetrate long distances through open underground channels. Pollution of municipal water supplies from this source is now an unusual occurrence; it can be anticipated if the water supply is safeguarded by proper and frequent chemical and bacteriologic tests.

Individual Household Water Supplies

Rain Water. Utilized frequently for household purposes in the tropics and in areas with high rainfall, rain water is practically distilled water, and if properly collected and stored, it is a safe but limited source of household water.

Springs. If completely protected from surface drainage and if the area does not have a limestone formation, springs are excellent sources of household water. The individual householder can secure directions from his local health department or from bulletins of the United States Public Health Service, Washington, D.C., concerning suitable procedures for protection of household spring water from surface pollution. Streams, rivers, lakes, and small reservoirs should not be utilized as a direct source for individual home water supplies because of the danger of pollution.

Shallow Wells. Although the most common source of water in the rural homes of America, shallow wells have the great disadvantage of being subject to pollution. If they are not very carefully protected from surface washing and drainage, they may become infected with pathogenic bacteria (Fig. 20).

Deep-drilled Wells. These are the safest and most reliable source of household water but have the disadvantage that the water frequently contains dissolved salts that are leached from the soil.

Excellent directions for the protection and safeguard of farm and

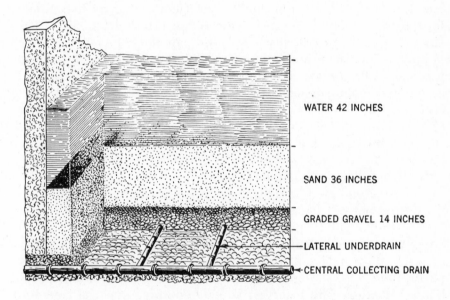

WATER 42 INCHES

SAND 36 INCHES

GRADED GRAVEL 14 INCHES

LATERAL UNDERDRAIN

CENTRAL COLLECTING DRAIN

Figure 19. A slow sand filter showing relation of sand, gravel, and under-drains. (Dunham, George C.: *Military Preventive Medicine*, 2nd ed., 1931. *Army Medical Bulletin 23*, p. 246.)

individual household water-supply systems can be obtained from local and state health departments. The U.S. Public Health Service bulletins on these matters, as well as farm bulletins from the Department of Agriculture, are splendid.

Community Water Supplies

Small cities and institutions can often obtain adequate and safe water supplies from deep-driven wells. This is the safest and best source of water that can be obtained.

Most cities must rely upon surface water from rivers, which is stored in large reservoirs. This source of supply is an intricate one, requiring careful supervision, and is always a potential source of danger. Various methods of filtration and purification of this source of water have been devised. These methods rely basically upon natural methods of water purification, supplemented by mechanical and chemical procedures.

Water Purification. Nature has devised a very successful method for water purification. It depends upon the catabolic portion of the nitrogen cycle. Organic matter in water is broken down by soil bacteria into NH_3 and CO_2. Further bacterial action changes the ammonia into nitrites, then to nitrates. This action occurs in the soil. Thus, when surface water slowly filters through the top soil, the animal pollution, including the pathogenic bacteria, is destroyed by natural processes, and the water again becomes pure and safe to drink.

Sanitary engineers constantly utilize this mechanism. They try to secure water that has been satisfactorily purified in the natural way (ground water); if ground water is not available, they filter surface waters from rivers and lakes through slow sand filters in order that the soil bacteria may purify the polluted water. A cross section of a slow sand filter is shown in Figure 19.

Other natural methods of water purification are sedimentation, and the destruction of bacteria by sunlight, by oxidation, and by reduction. Destruction of animal pollution also occurs by plankton, as well as by larger animals and plants that are found in still waters. Thus, storage of water for a sufficient period of time produces a high degree of purification and serves as an additional safeguard against water-borne infection. The reservoir and its environs must, of course, be carefully guarded against fecal pollution and cannot be utilized for bathing, fishing, or picnicking, in order to avoid the possibility of further pollution.

Chemical Methods of Purification. Various chemical methods have been applied to supplement natural methods of purification:

1. *Coagulants.* Sulfate of aluminum, sulfate of iron, lime, alum, and similar substances are used extensively to purify water. They have no bactericidal power. They are added to the water as coagulants. As the floc settles, it carries down bacteria together with other suspended matter. When settling has occurred, the water is then filtered rapidly through sand to remove the coagulant. Following this, other purification methods are employed as further safeguards. This chemical method is of special value where the source of water

supply is a turbid river with marked color and much suspended matter.

2. *Chlorination.* Chlorination of water has proved to be a most satisfactory method in the elimination of water-borne bacterial pathogens (see Table 9). Automatic devices are available which regulate the flow of the chlorine exactly in accordance with the need.

TABLE 9

Infections Transmissible through Drinking Water

	Infection	Susceptibility to Chlorination*
Metazoan		
	Schistosomiasis	?
	Ascariasis	?
Protozoan		
	Amebiasis	0
Bacterial		
	Cholera	+
	Bacillary dysentery	+
	Typhoid fever	+
	Leptospirosis	+
	Tularemia	+
Viral		
	Infectious hepatitis	0
	Coxsackie virus infection†	0
	ECHO virus infection†	0
	Poliomyelitis†	0

*For amounts of chlorine currently used in standard sanitation practice.
†Theoretically transmissible, but not proved.

The method has the disadvantage that an excess of chlorine imparts an unpleasant taste to the water. Heavily polluted water, with a high degree of turbidity, will require such an excess of chlorine that the taste of the water becomes disagreeable.

The great value of chlorine is that it can be used as a supplementary procedure, to be added after the other purification methods of storage and filtration have been employed. Thus the chlorine gives a further factor of safety.

Chlorination cannot be relied upon as an automatic and perfectly safe method of water purification. The method requires constant supervision, frequent testing of available chlorine by the use of the orthotoluidine test, together with daily bacteriologic checks of the efficiency of the procedures.

One fourth to one part per million of available chlorine represents the margins of safety that are ordinarily applied to water of low turbidity. An average installation provides 3 to 5 lb of chlorine gas per million gallons of water.

3. *Chlorinated Lime.* Chlorinated lime has been used extensively in protecting temporary water supplies intended for troops, concentration groups, campers, etc. A good general rule is to dissolve one-half teaspoon of chlorinated lime in 1 pt of water. Ten drops of this solution are added to 1 qt of water: or 1 teaspoon to 10 gal. The water is allowed to stand one-half hour before drinking. It will not have a pleasant taste, but it will be safe.

Analysis of Water. Two important methods are used for determination of the purity of water:

1. Supervision of the source of the water supply.
2. Laboratory analysis of the water.

Neither one of these methods is of great value unless supplemented by the other.

Inspection Service. It is the responsibility of the health department to provide for a constant supervision of community water supplies. Usually the state division of sanitary engineering has full control over all installations and modifications of community water-supply plants. A city cannot make any changes in existing plants, or new installations until the plans have been approved by state engineers. In some states, the state sanitary engineer provides for inspection service and also carries out all bacteriologic and chemical laboratory work on the municipal water supplies.

Each municipality has complete police powers for protection of the water supply and for prevention of all possible sources of pollution of community water supplies. The local health department also should have police power over all *individual* sources of water supply to which the public has access, such as the wells of roadside food stands, local picnic and recreation grounds, water supplies of rural schools, fair grounds, markets, camping grounds, and all other sources of water that may be consumed casually by an itinerant public.

Laboratory Analysis. The laboratory examination of water includes chemical and bacteriologic tests. *Chemical tests* are utilized to indicate the degree of pollution, and also to test the quality of the water.

The chemical analysis will reveal not only the intensity of pollution but the type of pollution; it will also indicate whether the nitrifying process has completed its cycle, i.e., whether the pollution is recent or not.

An example of a satisfactory chemical analysis of a filtered surface water is as follows:

Parts per Million

Albuminoid ammonia	0.15	
Free ammonia	0.02	
Nitrogen as nitrites	trace	
Nitrogen as nitrates	0.08	
Chlorine as chlorides	1.2	
Bacteria at 20° C		123.

Excess of chlorides may indicate proximity to the sea or animal pollution. Excess of nitrates, with no nitrites and low free ammonia, may indicate past pollution that has undergone complete nitrification. The engineer takes the results of the chemical analysis and after inspection of the water supply and the bacteriologic tests, he is able to interpret the results. He uses the laboratory data just as a physician does in making a clinical diagnosis.

Bacteriologic examination of water determines total numbers and types of bacteria present. The total number of bacteria present is an indication of pollution with organic material. Surface waters have a much higher bacterial count than ground waters. Sudden variation in total bacterial count in surface waters is usually due to rains, with an increase of organic pollution. Ground waters should have very low bacterial counts.

The most satisfactory index of fecal pollution of the water is the determination of the presence of organisms of the coli-aerogenes group. Pollution is estimated by utilization of gas formation in fermentation tubes of lactose broth (presumptive test). The organisms encountered in the fermentation tubes are studied further and if a Gram-negative nonspore-forming bacillus is found which forms gas in lactose broth, the test is considered complete.

It is practically impossible to find typhoid or dysentery bacilli in public water supplies by simple bacteriologic techniques, even in a water supply that is heavily polluted with community sewage. The presence of organisms of the coli-aerogenes group in the water is a satisfactory index of dangerous pollution: the higher the number of these organisms, the greater the danger. Absence of these organisms in a water supply is an index of safety.

Pollution of Water Supplies with Lead. Plumbism was frequently acquired in the past, through drinking water, but lead has not been used extensively in household plumbing in recent years. Pure water of a pH on the acid side is likely to dissolve the lead. The action seems to be an electrolytic one, and just the proper combination of circumstances is required to cause enough solution of the lead pipe to injure the consumer. The lead is slowly absorbed by the householders over a long period of time and eventually may produce serious symptoms of lead poisoning. At times household "epidemics" of lead poisoning have occurred from a faulty plumbing system. In recent years, lead poisoning is more frequently acquired as an industrial hazard than from faulty plumbing systems.

Ice. In past years, ice for domestic use was harvested from water sources that often were polluted. In addition, the ice was frequently harvested in a most unsanitary manner. Freezing does not destroy the organisms that produce intestinal disease. Thus, gastrointestinal outbreaks due to the use of polluted ice were not infrequent. This problem was greatly reduced with the introduction of systems of artificial refrigeration and with the innovation of ice manufacture.

Ice should be handled with the same sanitary precautions that are taken with other food; it should be manufactured only from water of unimpeachable quality. Individuals who handle ice should first wash their hands as carefully as any food handler; ice blocks should not be dragged over kitchen floors or left on sidewalks or doorsteps, common practice in many cities.

Outbreaks of acute gastrointestinal disturbance have frequently been traced to ice that has been polluted through careless handling. These have occurred most often in restaurants, institutions, and outing groups where large numbers of persons were fed. It is probable that individual and household icebox infections are frequent, but they go unrecognized. The opportunities for contamination of ice by ignorant and careless food handlers are numberless. The best domestic rule to follow with ice is the rule of the tropics: "Never put ice in food or drink; always put the food container in the ice."

Federal Standards of Water Supply

The U.S. Public Health Service has been instrumental in improving the quality of water supplies throughout the nation. The federal government has no direct jurisdiction in the various states but does have jurisdiction over interstate carriers. Standards of water purity have been set by the federal government for all supplies used on railroad trains, ships, and other vehicles of interstate traffic. These standards have been widely adopted by the various states for all municipal water supplies, as well as for other sources of water to which the public has access(2).

The Disposal of Human Excreta

Disposal of human excreta is one of the great preoccupations of civilized mankind. The primitive Eskimo of Greenland lives indiscriminately with his children, dogs, and household wastes; but the more civilized nomadic Indian of Labrador is very careful to take his drinking water from the upper reaches of the stream on which he is camped and to dispose of his feces on the lower side. With the advances in civilization, and as homes have become more permanent and living more complicated, the difficulties encountered in waste disposal, and the dangers therefrom, have multiplied enormously. Thus it has become a truism that the system for waste and sewage disposal encountered in any given community is a direct index of its stage of civilization and degree of development.

Nature has provided a very satisfactory system of safe excreta disposal in the nitrogen cycle, but this process takes time, requires much space, and is accompanied by very disagreeable odors. Engineering science has devised very ingenious procedures to remove household and community wastes and to enhance the natural process of disintegration.

About one third of the population of the United States lives in rural homes; the remainder in urban centers. The system of waste disposal is quite different in the two types of home. The rural family commonly uses the direct earth-disposal system for the disposal of all wastes, whereas urban homes utilize water carriage for the disposal of excreta, and many other community wastes. Practically all the household wastes of the city home, such as bath, dishwashing water, and excreta, together with the industrial wastes of the community, are disposed of by the water-carriage system.

The sanitary engineer is directly concerned with various modes of waste disposal from the point of view of community cleanliness, economy, and sanitation. The physician is directly interested in excreta and waste disposal largely because of the fact that unless the proper methods are employed in these matters, human infection and outbreaks of disease may result.

Human excreta, if not cared for suitably, quite frequently pollute the drinking water. They can also transmit disease in other ways, for example, by: (a) direct pollution of the surface of the soil, as in hookworm disease; (b) pollution of food, particularly oysters, clams, and other sea foods; (c) pollution of ice supplies that are harvested from ponds; and (d) pollution of places of recreation, such as fresh-water and salt-water bathing beaches. Thus, it is obvious that great care must be taken in formulating and effecting plans for the proper disposal of human wastes.

Excreta Disposal in Rural Homes

Two systems are commonly employed:

1. Direct disposal in the earth.
2. Septic tanks.

Direct Disposal in the Earth. The only household wastes that are of practical importance in producing infection in rural areas are human feces and urine. They may be disposed of very simply in a *pit privy*.

The pit should not be below ground-water level, otherwise it will breed culex mosquitoes. It need never be emptied, but when the sludge reaches almost to surface level, it should be filled and the superstructure moved to a newly dug pit.

Septic Tanks. A septic tank is a simple form of sewage disposal suitable for rural and suburban homes with an adequate water supply under pressure but which cannot be connected with a community sewage disposal system.

The sewage is discharged into a tank buried in the ground. After digestion of the material occurs, the effluent overflows and is distributed through the garden in the subsoil by loose jointed earthen tiles. The principles and the details of proper septic tank construction have been worked out carefully by sanitary engineers. Many of these details may seem unimportant, but successful operation of a septic tank system is dependent upon minute attention to all details of plan and construction. It is recommended that the experts of the sanitary division of the local health department be consulted in regard to septic tank installations, and all their suggestions should be followed to the least detail. The U.S. Public Health Service and state departments of sanitary engineering have excellent detailed plans for septic tank construction that can be obtained by writing for them. Kitchen wastes should never be discharged directly into the septic tank.

There should be an intervening "grease trap" or else the grease will interfere with the proper functioning of the system.

Sewage Disposal

The highly technical details of construction and operation of a municipal water-carriage sewage disposal system are the province of the sanitary engineer rather than of the physician. The chief interest of the physician in these matters is that improper handling of sewage will result in a widespread nuisance, with a possibility of great potential danger of community infection.

· For the most part, communities have discharged sewage into adjacent rivers, lakes, or into the sea, with the anticipation that self-purification of the sewage would occur. The heavier particles settle out, the organic material is oxidized, and the bacteria are killed by sunlight or by the lack of suitable environment. This method works very well if the body of water is very large and the volume of sewage very small and if other communities do not take their water supply from the lower reaches of the river or lake into which the sewage has been discharged. The dilution factor is great, and the time element for proper purification is not long. As the United States has grown in population and become more industrialized, the sewage from the rapidly growing communities now includes a great amount of industrial wastes. These cannot be handled satisfactorily on a self-purification basis.

Sewage Treatment Plants. In practically all the states with dense population and highly developed industries, it has been necessary to establish sewage treatment plants for each municipality in order to render the great bulk of sewage non-noxious before it is discharged into the outflow of the river or lake.

These various treatment devices for the purification of sewage are very ingenious and highly complicated. They are based on sound bacteriologic and chemical principles and employ natural methods as well for the breaking down of the complex nitrogenous products of sewage into their end products, when they can again be utilized by plants.

Cross Connections

Many epidemics of disease have been traced to a pollution of the public water supply through a faulty "cross connection."

Emergency water systems are frequently installed for fire protection or street cleaning. Many factories, storehouses, and other privately owned buildings may install a private water system for industrial processes and for fire protection. Usually these water supplies are obtained from polluted sources. In past years, these emergency water supplies often had a cross connection with the public water supply. If the emergency water supply was placed under a higher pressure than the municipal supply, then pollution of the public water supply sometimes occurred by leakage through a faulty cross-connection valve.

Most state sanitary codes now prohibit any cross connections between a private emergency fire-protection system and the public water-supply system.

Faulty plumbing systems may result in dangerous cross connections within the wall of large buildings such as hotels, apartment houses, and the like.

Ordinarily, the positive pressure in the water system will prevent leakage of pollution into the water system, even though there is a direct connection. But poor plumbing construction may result in heavy back pressure, or back siphonage, so that sewage and other household wastes may be forced directly into the water supply of the building. This situation actually occurred in the Chicago dysentery outbreak of 1933(3).

A suitable plumbing code, with a system of competent plumbing inspectors, will minimize the danger of outbreaks of illness due to cross connections. All direct water connections with waste pipes should be prohibited, and suitable specifications should be provided for check valves, flush valves, and vacuum breakers.

The Special Problem of Viruses and Water-borne Epidemics

Recently the hypothetical threat presented by human enteroviruses and the virus of infectious hepatitis has proved to be more than theoretical. There is now little doubt that water-borne outbreaks of infectious hepatitis can occur. Twenty-eight water-borne epidemics in 13 countries have been reviewed(4).

A particularly dramatic and well-studied epidemic occurred in Delhi, India, in 1955 (5). Following a flood of the Jamuna River in October of that year, the water receded and the river changed its course (see Fig. 20), resulting in the flow *upstream* of raw sewage that usually emptied below the water-purification plant. The raw sewage caused gross contamination of the city water supply as it entered the water pumping station. The situation was worsened by the absence of rain and storm water, so that the sewage entering the river from the *nalla,* or creek, was virtually undiluted. Study of the chloride concentration afforded a measure of the duration and degree

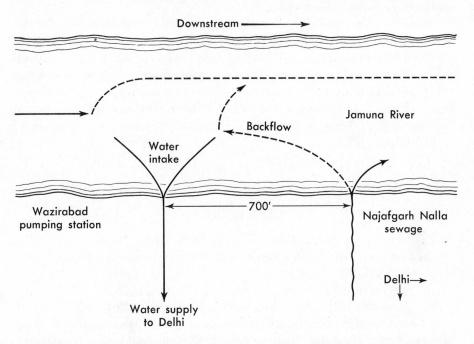

Figure 20. Contamination of Delhi water supply with sewage during back-flow in the Jamuna River. (Melnich, J. L.: *Hepatitis Frontiers,* ed., F. W. Hartman, *et al.* Henry Ford Hospital, International Symposium, No. 6. Boston, Little, Brown and Co., 1957.)

of contamination of the city water and demonstrated that contamination occurred during one week in mid-November. It was calculated that during the peak of contamination about *50 per cent of the water entering the pumping station was made up of sewage.* This contamination was promptly recognized, and the alum and chloride concentrations were immediately increased—the chlorine from 0.5 to 2.1 parts per million. This treatment of the water was apparently sufficient to prevent any significant increase in typhoid or other enteric bacterial diseases, but it did not prevent the extensive epidemic of 35,000 cases of infectious hepatitis which became evident six weeks later. The well-defined period of water contamination provided a unique natural experiment for the definition of the incubation period of the disease. This proved to be 22 to 60 days with a mode of 40 days—longer than is usual with infectious hepatitis. Other epidemics of infectious hepatitis which were clearly spread by chlorinated water have been reported(6).

Recent experimental studies have demonstrated not only the presence of poliomyelitis and other enteroviruses in raw sewage but also the resistance of certain enteroviruses to the concentrations of free and combined chlorine now recommended for sewage treatment. Although it is probable that water is a relatively unimportant vehicle for the spread of enterovirus infections, it is important to note that present-day sewage treatment does not truly "disinfect" or kill these pathogens.

REFERENCES

1. FRANK, L.: *Pub. Health Rep.*, Reprint 2185, 1940.

2. *Sanitary Manual for Land and Air Conveyances, Pub. Health Rep.*, 1944, **58**:159.

3. BUNDESEN, H., *et al.*: *J.A.M.A.*, 1933, **101**:1636.

4. MOSLEY, J. W.: *New England J. Med.*, 1959, **261**:703.

5. MELNICK, J. L.: *Hepatitis Frontiers*, ed. F. W. HARTMAN, *et al.* Henry Ford Hospital, International Symposium, No. 6. Boston, Little, Brown and Co., 1957.

6. POSKANZER, D. C., and BEADENKOPF, W. G.: *Pub. Health Rep.*, 1961, **76**:745.

10. THE CONTROL OF INFECTIONS TRANSMITTED BY MILK AND OTHER FOODS

The important infections transmitted by milk are brucellosis, group A (beta hemolytic) streptococcal pharyngitis, and bovine tuberculosis. Less commonly, typhoid fever, bacillary dysentery, and staphylococcal "food poisoning" are traceable to contaminated milk. Of the rickettsial infections, Q fever can be milk-borne and, recently, milk has been implicated in transmission of the virus of the Russian tick-borne complex of infections (see Table 10). Present methods of pasteurization are adequate for the destruction of any but the Russian tick-borne virus. The heat-stable enterotoxin of the staphylococcus also is not eliminated from milk by pasteurization if already present, although the staphylococci are destroyed.

If milk is not properly handled, it deteriorates rapidly as a food. It is an excellent cultural medium for bacteria and may act as a vehicle of pathogenic organisms. Thus, the procedures in the sanitation of milk are basically the application of simple bacteriologic principles to milk production. It has become a highly technical process, requiring the aid of skilled veterinarians, bacteriologists, sanitary inspectors, and other specialists in dairy technology.

It is obvious that the milk supply of the nation must be abundant, of pure quality, and perfectly safe to drink since it is a valuable food, particularly for babies and growing children. It must be produced at a low cost but with sufficient profit for both dairyman and distributor to maintain a permanent and safe milk supply for the community at all times. These rigorous requirements have been achieved, but the struggle has been a titanic one.

The results are one of the best examples we have of cooperative community planning. The agencies represented have been the departments of health (federal, state, and local), departments of agriculture (both state and federal), dairy farmers' associations, milk distribution companies, manufacturers of dairy equipment, and all others concerned in the production of milk.

The federal and state departments of agriculture, by concentrating chiefly on dairy sanitation and the improvement of dairy herds, have been responsible for the nation-wide campaign against bovine tuberculosis, brucellosis, and other cattle diseases. The U.S. Public Health Service has aided states in formulating satisfactory uniform laws of milk sanitation. The "Model Milk Ordinance," under federal sponsorship, has been widely adopted. Local health departments have been concerned chiefly with inspection of dairies and of milk pasteurization plants. Dairy associations and large milk distribution companies have aided the farmers in improving the sanitary conditions of their farms. Our milk sanitation program has indeed been a highly cooperative enterprise.

Dairy Sanitation

The production of clean milk requires intelligence and a real sense of cleanliness. The details of dairy hygiene are not the concern of this text and will not be enumerated. In brief, the cattle must be healthy and, particularly, be free from mastitis. The cattle and their surroundings must be kept scrupulously clean. The milking must be done in a clean manner, and the milk placed in containers that have been steam sterilized. It must be cooled immediately and kept at a temperature not higher than 50° F until it reaches the pasteurization plant.

TESTS OF MILK

Laboratory Tests

Adulteration of Milk. In years past, milk was frequently adulterated by the producer. The commonest procedures were: (a) removal of cream, (b) addition of water, with perhaps addition of limewater or other substances to give proper color and specific gravity, and (c) addition of preservatives. The older laboratory directors tell us that the chief activity of the milk laboratory during the early part of this century was devoted to tests for detection of fraud.

Chemical and physical tests have been developed to detect these adulterants very readily; the penalties have been so severe that the practice of milk adulteration has disappeared.

Bacteriologic Tests

Normally, milk as it leaves the healthy udder of the cow contains few bacteria. Thus a high bacterial count in a milk sample may indicate that (a) the milk was not cooled promptly, (b) the milk is dirty, or (c) the udder of the cow was infected.

Before the advent of good dairy practice, milk frequently reached the consumer with a count of 500,000 bacteria per cubic centimeter, and 100,000 bacteria per cubic centimeter was considered as allowable in samples collected from the delivery wagon. The Certified

TABLE 10

Infections Transmitted by Milk or Milk Products

Infection	Eliminated by Pasteurization
Brucellosis	+
Salmonellosis (especially typhoid fever)	+
Tuberculosis, bovine	+
Q fever	+
Streptococcal infections (group A)	+
Staphylococcal enteritis	0
Russian tick-borne complex (encephalitis)	0

Milk Commission set a standard of 10,000 bacteria per cubic centimeter as allowable for certified milk. Gradually dairy practice has improved to such a degree that market milk now often comes to the pasteurizing plant with a bacterial count of only 10,000 to 20,000 bacteria per cubic centimeter.

The bacteriologic laboratory is the best means we have of measuring the cleanliness and sanitary quality of milk. Standard practice requires the determination of the total bacterial count of the sample.

SANITATION METHODS FOR MILK

Pasteurization of Milk

The process of pasteurization is a final safeguard against milk-borne infection. It does not relieve the producer of the responsibility for employing cleanliness and all other proper dairy techniques: the milk must be clean and of good quality when it reaches the pasteurizer. Pasteurization, properly carried out, renders the milk *safe*.

Two common methods of pasteurization are used: the *holding* method and the *flash* method. The former method employs a temperature of 142 to 145° F for 30 minutes, with rapid cooling of the milk to 50° F and bottling by automatic machinery. Usually the milk is heated in large tanks with automatic temperature control and recording.

In the flash method there is a continuous flow of milk, with rapid heating to 160° F for 15 seconds, followed by rapid cooling.

The purpose of pasteurization of milk is to destroy all pathogenic bacteria in the milk without injuring the quality of the product or changing its flavor. Pasteurization does destroy some of the vitamin C of milk, but milk is not an important source of this vitamin. It should, in any case, be obtained from other sources of food. Other theoretical objections have been raised, but the advantages so overwhelmingly outweigh the disadvantages that milk pasteurization has become almost universal in the United States.

Phosphatase Test. The phosphatase test is used to determine whether or not milk has been suitably pasteurized. This enzyme is present in raw milk but is thermosensitive at pasteurization temperature. Thus a quantitative measurement of phosphatase in the milk is a good index of suitable pasteurization.

Boiling of milk is an unsatisfactory substitute for pasteurization. It renders the milk quite safe but changes the taste and even the quality of the milk. Boiling of milk is almost universal in the tropics; in many countries it is a household custom since it has been found empirically to be an important health safeguard.

Certified Milk

Certified milk was developed by a Medical Milk Commission at a time when the quality of market milk was very poor and it was necessary to secure a safe supply of pure milk for infants. This milk is produced under the supervision of an official medical board, with very rigorous restrictions which give assurance of a high-quality product. All certified milk should be pasteurized in order to be safe as well as of good quality. The cost of certified milk is usually more than that of market milk.

Grades of Milk

Formerly, milk was graded into different qualities in accordance with the fat content, the bacterial count, and other criteria. These grades included pasteurized and raw milk, grade A; and pasteurized and raw milk, grade B; together with other variable qualities of milk that brought confusion to the consumer and to the dairyman as well.

The general improvement in milk sanitation has almost nullified the necessity for the production of special grades of milk. The present tendency is to abandon the terms grade A, B, or C milk, and to produce one standard, high-quality, safe, pure milk which will be readily available to people in all walks of life at a reasonable cost. In promoting this standard of milk, primary insistence must be placed upon safety of the milk as an article of food.

Requirements for a Community Milk Supply

The basic requirements for a satisfactory community milk supply are:

1. Intelligent dairymen who are familiar with all the details of modern dairy practice. They should seek the guidance of the state department of agriculture in all matters relating to dairy sanitation.

2. The cows should be healthy and well fed, free from bovine tuberculosis, brucellosis, and mastitis.

3. Provision should be made to chill the milk immediately after milking, and to keep it at 50° F until delivered to the pasteurizer.

4. All milk should be pasteurized under carefully controlled conditions.

5. The milk should be placed directly after pasteurization into the container which will reach the consumer; it should be chilled at once and maintained at 50° F until it is delivered.

6. A uniform state-wide sanitary milk code(1) should be formulated, with provision for a proper system of inspection of dairies and of pasteurization plants.

7. Local laboratory service under health department auspices is essential, in order to act as a check on the purity, cleanliness, and safety of the milk.

Intestinal Infections

Milk is seldom infected with human intestinal discharges, but when this does occur through careless dairy technique, the results can be very serious. Many widespread milk-borne epidemics of typhoid fever and bacillary dysentery have been reported from this source of infection. In practically every instance, the milk was unpasteurized. There are exceptions to this rule.

Typhoid Fever Epidemic Due to Pasteurized Milk. Typhoid fever began to appear sporadically in a large Western city. It occurred over a large area and lasted for a considerable period of time. The health authorities investigated all possible common sources of infection without success. They were sure it could not be a milk-borne outbreak, since these epidemics are characteristically explosive in onset, limited in time, and usually confined to a small area.

All the persons affected used milk from one large distributor, but this source was ruled out, since the milk was pasteurized. The distribution of milk by this company was very extensive, and the incidence of the disease was small and scattered. The milk came to the distributor from many sources, but all were under sanitary supervision. The pasteurization plant was well managed, all automatic temperature records were in perfect order, and the milk was bottled automatically and distributed in individual quart bottles All employees of the pasteurization plant were examined, to be sure there were no typhoid carriers in the group.

The disease remained unchecked in the community, despite efforts to find a common source of infection. Fresh vegetables and fruits were studied, as well as butter and cheese, shellfish, and other possible modes of infection. Scattered cases of the disease continued to appear. The state epidemiologist was called into consultation, and on the basis of a statistical analysis of all the data, he made the following deductions:

1. The milk from one distributor was at fault.
2. The pasteurization process was working satisfactorily: otherwise the outbreaks would have been much more extensive, and would have occurred in spurts.
3. The delivery system was not at fault: else the cases would have occurred on a single or on individual delivery routes.
4. The infection must occur between the time the milk was pasteurized in bulk and the time it was placed on the wagons. This must be either in storage or in the operation of bottling.

The epidemiologist then studied the bottling operations, which were carried out automatically in a glass-enclosed room by two workers. He noted that the automatic capping machine failed, perhaps once in a hundred times; the two men at the bottling machines had a pile of caps nearby, so that they could cap the bottles by hand when the machine did not operate properly. Here was a possible source of contamination. One of these men was found, on repeated examinations, to be a typhoid carrier. He was an intermittent carrier—that is, only at times did he have large numbers of typhoid organisms in his stools. At other times they were difficult to find.

This outbreak had unusual characteristics because of the peculiar chain of circumstances that produced it, but it does illustrate the fact that milk may occasionally be infected even though it is properly pasteurized. The study also shows that a single negative stool examination is not sufficient proof that an individual is not a typhoid carrier.

Diseases Transmitted through Milk Products: Cream, Ice Cream, Butter, and Cheese

Numerous outbreaks of disease are recorded that have been traced to cream and to ice cream. These foods are highly susceptible to infection and must be handled with the same scrupulous care as milk itself.

The procedures that are employed in the manufacture of butter and cheese tend to eliminate infection with the hemolytic strepto-coccus and with staphylococcus, but epidemics of typhoid fever, as well as paratyphoid and dysentery, have been traced both to infected butter and infected cheese. The bovine tubercle bacillus also may not be destroyed in the process of butter and cheese manufacture.

Thus, milk that is used in the manufacture of any milk products should be pasteurized; it should be of as good a quality and handled with the same sanitary precautions as is the bottled milk that goes directly to the consumer.

Cheese that is properly ripened is safe. Many health departments require that cheese be aged for not less than 60 days before it can be sold.

The Control of "Food Poisoning": Acute Diseases Caused by Toxic Microbial Products Formed in Foods Prior to Their Ingestion

Although some acute illnesses derived from food are true infec-tions (i.e., salmonellosis), much so-called food poisoning is caused not by microbial invasion of tissue, but by the effects of toxins elab-orated in food before it is eaten. These entities have been described on preceding pages as botulism and staphylococcal enteritis (see Chap. 4). The prevention and control of these diseases are dependent to a large extent on public education concerning the handling and preparation of food.

Botulism has become a medical rarity in the United States because of the effective methods of sterilization introduced by the commercial canning industry. With home-canned products (especially beans) of dubious history, boiling of the food will destroy the heat-labile botulinus toxin. Specific antisera are available for the prophylaxis of infection in those exposed to toxin-containing food. These anti-toxins against the types A, B, and E toxins which affect man have also been used in therapy of the overt disease but have not proved valuable.

The prevention of the toxic enteritis caused by *Staphylococcus aureus* enterotoxin and the infective enteritis caused by *Salmonella* (see Chap. 5), and more rarely by other bacteria, may be considered together.

Prevention of Staphylococcus aureus and Salmonella Food Poisoning

Although the epidemiologic investigation of an outbreak of food poisoning is always interesting and usually revealing, it invariably leaves the investigator with a sense of complete futility, for the outbreak is over when it is discovered, and no preventive measures can be instituted.

The prevention of these conditions is a long, slow process of education of food handlers and enforcement of regulations relating to the handling, processing, and storage of all types of food, together with special emphasis upon improvement in methods of preparation and storage of protein foods.

Effort should be concentrated in those places where outbreaks most frequently occur. Large banquets are the chief offenders. The banquet often overtaxes the resources of the hotel or the caterer: food is prepared in large quantities, well in advance of the dinner hour, and placed in individual serving dishes in order to avoid a last-minute rush. Salads, shrimp cocktails, creamed foods, and the like are prepared and allowed to stand for several hours before they are served. Food is carelessly handled and is not stored at sufficiently low temperatures. The result is that conventions of all types, church dinners, fraternity picnics—in fact, all large gatherings of people—are very frequently accompanied by outbreaks of food poisoning.

Prevention depends upon the simple facts that the bacteria and their products are readily destroyed by heat and cannot develop at low temperatures. Even though the salmonella actually enter the protein foods through careless handling, no harm results if the food is kept at proper refrigerator temperatures. However, a good general household rule is to reheat all protein food to boiling if the food has been kept in storage for any length of time, i.e., 24 hours in the refrigerator or 3 hours at room temperature.

Antemortem and postmortem abattoir inspection is of some value since animals with obvious disease are condemned as unfit for food.

Scrupulous cleanliness in the preparation and handling of food, especially of meat and meat products, is an important safeguard. Pasteurization of milk and proper heating of milk products, such as ice-cream mix, custards, and all other such materials, are an essential part of the preventive program.

Constant supervision of restaurants, delicatessens, cold-storage plants, roadside eating stands, meat and fish markets, and all places that handle food in any way, is a laborious and uninspiring but very important service that the health department gives to the people. It is never wholly successful since carelessness and negligence are almost universal human failings, and unintelligent food handlers cannot be expected to maintain strict standards of cleanliness at all times, even under most careful supervision.

New Problems in the Control of Food-borne Infections

The increasing use of prepared foods and their processing in large quantities have increased the hazard of nontyphoidal salmonella infections. The major source of such infections is products made from raw or partially cooked dried eggs. The pooling of large numbers of eggs, including some contaminated with salmonella, inevitably increases the number of consumers at risk. The scattering of cases resulting from the wide distribution of such products may completely mask the relatedness of resulting cases of enteritis.

The prevalence of salmonella contamination of spray-dried egg powder is staggering. Almost 10 per cent of more than 7,000 samples of egg powder imported into England from the United States were contaminated with various salmonellae. The use of such powders by bakers and confectioners constitutes a special hazard, because cake and candy might not be sufficiently heated in their manufacture to kill the organisms. Perhaps related to the threat of raw-egg products and other processed foods, the incidence of salmonellosis has increased tenfold in Massachusetts between 1950 and 1956 and sevenfold throughout the United States at large in the period 1946 to 1955 (2). Concurrently, typhoid fever has gradually declined. There is recent evidence that paratyphoid B in addition to the food-borne salmonella enteritides may also be carried by processed chicken eggs.

The Prevention of Food-borne Infections Related to Fecal Contamination

It is obvious that all infections that can be acquired via ingestion of water or milk (see Tables 9 and 10) could be similarly acquired through food (Table 11). Therefore, the control of many of those infec-

TABLE 11

Common Infections Transmitted By Food

Infection	*Usual Sources*
Tapeworm infestations	
Taenia saginata	Beef
Taenia solium	Pork
Diphyllobothrium latum	Fish
Trichinosis	Pork
Amebiasis	Raw vegetables or fruit
Anthrax	Meat of sick animals (rare)
Brucellosis	Meat of sick animals (rare)
Bacillary dysentery	Meat products
Cholera	Raw vegetables or fruit
Streptococcal infections	Meat products
Salmonella enteritis	Meat and egg products
Typhoid	Shellfish
Tularemia	Rabbit meat
Tuberculosis, bovine	Meat of sick cattle
Staphylococcal enteritis (toxic)*	Milk and egg products (custards, mayonnaise, etc.)
Botulism*	Sausage, fish, home canned legumes (beans)
Infectious hepatitis	Oysters,? clams

* Not true infections but intoxications.

tions classified literally as "food-borne" depends finally upon the elementary principles of sanitary sewage disposal and water purification. Thus the hazard of food-borne amebiasis results from the grossest type of contamination of leafy vegetables with human feces (night soil) used for crop fertilization in the Orient. Other infections of the type in which uncooked vegetables are essentially a passive vector of human feces include schistosomiasis, ascariasis, and whip-worm infestation. In the absence of effective sanitation, infections of this type can be prevented by the cooking of contaminated veg-etables.

The Control of Infections Carried by Meat and Fish

Unrefrigerated and improperly handled meat and fish provide, as milk does, a fertile culture medium for many bacteria. In the natural course of events, bacterial growth leads to the hydrolysis of proteins and to the "putrefaction" or "decay" of the animal flesh. Despite its stench and esthetically forbidding aspect, "rotten" meat is not intrinsically dangerous to the human organism unless the bacteria which have initiated decomposition include (a) enteric pathogens (salmonella or shigella) or (b) producers of toxins (staphylococci or clostridia). Putrefied seal meat is valued by the Eskimo as a delicacy and the hundred-year-old eggs of the Chinese are essentially a cheese produced by protein denaturation. In western culture the hanging of beef or venison fosters protein and collagen breakdown through endogenous enzymatic action which increases the meat's tenderness and palatability. For centuries man has devised many methods for delaying the decay of meat, all of them inadvertently directed at the suppression of bacterial growth.

There has been a tremendous improvement in the diet of man within a period of 25 years, due to engineering advances in methods of preservation of foods. Formerly the diet of the average family was limited to certain staple foods: salted or dried meat and fish, potatoes, bread and other cereals, milk and milk products, with fresh meat at intervals, and vegetables and fruits only in their seasons.

The development of cold-storage facilities by the use of refrig-erator railway cars on a large scale, the establishment of enormous community refrigerator plants, and the invention of simple family cold-storage units have revolutionized food habits and made most fresh foods, such as fruits and vegetables, fresh meat and fish, avail-able to all people at all times of the year.

The principles of good food preservation are very simple. They depend upon the facts that:

1. Food spoilage is due largely to bacterial action. Thus, bacte-rial control results in food preservation.

2. Bacteria require certain favorable conditions for development. In general, they require: (a) a suitable—usually warm—temperature,

(b) moisture, (c) protein food, and (d) a favorable medium for growth. For example, a high concentration of salt or sugar will check the growth of many bacteria.

Air is required for the growth of some organisms; others do not require it. Many bacteria require very special conditions for development, including a favorable hydrogen ion concentration and exact temperatures. Thus food preservation, developed for centuries on an empirical basis, has now become an exact science. It is, in great part, an application of simple bacteriologic principles to the processing of foods.

Refrigeration. Most bacteria which destroy food, and most pathogenic bacteria as well, do not develop at low temperatures, though few organisms are killed by freezing. (Trichinae and cysts of the tenias are killed at −10° F in a 20-day period.) Some foods, such as meat, fish, and fowl, are well preserved by being kept at temperatures below freezing, while other foods such as oranges, tomatoes, and potatoes are well preserved at low temperatures but injured by freezing.

The quick-freezing process, which is carried out at very low temperatures (−35° F), with a holding temperature of −10° F, has proved to be a very successful and safe method of preserving many fruits, vegetables, meats, and other farm products.

Cold-storage foods lose little of their nutritive qualities, but they decompose rapidly when removed from storage and therefore should be consumed immediately.

Canning. This process applies the bacteriologic principles of the autoclave, or of fractional sterilization, and is a very safe and satisfactory method of food preservation. Commercial canning of food is done on a scientific basis and under health department supervision. This food may be stored for long periods at room temperature without spoilage. Gas formation, with bulging of the can, is a good index that this type of food is unfit for use.

Home-canned foods are often prepared under rough-and-ready conditions by unskilled hands. There is always a possibility of food contamination. Thus, home-canned foods—particularly meats and vegetables—should always be heated before use. (See the discussion on botulism, pp. 155-56.)

Salting, Drying, Corning, and Pickling. These are methods of preservation of foods that utilize the principles that bacteria cannot develop without moisture and that they fail to grow in high concentrations of sugar, salt, or acids such as vinegar.

Cooking. This process is an invention of civilization which is, by far, the most important factor in the destruction of bacterial products and the preservation of food. Cooking frequently injures the flavor of food and destroys some of its nutritive value, but its advanage as a mode of health protection greatly outweighs its disadvantages. The use of heat in the preparation of food is one of the greatest methods of health conservation.

In areas or at times of economic duress, meat animals which are obviously sick are slaughtered and used for food. Under these conditions, certain unusual types of food-borne infection have occurred, including brucellosis, botulism, anthrax, and tuberculosis. Even this type of infection might be prevented by adequate cooking of the meat.

The principal hazard of meat that is obtained from manifestly healthy animals or fish and properly handled and refrigerated is from certain helminthic parasites in which the larval form encysts in the skeletal muscle. These infections are the tapeworm infections (see p. 113) and trichinosis. Intervention at any point in the life cycles of these parasites could control these diseases, but economic and political considerations make such attempts unrealistic. For example, if only cooked garbage were fed to hogs and if rats were excluded from their enclosures, trichinosis could be abolished by eliminating the sources of swine reinfection.

Inspection of meat is a virtually hopeless method of control because:

1. Even costly microscopic inspection cannot guarantee the safety of the entire carcass.
2. The consumer might be sold uninspected meat.

Therefore, the definitive and realistic control of these infections is based on accepting their probable occurrence and utilizing the principle of "terminal disinfection" by adequate cooking of the meat. In the case of trichinosis, recent studies have demonstrated that X-irradiation as well as freezing is also effective in killing encysted larvae in the meat. Interesting experiments with ionizing radiation for the preservation and microbial sterilization of food are now being conducted. At the present time, however, the final responsibility for avoiding meat-borne infection rests with the cook.

REFERENCES

1. Milk Ordinance and Code. *U.S. Pub. Health Service Bull. 220.* Government Printing Office, Washington, D.C., 1936.

2. BLACK, P. H., KUNZ, L. J., and SWARTZ, M. N.: *New England J. Med.*, 1960, **262**:811.

11. THE CONTROL OF ANIMAL RESERVOIRS AND ARTHROPOD VECTORS OF INFECTION

The Control of Infections of Domestic Animals as Related to Infections in Man

Infections of domestic animals that are transmitted to man (Tables 6 and 7) could obviously be eliminated by the detection, then cure or elimination of all infected animals. In the United States the virtual elimination of bovine tuberculosis has contributed less to the control of enteric tuberculosis (which is preventable by milk pasteurization) than to economic and nutritional welfare by ensuring healthy herds of cattle. The problem of brucellosis is similar, and the trichinosis problem has been discussed in Chapter 10. Therefore, it can be said, in brief, that regulation of disease in domestic food animals is critically important only in relation to the economic and nutritional importance of the animals. This is also true with respect to domestic animals which may serve as intermediate hosts for human parasites (e.g., African trypanosomiasis). Such infections are more readily controlled by attack upon the insect vector or by chemoprophylaxis in man himself.

An exception to the foregoing statement is the case of *psittacosis* in which careful supervision and control of the avian host are essential for the prevention of human infection. Such control is now aided by treatment of infected flocks with antimicrobial drugs (i.e., tetracycline).

Another exception is *rabies* in which there is now no substitute for strict supervision and control of domestic canines through licensure and rabies immunization. The hazards of currently available vaccines interdict routine immunization of any but certain high-risk groups of the human population (see Chap. 17).

In the case of wild animals and birds infected with viruses transmissible to man by arthropods (see Table 6), prevention of such transmission is obviously best directed at the vector.

The Control of Arthropod Vectors of Infection

Among the more dramatic accomplishments of modern medicine has been the control of certain arthropod-borne diseases by assaults upon the vector. The conquest of urban yellow fever in the West Indies by the elimination of the town-dwelling *Aëdes aegypti,* and the reduction of malaria in Europe and the United States by control of swampy anopheline breeding places were followed by the truly revolutionary discovery of DDT. This remarkable chlorinated hydrocarbon is relatively inexpensive, has low toxicity for man and other mammals, is effective against a wide variety of arthropods, and has residual killing activity long after it is applied to walls or other surfaces. Shortly after the discovery of its insecticidal potency in 1939, it was shown to be remarkably effective in controlling louse-borne epidemics of typhus in Italy during World War II by its direct application as dusting powder to the clothing and persons of those at risk.

In the winter of 1943 and 1944 the siege of Naples had driven people into large caves where they were crowded in indescribable filth and confusion. Typhus broke out in the city, and the danger of a serious widespread epidemic of the disease was apparent. The army in conjunction with the Typhus Commission organized a delousing campaign. Each person was deloused without removal of clothing. A simple technique was instituted of spraying the fine DDT powder into the hair and at the neckband. The "hand-operated powder duster" also sprayed the dust up each sleeve and at the waistband, front and back. About one ounce of powder was used for each person. The DDT powder impregnated the clothing so thoroughly that the individual was rendered louse-free for about four weeks. In many thousands of persons treated there were no reports of dermatitis or other intoxication. The epidemic was promptly brought under control.

In recent times a serious effort is being made by the World Health Organization to eradicate malaria by intensive, carefully planned nation-wide cycles of DDT spraying. Typical examples of such programs have been cited in the *WHO Chronicle*(1):

The delegate of Afghanistan stated that malaria was the greatest public health problem in his country. The eradication campaign there had started 18 months earlier, and more than 4 million persons were now protected in areas where malaria prevalence had been almost 75 per cent.

The malaria eradication programme in Colombia is considered to be the most successful of the country's health activities. An agreement on the programme of the campaign was concluded with WHO in 1956, and spraying started in 1958. The fourth spraying cycle has just ended, and it is hoped to finish the fifth cycle, thus completing the first stage of eradication, in March 1961. Eradication is expected to be achieved by 1962. Insecticide resistance has developed in some localities among certain *Anopheles,* but the question has been studied thoroughly by experts and it is hoped to overcome this difficulty. Evaluation of the campaign started with the end of the first spraying cycle and every care is being taken to ensure that it is as complete as possible. Technical staff for the Colombian campaign has been trained with WHO assistance, and 25 per cent of the national health budget is being devoted to the campaign. Agreements have been concluded with neighbouring countries—Venezuela, Peru, Ecuador and Panama—for joint eradication efforts, aimed in particular at freeing the Pan American Highway from malaria hazards.

In India, practically the whole population of 400 million is being protected by spraying, and complete eradication of malaria is one of the aims of the country's third five-year plan which starts next year. "The plan for (malaria) eradication," said the chief of the Indian delegation, "will go down in history as one of the most fascinating endeavours on a global scale for the welfare of mankind."

Such bold campaigns for the reduction or elimination of biological species require not only the international political cooperation reflected in the foregoing citation, but also detailed knowledge of geography, topography, and climate, as well as of the biology of the mosquito and its habits. This indeed is true of any type of vector or vermin control. As pointed out in "Insecticide Resistance and Vector Control"(2):

Application of pesticides by routine methods and on a nonselective basis often leads to unsatisfactory and costly results. Frequently, the period of activity of an insect is restricted, so that effective use of a chemical measure is limited to that period. For example, the application of insecticidal fogs before dusk is unsuccessful in controlling infestations of certain species of mosquitoes, whereas, the same treatment at dusk, or shortly thereafter gives excellent results. Some species of anophelines (e.g., *Anopheles sergenti* in Israel and Jordan) are semi-domestic in their habits, and residual treatments are only partially effective in reducing or interrupting malaria transmission. In contrast, in the same countries a domestic species (*A. sacharovi*) has been almost completely eradicated by similar applications.

But the greatest deterrent to eradication campaigns is the selection, by widescale use of a chemical insecticide, of genetically resistant insects within a species. This problem has become of great practical importance recently, and it is reported that at least 50 arthropod species of public health importance (including flies, mosquitoes, lice, and ticks) are resistant to one or more of the commonly employed insecticides, including DDT. This problem, which is similar to microbial resistance to antibiotics, has been partially circumvented by the development of other chlorinated hydrocarbon insecticides (dieldrin, Chlordane, and lindane) which may be effective against DDT-resistant flies or mosquitoes. The inevitable development of resistance to these newer compounds has already occurred and emphasizes the need for "saturation" eradication programs to forestall the gradual genetic development of resistance in arthropod populations.

A Summary of Methods for the Control of Arthropod Disease Vectors. The important human infections borne by arthropods are listed in Table 12 together with chemical methods for their control. This highly simplified summary emphasizes the diversity of approach to the chemical (insecticidal) control of arthropod disease vectors. Although this chemical approach is of major importance in disease eradication programs, it must be supplemented by the older methods of arthropod control, which include:

1. Elimination of breeding sites.
2. Control of infected animals which may carry fleas, mites, or ticks.
3. Use of insect repellents for personnel exposed in the field.

Control of ticks, mites, and culicine mosquitoes which inhabit rural, forest, or jungle areas is obviously difficult or impossible at times. In such areas, special ecologic problems are encountered because the use of toxic residual insecticides could kill birds, fish, and game animals. In these circumstances it is more reasonable to protect man by immunization or chemoprophylactic procedures. Such prophylaxis is indeed used and includes vaccines against yellow fever, as well as quinacrine (Atabrine) and chloroquine for malaria, and broad-spectrum antibiotics for scrub typhus.

The Control of Disease-carrying Rodents

The basis of rodent control is proper environmental sanitation with respect to food handling, garbage disposal, and adequate human dwelling places. In addition, relatively specific and powerful poisons have been developed which, when ingested, kill rats or mice rapidly.

TABLE 12 **Important Diseases Transmitted by Arthropods: Chemical Control of Vectors**

Arthropod	Disease Transmitted	Chemical Control*	How Applied
Lice	Epidemic typhus, relapsing fever, plague (rare)	DDT, lindane	To person
Fleas	Plague, murine typhus	DDT	To rat runs and harborages
Ticks	The spotted fevers, plague, tularemia, Russian tick-borne encephalitis, relapsing fever	DDT, chlordane, dieldrin, parathion	Area control by sprays and dusting
Mites or chiggers	Scrub typhus, rickettsialpox	Dieldrin	Area treatment
House flies	Enteric infections, especially typhoid and bacillary dysentery	DDT, dieldrin, lindane (organophosphorus compounds)†	Residual spray (dwellings)
Biting flies			
Tsetse fly	Trypanosomiasis	DDT	Area control
Black fly	Onchocerciasis	DDT	To watercourses for larva control
Sand fly	Leishmaniasis	DDT	Residual spray (dwellings)
Cone nose bugs (triatoma)	American trypanosomiasis	Dieldrin	Residual spray (dwellings)
Mosquitoes			
Anophelines	Malaria	DDT, dieldrin, BHC‡	Residual spray (dwellings), larva control
Culicines	Yellow fever, filariasis, dengue, encephalitis	DDT	Dwellings (yellow fever)
		DDT, dieldrin, BHC‡	Area and larva control (filariasis encephalitis)

* For complete information on chemical names and other data see WHO Technical Report Series, No. 191.
† Other DDT-like compounds are chlorinated hydrocarbons.
‡ The insecticide benzene hexachloride (hexachlorocyclohexane).

These poisons include:

1. Warfarin, a dicoumarin derivative.
2. Pival (2-pivaloyl-1-3-indandione).
3. ANTU (α-naphthyl thiourea).
4. 1080 (Sodium monofluoroacetate) — the most potent compound, but also extremely toxic for man and other animals.

As with the insecticides, knowledge of the biology and habits of the species is needed so that baits will be taken. Actual eradication of rodents is almost impossible.

REFERENCES

1. *WHO Chronicle,* **14**(8):297. World Health Organization, Geneva, Switzerland, August, 1960.

2. *Insecticide Resistance and Vector Control,* WHO Technical Report Series, No. 191, p. 98. World Health Organization, Geneva, Switzerland, 1960.

Man as an Infectious Hazard to Man (the "contagious" or "communicable" infections transmitted directly from man to man)

There is a large group of infections whose perpetuation depends on the direct transmission of their infective agents from man to man *without the necessary intercession of intermediate hosts, arthropod vectors, or prolonged survival in the environment.* These are truly human infections and are caused only by the smaller parasites — bacteria and viruses — which are obligate and specific parasites of man. Intimate human association and contact are required for the spread of these infections, and certain of them (smallpox, measles) have been recognized as contagious for centuries on the basis of circumstantial evidence and high clinical attack rates. Others of these infections such as poliomyelitis have only recently been recognized to be equally contagious because the clinical attack rate or incidence of manifest *disease* is low, although the incidence of inapparent *infection* is high in susceptibles.

It is appropriate to consider together in this section infections as manifestly dissimilar as cholera, syphilis, and influenza because the problems concerning their spread and, conversely, their containment are basically similar.

169

12. INFECTIONS THAT ARE PRIMARILY ENTERIC

The so-called enteric infections are those in which the parasite primarily invades and multiplies in the gut, usually the small intestine. Such infections are almost invariably acquired by ingestion; therefore it is predictable (and a matter of fact) that the infective agents are hardy enough to pass the acid barrier of the stomach and that they possess the ability to survive for a time outside the host. It is also apparent that all those agents potentially could be borne and spread by food and water in the absence of direct human-human contact (see Table 8).

Bacterial Infection

The evidence that the bacterial enteric infections (Table 13) are spread directly by fecal-oral contact is for the most part epidemiologic. In the case of bacillary dysentery, outbreaks of the so-called asylum type have occurred in the absence of food or water contamination and have been correlated with the grossly poor sanitation of inmates in institutions and with bacteriologic evidence of fecal contamination of doorknobs, etc. The epidemiology of cholera and shigellosis is influenced by the fact of subclinical or inapparent infection; in the case of typhoid the epidemiology is affected by the occurrence of a protracted carrier state in almost 3 per cent of cases. These factors result in the shedding of organisms into the environment in the absence of diarrheal disease. In areas of poor sanitation and high population density, a relative immunity develops in survivors of infection, thus complicating further the accurate assessment of endemic infection. Furthermore, typhoid in infants and young children can be so mild as to be unsuspected and thus constitutes an unrecognized infection focus. The more prolonged course of typhoid coincides with protracted (one to eight weeks) excretion of bacilli in the feces, so that the recognized case is a constant hazard.

170

The Enteroviruses

In a little more than a decade the development of revolutionary approaches in virology has resulted in the recognition of more than 50 "new" viruses and a completely altered concept of the previously recognized diseases, which they have since been found to cause. Among these viruses, the 30 Coxsackie viruses and 28 antigenic types of ECHO viruses comprise (together with the 3 polioviruses) the biologically related enteroviruses which cause varying disease states in man but primarily infect his intestinal tract. The neurotropic potential of these viruses, especially the polioviruses, initially obscured their relationship to non-neurotropic disease and complicated the understanding of their epidemiology. It is now clear that the viruses of this group are epidemiologically not unlike typhoid in their primary invasion of the enteric tract, their subsequent spread to other organs, the mildness of their disease if engendered in childhood, and their protracted persistence in the gut.

The formulation of new laboratory methods (tissue culture, use of infant mice) for virus isolation and antibody studies has led to recognition of the importance of clinically inapparent infections and to the concept that the enterovirus infections are among the most contagious of diseases.

Coxsackie Virus Infections

In 1948 a "new era" in modern medical virology began when Dalldorf and Sickles(1) isolated a virus from the stool of a poliomyelitis patient from Coxsackie, N.Y., which paralyzed infant mice — animals not previously used in the study of poliomyelitis. Similar viruses were soon isolated from patients without paralytic poliomyelitis, so that quite early it was clear that the new virus was the agent of nonpoliomyelitic infections.

In the past decade, 24 distinct types of group A and 6 of group B Coxsackie virus have been categorized. The Coxsackie viruses of both groups A and B have pathogenicity for the infant mouse in common but differ in their pathologic effects. The group A and B viruses differ also in the diseases which they induce in man. Although viruses of both groups can cause lymphocytic (aseptic) meningitis, the group A strains cause herpangina and also an exanthematous fever, whereas the group B strains cause epidemic myalgia or pleurodynia, pericarditis in adults, and fatal myocarditis in infants.

TABLE 13

Infections Directly Transmitted from Man to Man: the "Communicable" or "Contagious" Diseases

I. Infections That Are Primarily Enteric

Infection	Infective Agent	Nonenteric Sites of Infection	Persistence of Agent in Stool
Bacterial			
Cholera*	*Vibrio comma*	—	One or 2 days, or duration of illness (carried 30 days)
Bacillary dysentery*	*Shigella* species		Duration of illness (occasional carrier state)
Infantile diarrhea	*E. coli* (certain species, e.g., 0111, 055), possibly viruses		?
Typhoid*	*Salmonella typhosa*		Thirty days or more; carrier state in 3 per cent for 1 year
Viral			
Enteroviruses			
Coxsackie group A Herpangina, summer grippe, meningitis, exanthem	Coxsackie A, types 1-24	Pharynx, vagina	Up to 30 days
Coxsackie group B Pleurodynia, summer grippe, meningitis, pericarditis	Coxsackie B types 1-6	Pharynx	Variable
ECHO virus infections Pharyngitis, meningitis, exanthem, diarrhea, colds	ECHO virus, types 1-28	Pharynx	Variable
Poliomyelitis	Poliovirus, types 1-3	Pharynx	Pharynx: 10 to 14 days; stool: 7 to 123 days
Reovirus infections	Reoviruses	Pharynx	?
Infectious hepatitis	Hepatitis, virus A	?	Unknown, but occasionally 5 months
"Viral" or nonbacterial gastroenteritis	Two or more filter-passing agents	?	?

*Rarely transmitted directly man to man. Controllable by environmental sanitation.

172

The Coxsackie viruses are isolable from the pharynx but are present in highest concentration in the gut. Virus can be carried for as long as 30 days after acute infection.

The ECHO Viruses

Whereas the Coxsackie viruses are separable from other enteroviruses by their pathogenicity for infant mice, the ECHO viruses (with few exceptions) are pathogenic only in primate tissue culture. Indeed, their recognition is a direct outgrowth of the use of tissue cultures in poliomyelitis research. When tissue culture became widely used for the isolation of poliovirus from suspected cases of poliomyelitis, pathogenic agents which were not polioviruses were found in increasing number. Because some of these agents were initially recovered from patients without apparent disease, they were originally known as orphan viruses or "viruses in search of disease," then, more definitively, as enteric cytopathogenic human orphan (ECHO) viruses(2).*

The 28 types of ECHO virus have been implicated as have the Coxsackie agents in lymphocytic meningitis, but more frequently than the other enteroviruses in illnesses associated with rash (ECHO types 4, 9, 16). The indication that certain types cause diarrhea is the first evidence that a virus propagable in the laboratory can cause that syndrome. It is remarkable, in fact, that the *entero*viruses do not usually cause *enteric* symptoms.

Poliomyelitis

Only 15 years ago poliomyelitis loomed as a virtually unassailable fortress on the medical horizon. At that time research was tremendously handicapped by the lack of convenient and reliable methods of cultivating the virus and measuring antibody against it. The inadequacy of earlier methods had led to the erroneous concept that poliomyelitis was a unique type of viral disease, a disease of low contagiousness (as indicated by paralytic cases), a disease which defied the usual laws of immunology, an infection predominantly of "civilized" society which produced "infantile paralysis." Because the virus was neurotropic in the chimpanzee and monkey, it seemed unlikely that it could ever be propagated in tissue cultures of non-

---

*Cattle, swine, and other species have been found to have orphan viruses of their own: ECBO (enteric cytopathogenic bovine orphan) viruses, etc.

neural cells. The enormous progress within the past decade in the understanding of the true nature of poliomyelitis is attributable to the brilliant and painstaking work of many research scientists and field workers; it is specifically related to the acquisition of evidence that:

1. Poliovirus is excreted in human feces.

2. There are three separate types of poliovirus which induce little or no immunity to one another.

3. Most infections with poliovirus are nonparalytic.

4. Most so-called nonparalytic poliomyelitis is caused by other enteroviruses.

5. Certain other enteroviruses cause paralytic poliomyelitis.

6. Poliovirus can be cultivated in cultures other than neural tissues.

7. Virus so cultivated can produce effective immunity to paralysis in man.

The cornerstone of much of this evidence is the Nobel prize-winning discovery by Enders, Weller, and Robbins that the polio viruses could be cultivated in non-neural tissue cultures(3). There is no stronger argument for the "practical" importance of basic research than the poliomyelitis story. Epidemiologic research, no matter how brilliantly conceived or logically executed, is finally dependent upon the specificity and precision of its methods.

Renewed investigation of poliomyelitis soon confirmed earlier suspicions that poliomyelitis was not an infection principally of civilized countries. On the contrary, infection with poliovirus – as with other enteric pathogens – is more common in areas of poor sanitation where it occurs at an earlier age. Because infection in infancy is less often associated with manifest disease or paralysis, the paralytic *disease* is less common in poor areas, although, paradoxically, *infection* is more widespread. The emergence of the apparently "new" disease of infantile paralysis in this century has occurred initially in nations with the highest level of sanitation (the Scandinavian countries, the United Kingdom, and the United States) and closely parallels the decline of other enteric infections such as typhoid. The postponement of poliovirus infection until later childhood or even adulthood resulted more frequently in the paralytic effects of the infection (poliomyelitis) in the older host, which is *more vulnerable to the effects of the infection* than the very young infant. The studies of

Gelfand and his associates(4) have shown that infection in the early months of life is rarely symptomatic. Thus poliomyelitis is in a sense a disease of civilization—a price paid for a cleaner environment, but a small price for the concomitant reduction in bacterial enteric infections and their attendant high infant mortality.

Among the myths about poliomyelitis which have been dispelled by recent research are the ideas that (a) it is necessarily a disease of the summertime, and (b) it is not very contagious and spreads

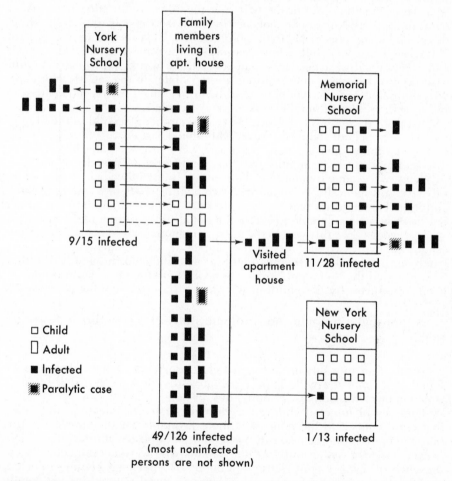

Figure 21. Lines of midwinter transmission of poliomyelitis virus from York Nursery School to hospital apartment house and the other two nursery schools. (McCarroll, J. R., Melnick, J. L., and Horstman, D. M.: *Am. J. Pub. Health*, 1955, 45:1541.)

erratically through the community. A thoroughly studied outbreak caused by type 1 poliovirus in midwinter in New York City provides effective refutation of both ideas. A brief description of the epidemic follows (see also Fig. 21):

The first sign of poliomyelitis occurred when a three-year-old girl in the York Nursery School developed paralytic disease on January 7, 1955. She lived in the apartment house containing eight of the families with children in the York Nursery School, and one child in the New York Nursery School. Ten days after the onset of the first case the 29-year-old father of a second child in the York Nursery School, and living in the same apartment building, developed symptoms of paralytic poliomyelitis. This second nursery school child had been well but a four-year-old brother not attending the school had complained of a headache and fever three weeks previously. A third case occurred in the same building ten days later in the mother of a child who did not attend the school but had been in contact within the apartment house with children from the York Nursery School.

Just prior to the onset of the initial case, a mother of a child in the Memorial Nursery School living in the neighborhood visited two families living in the apartment house where the cases were to occur. She had lived in this building until six months previously and was on friendly terms with two housewives now living there. The mother brought two of her children on this visit and spent the afternoon with two families, both of whom had young children. The children who were visited did not attend any nursery school but there was considerable intermingling of all the children in the building.

Two weeks after this visit to the apartment house a child not attending any school but with two brothers in the Memorial Nursery School, developed paralytic poliomyelitis. He apparently became infected through his brother who attended the Memorial Nursery School where the virus had presumably been introduced by the children who had visited the apartment house(5).

A thorough virologic and serologic study of this outbreak revealed that:

In the first two schools investigated 60 per cent of the children were found to be infected with Type I poliomyelitis virus, as revealed by virus isolation or possession of CF antibodies, or both.

Families of infected children gave higher rates of infection, indicating that close contact in the home was more favorable for the spread of virus than the more limited contact in the school. *All siblings of infected children became infected* (italics ours). Of the parents who were not protected by the presence of Type I neutralizing antibodies, 93 per cent became infected, confirming the high invasiveness of the virus usually noted in such family groups.

Investigation of a third school in which a known carrier of the virus was found, however, failed to reveal any spread of the virus, indicating that the usual high invasiveness of the virus may be modified under some circumstances(5).

Reovirus Infections

A newly recognized group of viruses that apparently cause disease of both the respiratory and enteric tracts has recently been separated from the ECHO viruses and termed the "reoviruses"(6).

It is too early to assess the importance of these viruses as agents of human disease, but it is interesting that at least one such virus has been associated with a steatorrheic enteritis in adults and diarrhea in children. These or related viruses apparently infect many animal species as shown by serologic methods.

"Viral" or Nonbacterial Gastroenteritis

Often called "intestinal flu" but having no relation to true influenza, "viral" enteritis causes an immense morbidity in the winter months of the year. The acute onset and brief but prostrating course can be mistaken for the vomiting and diarrhea of food poisoning. However, the sequential onset of cases within family groups aids in the differential diagnosis.

Two clinical patterns of illness are recognized:

1. An afebrile diarrheal disease attended by nausea and vomiting.
2. A febrile disease with abdominal pain but usually without diarrhea.

The two diseases appear to be immunologically distinct. The etiologic agents of "viral" enteritis have not been cultivated in the laboratory so that evidence for its viral etiology comes from studies in human volunteers.

Infectious Hepatitis

Infectious hepatitis is an infection of widespread prevalence with a peak incidence in childhood. On the basis of human volunteer studies, the infective agent appears to be a filter-passing virus (termed hepatitis virus A) which is remarkably resistant to thermal and chemical inactivation, withstanding exposure to 1 residual part per million of chlorine for 30 minutes or more (see Chap.10).

Study of this disease has been badly handicapped by the lack of laboratory methods for isolating and cultivating the causative virus. Nevertheless, clinical and epidemiologic studies have drawn a tentative picture of the natural history of hepatitis. It is probable that infection by the fecal-oral route is prevalent in childhood, particularly in areas of poor sanitation. Such infection is often without jaundice and is sometimes completely inapparent in infants and young children. Certain geographic areas such as the Middle East and Mediterranean Coast seem to have an unduly high endemic prevalence. In Denmark, a country of good sanitation where accurate disease reporting has been carried out, seasonal trends of incidence have been noted with increases beginning in late summer and peaks in midwinter; yearly variation in "epidemic waves" was also observed.

The presence of antibody against the virus in gamma globulin from pooled human blood suggests that most adults have had infection and have developed immunity. However, as with poliomyelitis, the overt, severe *disease* is more common in older children and adults and is *less* common in the areas of poor sanitation where the incidence of inapparent childhood infection (and consequent adult immunity) is high. Here again is the misleading clinical suggestion that in underdeveloped areas there is "no polio" and "no hepatitis." It is probable that the asymptomatic infant (who carries virus for months in his stools) could be an important source of infection in all areas.

The epidemiology of infectious hepatitis is further confused by the existence of the virus of serum hepatitis (virus B). That virus produces a similar clinical picture but may be immunologically different and it is probably not spread by the fecal-oral route (see Chap. 15).

REFERENCES

1. DALLDORF, G., and SICKLES, G. M.: *Science*, 1948, **108**:61.

2. Committee on the ECHO Viruses: *Science*, 1955, **122**:1187.

3. ENDERS, J. F., WELLER, T. H., and ROBBINS, F. C.: *Science*, 1949, **109**:85.

4. GELFAND, H. M., LeBLANC, D. R., FOX, J. P., and CONWELL, D. P.: *Am. J. Hyg.*, 1957, **65**:367.

5. McCARROLL, J. R., MELNICK, J. L., and HORSTMANN, D. M.: *Am. J. Public Health*, 1955, **45**:1541.

6. SABIN, A. B.: *Science*, 1959, **130**:1387.

13. INFECTIONS PRIMARILY OF THE RESPIRATORY TRACT

The most common and troublesome of human infections are those in which the infective agents multiply primarily in the respiratory tract. These agents, which almost invariably are spread by intimate human contact, are specific and demanding in their requirements, and thus cannot exist for long in the external environment, in contrast to the enteric pathogens (see Tables 8 and 13). They are thus unaffected by environmental sanitation so that by exclusion they become relatively more important in contemporary "civilized" societies. The causes of many of these infections have only recently been identified, and the causes of most minor infections of the respiratory tract are still unknown.

Diphtheria

In almost all countries diphtheria remains an important medical problem despite the fact that it is one of the best studied of microbial diseases. In underdeveloped areas in which immunization is not practiced, *Corynebacterium diphtheriae* is a killer of infants and children; in countries such as the United States in which childhood immunization is widespread, the disease is a constant threat to the increasing number of adults who lose their artificially induced childhood immunity. The continuing immunity of adults in impoverished areas is related to endemic prevalence of *C. diphtheriae* among carriers in the population, so that immunity is continually reinforced by re-exposure and latent reinfection.

Diphtheria is primarily a local infection of the upper respiratory tract by one of three types of *C. diphtheriae: gravis, mitis,* and *intermedius,* which apparently cause disease of the varying severity indicated by their names. The exotoxin liberated by bacilli growing superficially in the mucous and dead epithelial cells of the upper respiratory tract destroys adjacent living cells, which in turn become the sites of further bacterial multiplication and local "membrane" formation. Unless the infected individual possesses appropriate blood concentrations of specific antitoxin, systemic absorption of toxin may result in toxic damage to peripheral nerves and heart muscle — much of which is reversible with time.

Because the immunity of artificial immunization is specifically antitoxic and not antibacterial, it is interesting that nevertheless *Corynebacterium diphtheriae* has almost disappeared in communities in which childhood immunization is prevalent. It seems probable that perpetuation of the bacterium in the population depends in part on its capacity to injure the host with its toxin sufficiently to permit its further local multiplication and subsequent dissemination.

Hemophilus Influenzae Infections

The importance of *H. influenzae* in human disease remains controversial. In the sense that the bacillus is not etiologically related to influenza, it is misnamed. Although studies during the pandemic of 1918 suggested an association of *H. influenzae* (Pfeiffer's bacillus) and influenza, other studies indicated the equal or greater importance of pneumococci, streptococci, and staphylococci in secondary bacterial invasion. It has since been learned that many (up to 50 per cent) normal people carry *H. influenzae* in the respiratory tract in the winter months. However, most of these organisms are "untypable," nonencapsulated, and nonpathogenic.

Nevertheless, there is no question that *H. influenzae*, especially type B, causes primary pyogenic respiratory tract infections, which are often complicated by otitis media, pneumonia, septicemia, and meningitis — especially in young children.

Pertussis (Whooping Cough)

Pertussis is a highly contagious and potentially fatal air-borne infection of childhood caused by *Hemophilus pertussis*. A related bacterium, *H. parapertussis*, causes a similar but milder clinical syndrome, which includes the classical symptom of "whooping cough" and evidence of peribronchiolitis.

Pertussis is endemic throughout the world and occurs at any season. In the United States, peak incidences occur in early winter in the North and in the spring in the South. The spread of the infection seems to be related to cases of clinical disease; healthy carriers are not considered important in this regard. However, the prevalence of partial immunity from vaccination may so modify the disease that it is misdiagnosed; such undiagnosed cases could become unrecognized sources of infection.

Mortality from pertussis occurs principally in patients less than one year of age. The mortality has progressively declined in the United States since 1920.

Meningococcal Infections and Meningitis

As in the case of poliovirus infections, meningococcal infections are frequent, but they are only rarely associated with manifest disease or central nervous system involvement. During epidemics the carrier rate can reach 95 per cent. Although the interepidemic carrier rate is 5 to 15 per cent, examination of a given population over a winter period has disclosed that most of the population have carried meningococci at some time during the observation period. In temperate climates, minor epidemics occur yearly with fluctuations to major epidemics at five- to twelve-year intervals.

In most individuals, meningococcal infection of the nasopharynx is either wholly asymptomatic or attended by mild rhinitis or pharyngitis. The next most common manifestation is a subacute septicemia with recurrent fever, rash, and polyarthritis. Least common are the severe and potentially fatal manifestations of fulminating septicemia or meningitis. Acute septicemia and meningitis with their fatal sequelae are most common in infants and children. In contrast to *H. influenzae* meningitis, which is more common in girls, meningococcal disease appears to be more common in boys.

Crowded living conditions seem to foster the dissemination of organisms, for the incidence is higher in crowded urban areas and in army barracks and institutions. Undiseased carriers are important in the spread of infection, and one clinically apparent case is rarely traced to another.

Pneumococcal Pneumonia

It is estimated that in adults 95 per cent of primary bacterial pneumonia is caused by the pneumococcus (*Diplococcus pneumoniae*). Even in the so-called secondary or bronchopneumonias, which may complicate chronic lung diseases or surgery, the pneumococcus is the most common etiologic agent. In view of the fact that 40 to 70 per cent of the healthy population may carry pneumococci, many of them virulent types, it has long been evident that

[*Text continued on p. 184.*]

TABLE 14

Infections Directly Transmitted from Man to Man: The "Contagious" Diseases

II. INFECTIONS PRIMARILY OF THE RESPIRATORY TRACT

Infection	Infective Agent	Nonrespiratory Sites of Infection	Persistence of Infective Agent in Respiratory Tract
Bacterial			
Diphtheria	*Corynebacterium diphtheriae*	Skin, myocardium, nervous system	2 to 4 weeks
Hemophilus influenzae infections	*Hemophilus influenzae*	Meninges	6 to 8 weeks
Pertussis	*Hemophilus pertussis*		
Meningitis (epidemic)	*Neisseria intracellularis*	Meninges, skin, joints	
Pneumonia	*Diplococcus pneumoniae, Klebsiella pneumoniae*	Meninges, urinary tract	Variable
Staphylococcal infections	*Staphylococcus aureus*	Skin, endocardium	
Streptococcal pharyngitis and scarlet fever	*Streptococcus pyogenes*	Skin	2 to 4 weeks
Tuberculosis	*Mycobacterium tuberculosis* (var. *hominis*)	Multiple	Variable
Leprosy	*Mycobacterium leprae*	Multiple	?

182

Viral

Adenovirus infections ("ARD," pharyngitis)	Adenoviruses (types 1-18)	Eye, gut	4 days or less
Common cold cough, rhinitis, and fever	? Respiratory syncytial virus (CCA)	? ?	? ?
Parainfluenza (croup, colds)	Parainfluenza viruses 1-4	?	?
Influenza	Influenza viruses A,B,C	?	1 to 7 days
Mumps	Mumps virus	Meninges, central nervous system, salivary glands, gonads, pancreas	Up to 9 days
Smallpox	Variola virus	Skin, viscera	? 14-21 days
Chickenpox and herpes zoster	Varicella virus	Skin, posterior roots	7 to 14 days, lifelong*
Herpes simplex	Herpes simplex virus	Skin, eye	Lifelong*
Measles	Measles virus	Skin, C.N.S.† (P)	Up to 9 days?
Rubella	Rubella virus	Skin, C.N.S.† (P)	?
Primary atypical pneumonia	PPLO	?	?
Infectious mononucleosis	Virus ?	Liver, spleen	?

*In latent, noninfective form.
†Central nervous system.

factors other than the presence of pneumococci in the nose and throat are important in the pathogenesis of pneumococcal pneumonia. Epidemiologic studies of man and experimental observations in animals suggest that damage to the respiratory mucosa by noxious agents (especially viruses) and factors which depress the defenses of the lower respiratory tract (alcohol, pulmonary edema, etc.) lead to aspiration of pneumococci so that they reach the alveoli.

Although pneumococcal pneumonia is so sporadic in occurrence that it is not considered to be a "contagious" disease, it may become epidemic if: (a) the pneumococcal carrier rate of a population becomes high and (b) the concomitant incidence of viral respiratory disease is high. Such conditions are sometimes seen in institutional groups or military populations.

Although more than 75 antigenic types cause human disease, most cases of pneumonia are caused by the "lower-numbered" types of pneumococcus, types 1, 2, and 3. Of these types, 1 and 2 are not commonly carried by normal subjects. The type-specific immunity associated with recovery from pneumonia appears to reduce the chance of a subsequent carrier state in the convalescent.

Primary pneumococcal pneumonia is most common in young adults, in males (perhaps because of occupational exposure), and in workers in steel mills and coal mines.

Primary pneumonia caused by *Klebsiella pneumoniae* (Friedländer's pneumonia) may be confused diagnostically with pneumococcal pneumonia. The ecology of this infection is very different, however. *Klebsiella* is found both in the throat and in the normal intestinal tract, and can be naturally carried by species other than man. It rarely causes pneumonia in the absence of obvious general debility, previous infection, or alcoholism. It is a rare cause of pneumonia.

Staphylococcal Infection

Among bacteria which cause respiratory tract infection, the staphylococci are unique in their capacity to resist environmental stress and in their apparent capacity for mutation to withstand such stresses. Thus while meningococci, group A streptococci, and pneumococci remain susceptible to most antibiotics, increasing numbers of antibiotic-resistant staphylococci have appeared. Basic knowledge of the pathogenesis and immunity of staphylococcal disease is less advanced than with most other bacterial infections; this fact also contributes to emergence of staphylococcal infection as a current problem of modern society.

It is *Staphylococcus aureus* strains of certain types (coagulase positive) that are of principal importance in human disease. Such strains can be carried nasally and cutaneously by 30 to 50 per cent of the general population. Yet overt disease as evidenced by furuncles, osteomyelitis, or pneumonia is relatively uncommon. In recent years it has become apparent that *epidemic* staphylococcal disease (as in hospitals and nurseries) seems to be engendered by relatively few types of staphylococci. Most such strains are of bacteriophage group III; coincidentally they are antibiotic resistant. Of group III, the phage subtype 80-81 has caused most hospital infections in the United States in the last decade; in the United Kingdom and Australia, phage types 80 and 52A have been responsible. Because typing staphylococci has not been done routinely until recently, it is not clear whether the ostensibly "virulent" strains of today differ from those of the past. Another question is whether or not staphylococcal infections are becoming more numerous and more serious as the proportion of antibiotic-resistant strains increases.

Staphylococcal infections are most common in infancy and childhood. However, they are a constant threat to the debilitated or organically damaged host of any age, e.g., the diabetic or the patient with influenza.

Although the epidemiology of staphylococcal infections has not been definitively established, it appears that nasopharyngeal carriage of the organisms is of major importance in spreading infection. The staphylococcal type carried cutaneously is usually the same as that in the nose of the carrier.

Streptococcal Pharyngitis and Scarlet Fever

Only hemolytic streptococci categorized serologically as group A are important in the causation of respiratory disease in man. The usual manifestation of such infection is acute pharyngitis. If a rash occurs concomitantly, the disease is termed "scarlet fever," although epidemiologically it does not differ from pharyngitis without rash. Erysipelas was once thought to be a different disease, but now it is recognized as a cutaneous manifestation of streptococcal infection.

Group A streptococcal infections represent a special problem among infectious diseases because of the serious and sometimes permanent damage which may occur as late sequelae in some patients. These sequelae of infection include acute rheumatic fever and the permanent cardiac damage which may occur during its course. Another sequela is a form of acute glomerulonephritis, which is initiated only by specific group A streptococcal types, particularly type 12; this rarely leads to permanent renal damage.

Although immunity following streptococcal infections is type-specific, there are indications that general nonspecific immunity to streptococcal disease may develop with age. Infections in infants and young children may be mild and protracted and difficult to diagnose clinically. Apparently healthy individuals, as well as convalescents, may harbor pathogenic streptococci during epidemic seasons in the winter and spring. A rise in this carrier rate may herald an epidemic. Streptococcal infections are world-wide in distribution, but the incidence of disease is higher in cold climates. Infection is spread by intimate association of a susceptible person with one carrying streptococci in his upper respiratory tract. Although the clothing and adjacent environment of such a carrier may contain organisms, spread probably occurs directly from one respiratory tract to another.

Tuberculosis

Most human tuberculosis is caused by the human type of *Mycobacterium tuberculosis*. Ten per cent or less may be caused by bovine or avian variants of this bacterium. In the United States, tuberculosis caused by the bovine strain has been essentially eliminated through pasteurization of milk and careful supervision of dairy herds.

The spread of tuberculosis from man to man is dependent upon close human contact and presumably occurs as an air-borne infection. The genesis of most tuberculosis is within the family, and the incidence of tuberculosis within family groups in which an adult has an open or cavitary lesion is extremely high. Indeed, the demonstration of a positive tuberculin test in an infant or a young child may serve as a case-finding method for "open" disease in an adult with whom the child has been in close contact.

Tuberculosis differs from most infections of the respiratory tract in its chronicity and in the limited efficacy of both the healing process and the immunity engendered by the infection. These circumstances influence the epidemiology of the disease. Thus, supposedly cured or arrested tuberculosis may be endogenously reactivated in the absence of external reinfection, and the patient may become a threat to society years after the primary infection.

Because primary (or childhood) tuberculosis and reinfection (or adult) tuberculosis behave like two different diseases, they are often considered separately with respect to their pathogenesis and epidemiologic significance. Man is intrinsically quite resistant to infection with *Mycobacterium tuberculosis,* and most such infection does not result in disease. However, the initial invasion by tubercle bacilli, whether in the child or in the adult, may be followed by an acute illness associated with caseation of the lymph nodes and by rapid progression of healing within a brief period of time. If hematogenous spread of the organism occurs, generalized or miliary tuberculosis or tuberculous meningitis may result. Paradoxically, this more acute form of the disease is rarely contagious because of the absence of necrotic lesions, which permit the egress of mycobacteria into the bronchi.

In the postprimary or reinfection type of disease, the prior development of significant but incomplete immunity causes the disease to be localized to the lungs and bronchi and to their lymphatics, and the disease has a less acute and more protracted course. Disease of this sort is of paramount importance in the spread of pulmonary tuberculosis.

The Influence of Age, Race, Sex, and Environmental Factors on the Epidemiology of Tuberculosis. No infection is more influenced by the environmental conditions of the host and his physiologic state than is tuberculosis. It is notable that significant decline in the incidence and the death rate of tuberculosis occurred long before the advent of chemotherapy. Nevertheless, in the world at large, tuberculosis is still the most frequent cause of death in those between the ages of 15 and 45. It is significant that in the United States a declining *mortality rate* from tuberculosis has not been paralleled by an equal decrease in *morbidity and prevalence* of infection. Outside of Western Europe, North America, and Australia, both morbidity and mortality rates are still very high.

In the United States, the characteristic peak mortality previously observed in the third decade of life has changed; now the highest mortality rate from tuberculosis is in elderly males. In underdeveloped countries, however, the peak mortality is still observed in the third decade.

The occurrence of severe disease and death is generally higher in very young infants, in males, in nonwhite races, in poorer economic groups, and in the malnourished. It is obvious that there is a considerable overlap of these various parameters. For this reason it is not clear whether the apparent racial differences in susceptibility to serious tuberculous disease are on a genetic basis or are coincidentally related to environmental factors. Physiologic and psychologic stresses, such as pregnancy and mental illness as well as intercurrent disease or infection, appear to predispose to postprimary tuberculosis.

The Changing Pattern of Tuberculosis. The differences in mortality rate and its pattern are similarly reflected by a changing age of acquisition of primary tuberculosis in the United States and other highly developed countries. These age differences of initial tuberculous infections are most easily detected by tuberculin skin testing and an assessment of the percentage of individuals in a group who are

TABLE 15

The Changing Incidence of Tuberculin Reactors among Students
Entering Cornell University Medical College, New York*

Year	Number Positive	Per Cent
1952	18	21
1953	14	17
1954	5	6
1955	3	4
1956	6	7
1957	6	7
1958	4	5
1959	8	10
1960	8	10
1961	5	6

*Unpublished data, courtesy Dr. J. R. McCarroll.

positive reactors to tuberculin (i.e., have developed cutaneous hypersensitivity following infection, the latter usually inapparent). In Table 15 is shown the marked change in the percentage of tuberculin reactors in Cornell University Medical College students (New York City) in different years. Even in urban areas in the United States, primary infection with tubercle bacilli is frequently postponed beyond childhood. Because specific immunity from previous infection, rather than age per se, is most important in modifying the character of tuberculosis, it is evident that the clinical picture of tuberculosis in the adult (when infection results in disease) will be increasingly like the primary or childhood type.

Epidemiologic Implications of Disease Caused by Chromogenic or Atypical Mycobacteria

Within the past decade there has been increasing recognition of the pathogenic potential of so-called atypical or chromogenic mycobacteria. Because some of these organisms appear to be geographically restricted in their distribution and may come more from the environment than from human beings, they can confuse considerably the picture of tuberculosis unless their existence is recognized. These mycobacteria confound epidemiologic surveys because some are of low pathogenicity and cause virtually no disease; yet they may induce hypersensitivity to tuberculin in a majority of the population. The role of most of these organisms in human disease is only now being explored.

Viral Infections of the Respiratory Tract

Since 1950, tremendous progress has been made in the study of acute infections of the upper respiratory tract. Many new viruses have been isolated, categorized, and related to specific disease processes. Although the cause of most minor infections (the common cold) remains unknown, viruses have been recently isolated from certain patients with the common cold syndrome—usually defined as an acute, brief, benign illness which is afebrile and predominantly manifested by rhinitis.

The importance of minor respiratory tract infections lies in the enormous incidence of illness they occasion rather than in their threat to life. Nevertheless, it is probable that even the most minor of these infections may pave the way for secondary bacterial infections and their sequela of chronic pulmonary disease. It is also true that such "minor" infections in the aged or those with underlying cardiopulmonary disease occasionally result in severe and even fatal illness. In addition, it is apparent that respiratory symptoms of presumed viral etiology comprise a surprising burden to ostensibly healthy people even when the symptoms are not severe enough to cause absenteeism from work.

An intensive study(1) of ten "healthy" young adults during a nine-month period has demonstrated:

1. A surprisingly high frequency of minor symptoms, as revealed by careful daily questioning.
2. The occurrence of approximately seven discrete minor illnesses per person, the majority of them involving the upper respiratory tract.

3. The afebrile nature of these illnesses and the low rate of absenteeism associated with them.

4. A failure to categorize by the best of the then current virologic methods any but two of these illnesses.

The striking contribution of respiratory symptomatology to total symptoms is graphically shown in Figure 22.

Adenovirus Infections

Eighteen types of adenovirus have been identified since the discovery of this group in 1953. However, the importance of these

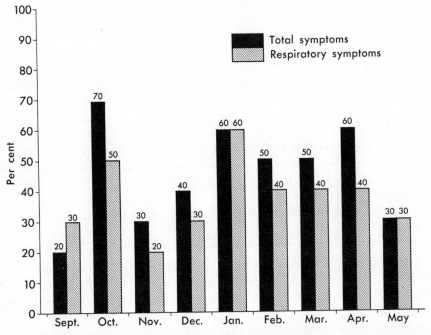

Figure 22. The concordance of respiratory and total symptomatology. The proportion of subjects who manifested undue prevalence of respiratory and total symptoms in each month. Percentage of subjects with above-average number of symptoms per month compared with percentage with above-average respiratory symptoms, 1958-1959. (McNamara, M. J., *et al.: Am. Rev. Resp. Dis.*, 1960, 82:469.)

viruses in human disease is only now being established. It is apparent that certain specific types (types 3, 4, and 7) are important causes of illness under certain restricted conditions. For reasons that are not clear, these viruses cause a very high incidence of infection and disease in military recruits in training camps. These viruses, with the exception of type 3, seem to be of little importance in causing disease in the civilian population at large.

In civilian populations, other virus types (including types 2 and 5) may cause outbreaks or sporadic cases of acute pharyngitis or pharyngoconjunctival fever and "pink eye" or swimming pool conjunctivitis. Type 8 adenovirus has been clearly related to *epidemic keratoconjunctivitis.*

The adenoviruses of greatest biologic interest are those that appear to be truly latent in the adenoidal and tonsillar tissue of man. The adenoviruses may persist for years within those tissues without inducing disease, as is true of herpes simplex and herpes zoster viruses in other sites. Such adenoviruses are detected only when the tissue is removed and cultivated *in vitro.*

The Common Cold

Because of its mild and poorly defined characteristics, as well as its obvious association with changing climates and temperatures, there has been question in the past whether the common cold was indeed a contagious and infectious disease.

Until recently, the best data have been provided by studies of isolated communities such as Spitsbergen (see Fig. 12, p. 81) in which the common cold occurred as an epidemic disease after its apparent introduction by people from outside the community. For many years there has also been evidence that the common cold could be induced in human volunteers by inoculation of nasopharyngeal washings from patients with the syndrome. Within the past five years there has been more conclusive evidence for a virus etiology. It has been shown that certain agents capable of causing the common cold syndrome can be propagated in tissue culture and that they are, in fact, viruses. These agents include the JH or 2060 virus, which appears to be a type of ECHO virus(2), and other agents with even more fastidious growth requirements that have been isolated in the common cold studies in Salisbury, England(3). In order to propagate some of the "common cold" viruses it has been necessary to maintain the human embryonic tissue at temperatures and pH comparable to the human nasal mucosa. Evidence from continuing human volunteer studies indicates that there is probably more than one virus capable of causing the common cold and that specific immunity to these viruses follows infection(4).

Parainfluenza Viruses

The parainfluenza viruses are so named because they fit biologically into the myxovirus group, of which influenza viruses are the original prototypes. Again, as with the adenoviruses and the common cold viruses, the importance of these agents in human disease is only now being defined. However, it is clear that the four types of parainfluenza virus thus far identified in man are associated with acute upper respiratory infection in infants and children, which may be attended by laryngotracheitis or croup; it is also probable that a milder "common cold" type of disease may occur in adult infection. The limited data now available suggest that a considerable percentage of croup and acute respiratory infections in young children may be accounted for by these viruses (at least in certain years).

The identification of similar viruses in nonhuman species, including the monkey and the bovine, has suggested a possible animal reservoir of infection, but this possibility remains unproved.

Respiratory Syncytial Virus

The respiratory syncytial virus was first isolated in 1956 from chimpanzees, and originally termed the chimpanzee coryza agent (CCA). Its current name reflects the cytopathic effect it induces in tissue culture. It has been demonstrated that the virus is important in causing febrile illness in children. The disease may be related to involvement of either upper or lower respiratory tracts. The highest incidence of infection appears to be in children one year of age(5). Confusion with influenza is possible because fever and cough are the principal presenting signs(6).

Influenza

The virus of influenza appears to be unique among the infectious agents of man in its capacity for undergoing mutation so extreme that it can circumvent immunity produced by its pre-existing forms. This fact, together with the relative brevity of even its specific immunity, has allowed it to persist in modern times as the last great unconquered plague.

It is unlikely that bubonic plague or smallpox will ever recur as pandemics because of (a) the advances of environmental sanitation and chemotherapy for the containment of plague, and (b) the triumph of smallpox vaccination. The "white plague" of tuberculosis is also yielding to improved environmental conditions and newer chemotherapeutic measures. Yet even with our ability to produce a specific vaccine rapidly, influenza occurred again in pandemic form in 1957 and 1958. Specific immunization did prevent the disease in a minority of the world's population, and the fatal effects of secondary bacterial pneumonia were appreciably curtailed by modern antibiotics. Nevertheless, the impact of this brief but prostrating infection was felt throughout the world.

Although there are three distinct types of influenza virus (A, B, and C), only influenza A virus is an important cause of epidemic disease in the general population. Since the original isolation of

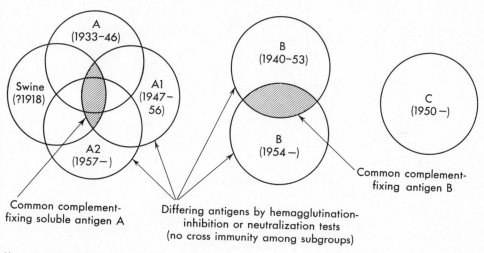

Note: <u>No</u> antigens are common to influenza A, B, and C viruses

Figure 23. Antigenic character of influenza A, B, and C viruses and their subgroups.
Note: A third distinct group of B strains appears to have evolved since 1955.

influenza A virus in 1933, two major antigenic changes have occurred — the first in 1947 and the second in 1957, when the first pandemic in the era of modern virology occurred. Although the virus was still recognizable in the laboratory as influenza A, its mutations were so great that members of the population who had been vaccinated with pre-existing strains of virus had no immunity to the new variants (the problem which such mutation poses with respect to control of the disease is discussed fully in Chap. 17).

In light of the evidence that an influenza virus can demonstrably cause pandemic as well as sporadic epidemic disease, the inference that the great 1918 pandemic was caused by a similar virus seems more and more justifiable. Although no virus was isolated from human beings in 1918, a virus causing influenza in swine at that time was subsequently isolated from those animals and shown to be closely related to the human influenza A viruses which were later discovered. The relation of these viruses is schematically shown in Figure 23.

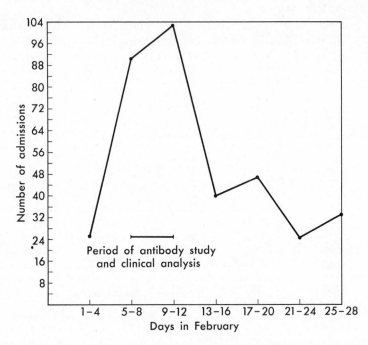

Figure 24. Number of admissions for upper respiratory infection for each of seven four-day periods. (Data derived from 60 per cent of all respiratory disease admissions for February, 1947.) (Kilbourne, E. D., and Loge, J. P.: *Ann. Int. Med.*, 1950, 33:371.)

When influenza appears in the community, the two major public health problems are:

1. A sometimes explosive onset of morbidity which involves large numbers of the population with a brief, usually benign, but prostrating disease.

2. Increased mortality in certain members of the population— principally those with underlying cardiopulmonary disease or pregnancy.

The impact of influenza in a military population is shown in Figure

24. This curve, which traces the admission rate to an army station hospital, is illustrative of the acute nature of influenza in semiclosed populations of susceptible people.

The rapid spreading of what was then a "new" virus, to which everyone was susceptible, is illustrated in Figure 25 showing the extremely rapid dissemination of A2 (Asian) influenza within a

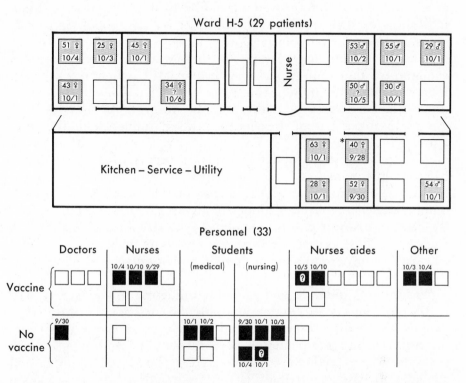

Figure 25. An influenza epidemic on a hospital ward (A2 [Asian] influenza in 1957). Topography of ward H5 and make-up of ward personnel. Shaded blocks represent individual patients and personnel who developed influenza symptoms. The date of appearance of symptoms is indicated within or above the blocks. The location of the initial case is indicated by an asterisk. (Blumenfeld, H. L., *et al.*: *J. Clin. Investigation*, 1959, 38:199.)

hospital ward. The protective effect of vaccination of attending personnel is shown in the lower part of Figure 25. It must be emphasized, however, that the spread of influenza is sometimes puzzlingly slow; within family groups it may not have a uniformly high attack rate, and secondary cases may appear only after six or seven days(7). Factors of virus dose, environment, and differences in age may influence markedly the incidence of influenza even in populations without any specific immunity to the virus.

Influenza virus alone may induce a fatal pneumonia in elderly or cardiac patients(8), but it more frequently increases mortality indirectly by preparing the way for secondary bacterial pneumonia. Indeed, so constant is this relationship that an excess mortality related to pneumonia is widely used by public health officers as a subtle indication of the presence of influenza in the population. This mortality occurs chiefly in those over 45 years of age. Because older, less active people may escape the first wave of infection in the community, their infections may occur later, when evidence of influenza morbidity in the population at large has disappeared. Thus, a puzzling increase in mortality may be observed in the older age groups in the apparent absence of clinical influenza in the community.

It is possible that influenza not only predisposes to secondary bacterial infections in the individual patient but that it also increases the carrier rate and prevalence of pathogenic bacteria in the community. A remarkable coincidence of high incidence of influenza and an increased carrier rate for beta-hemolytic streptococci is shown in Figure 26. This occurred in the same epidemic illustrated in Figure 24. In this army camp a major epidemic of streptococcal pharyngitis followed during the subsequent month.

Pandemic, Epidemic, and Endemic Influenza. Influenza may exist in the community in pandemic, epidemic, or endemic form. Pandemics of the disease are rare and occur at roughly 30- to 40-year intervals. During interpandemic periods, the virus continues to cause sharp localized epidemics in closed or isolated communities and sporadic disease (sometimes fatal in the elderly) in larger open population groups. The question of "what happens to the virus between epidemics" has not been completely answered. It seems reasonable to surmise, however, that as population immunity rises, *continuing infection is less frequently evidenced by disease*. Therefore, the disappearance of epidemics of disease does not necessarily reflect the absence of virus in the community. There is already evidence of such "endemic" persistence of influenza virus following the 1957 pandemic(9).

Mumps

Mumps or epidemic parotitis is caused by a virus biologically similar to the influenza and parainfluenza viruses. It is a myxovirus

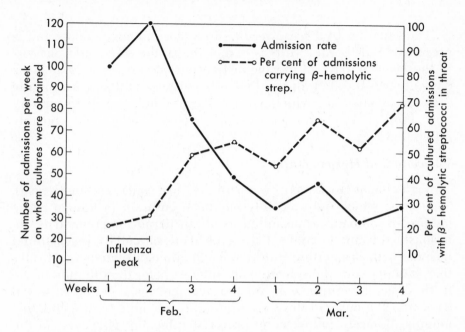

Figure 26. Increase in the proportion of patients carrying streptococci following an influenza epidemic in a military population. (Kilbourne, E. D., and Loge, J. P.: *Ann. Int. Med.*, 1950, *33*:371.)

which apparently does not vary in its antigenic constitution. For this reason, one attack of infection appears to confer lasting immunity, although second or even third attacks have been reported. In view of the fact that other infections, including group B Coxsackie virus infections, occasionally cause disease of the salivary glands, it is not surprising that alleged recurrences of mumps have been reported.

The disease is acute and incapacitating; however, in children (the usual victims), it is almost always benign. In adults a painful and feared complication is orchitis, which occurs in 20 per cent of male cases. However, sterility or sexual abnormality after such a complication is rare.

Although case histories indicate that only 60 per cent of adults have had mumps in childhood, serologic studies indicate a much higher percentage of infections. This evidence of past occurrence of clinically inapparent infections has been confirmed by human volunteer studies. These studies have shown that subjects may excrete virus in the total absence of symptoms. Such inapparently infected people undoubtedly contribute to the spread of infection.

Transmission of disease results from close human contact and is presumably air borne. Virus is detectable in the saliva and pharynx in the last few days of the incubation period and for as long as six days after the onset of illness. Probably because mumps is essentially a systemic infection which does not cause necrosis of respiratory tract epithelium, secondary bacterial complications are notably infrequent.

Varicella and Herpes Zoster

Varicella, or chickenpox, is one of the most contagious of diseases. The virus, which only recently has been cultured in human tissue culture, is probably transmitted as an air-borne infection. It is notoriously difficult to prevent the spread of varicella virus within a hospital with susceptible children. Epidemiologic evidence indicates that patients with the infection are infectious for the duration of the fresh vesicular eruption or, on the average, for a period of seven days after the onset of illness. Chickenpox is a mild disease and, like mumps, is rarely followed by bacterial infection. However, in the adult it may cause a severe and sometimes fatal illness characterized by extensive viral pneumonia.

It has long been suspected on epidemiologic grounds that herpes zoster or "shingles" was caused by a virus similar, if not identical, to that of varicella. Thus the appearance of herpes zoster in an adult has sometimes been followed by chickenpox in his children. Culture of both viruses has proved their biologic and immunologic identity. There seems to be little doubt that herpes zoster represents the reactivation of pre-existing latent varicella virus in posterior nerve roots or their dermatomes.

Herpes Simplex

Herpes simplex is a perfect illustration of the differing pathogenic potentials in a given infectious agent under varying circumstances. In premature infants, the virus may cause a fatal generalized infection characterized by visceral necrosis. In some infants it assumes its more usual manifestation of acute stomatitis with fever; in other infants, it causes clinically inapparent infection. In older children or adults, it may be present as an acute pharyngitis or aseptic meningitis; in younger children, it may cause fatal encephalitis. Its recurrent manifestations may be asymptomatic or may be evidenced as the common fever blisters or cold sores, which attend other acute infections. The wide range of host-virus relationships illustrated in Figure 16, page 88, demonstrates that the relatively narrow focus of the practitioner of internal medicine cannot permit a true view of the spectrum of infection with this virus. A similar figure could be drawn for almost any other infectious disease.

Herpes simplex per se is not an important infection; however, it is a fascinating prototype of the latent viral infection which can be reactivated in later years in spite of demonstrable and persisting serologic immunity. It could therefore serve as a model for studies of virus in the etiology of tumors.

Smallpox

One of the plagues of ancient times, smallpox is endemic throughout most of the world with the exception of North America and Australia, but remains a constant threat to all people. The virus of smallpox is unique among respiratory-borne viruses in its hardihood and, as indicated elsewhere (p. 123), may exist in the environment for significant periods of time. However, such extra-human residence is of little importance in the epidemiology of the disease since most cases originate from an actively infected patient with a discernible skin rash.

Sustained immunity to the disease seems to depend on its endemic prevalence in the community. In endemic areas, mild or inapparent infections in partially immune persons may contribute to the spread of the disease.

Two types of smallpox have been described: (a) variola major, the classical severe type attended by a high mortality, and (b) variola minor or alastrim, a relatively benign disease, which has appeared in Africa, Western Europe, and America during the last 60 years. The high mortality of approximately 30 per cent which can result from variola major is not due to secondary bacterial pneumonia per se, although this may occur as a complication.

Measles

This ubiquitous and highly contagious virus disease is worldwide in distribution. It is chiefly a childhood disease except in populations which remain isolated for long periods of time. When isolated communities such as the Faroe Islands or Greenland are infrequently attacked by measles, the attack rate of clinical disease is close to 100 per cent, and the disease involves all age groups.

In this situation, mortality from pneumonia occurs in the very young and the very old, as is the case with influenza.

Measles occurs at any time of year, but most outbreaks take place in the late winter and early spring. The disease occurs in epidemic cycles of two- to three-year intervals. This epidemic periodicity has been explained as the result of introduction of new susceptibles into the population by birth or immigration.

Unlike most other viral infections, infection with measles virus appears to provoke manifest disease in almost all patients; i.e., the clinical attack rate is extremely high, and inapparent infection is virtually unknown. Therefore, new epidemics must result from the exogenous introduction of virus in the communities into which new susceptibles have also been introduced.

Secondary to viral multiplication and damage in the respiratory tract, bacterial invasion may occur so that as many as 15 per cent of patients could suffer otitis media or pneumonia related to pneumococcal or streptococcal infection. As with influenza, most mortality (particularly in primitive populations) is the result of secondary bacterial pneumonia. Encephalitis is a dangerous but relatively infrequent complication, occurring in fewer than 1 per cent of cases.

Rubella

(See also congenital and neonatal infections, page 216.) This mild exanthematous viral infection (also known as German measles) is almost always benign in children but can produce a more serious illness in young adults who have escaped childhood infection. It has the potential for causing serious congenital malformation if contracted during pregnancy. The virus of rubella has not yet been isolated in experimental animals or tissue culture, and therefore knowledge of the epidemiology of this infection is limited. Because the clinical syndrome is essentially that of a low-grade febrile disease with transient erythematous rash, it is probable that many other infections have been confused with it, including the recently recognized enteroviruses which may produce rash (see Chap. 7)

It may be inferred that rubella is not as widespread nor as contagious as measles because many adults escape childhood infection only to suffer the disease in later life. Transmission of the infection is presumably via the respiratory tract. Secondary bacterial infection is rarely encountered. The major importance of this disease is as a cause of congenital malformation.

Primary Atypical ("Viral") Pneumonia

During World War II, an atypical type of pneumonia emerged to prominence. This pneumonia differed from the acute bacterial pneumonias in: (a) its relative indolence of course, (b) its lesser severity, and (c) its failure to respond dramatically to sulfonamides and penicillin. This disease was only sporadically encountered in civilian practice, but it often became epidemic in military camps or in institutions such as boarding schools. Bacterial pneumonic pathogens such as pneumococci or group A streptococci were rarely isolated from patients with this disease. The only laboratory tests of value in categorizing patients with this syndrome were tests for the presence of increasing amounts of "cold agglutinins" for human erythrocytes or agglutinins for a nonhemolytic streptococcus (streptococcus MG) inconstantly isolated from patients with the disease and from normal people.

Human volunteer studies during World War II by the Commission on Respiratory Diseases suggested the possibility that the disease was caused by a virus. A filter-passing agent was isolated in cotton rats by Eaton(10). In the last few years, newer techniques involving fluorescent antibodies(11) have demonstrated the association of Eaton's agent with cases of "viral" pneumonia. The nature of the agent is not yet clear, however, it may prove to be a small form of bacterium—a pleuropneumonia-like organism (PPLO)(12). Should this be the case, then the claims of some investigators that tetracycline antibiotics are effective in the disease will gain support, as the PPLO are susceptible to broad-spectrum antibiotics. In any event, the agent is susceptible to antibiotics when cultivated in the chick embryo.

REFERENCES

1. MCNAMARA, M., *et al.: Amer. Rev. Resp. Dis.*, 1960, **82**:469.
2. PELON, W.: *Am J. Hyg.*, 1961, **73**:36.
3. TYRRELL, D. A. J., *et al.: Lancet*, 1960, 1:235.
4. JACKSON, G. G., and DOWLING, H. F.: *J. Clin. Invest., 1959*, **38**:762.
5. MCCLELLAND, L., *et al.: New England J. Med.*, 1961, **264**:1169.

6. REILLY, C. M., *et al.: New England J. Med.*, 1961, **264**:1176.

7. JORDAN, W.: *Am. Rev. Resp. Dis.*, 1961, Part 2, **83**:29.

8. LOURIA, D. B., *et al.: J. Clin. Invest.*, 1959, **38**:213.

9. HAYSLETT, J., *et al.: Am. Rev. Resp. Dis.*, 1962, **85**:1.

10. EATON, M. D., MEIKLEJOHN, G., VAN HERICK, W.: *J. Exp. Med.*, 1944, **79**:649.

11. LIU, C.: *J. Exp. Med.*, 1957, **106**:455.

12. CHANOCK, R. M., *et al.: Proc. Nat. Acad. Sci.*, 1962, **48**:41.

14. VENEREAL AND OTHER INFECTIONS ACQUIRED BY DIRECT CONTACT

The human infections that are spread by direct contact of untraumatized skin or mucous membranes include the venereal diseases:

Syphilis *(Treponema pallidum).*
Gonorrhea *(Neisseria gonorrhoeae).*
Chancroid ("soft chancre") *(Hemophilus ducreyi).*
Lymphogranuloma venereum (LGV virus).
Granuloma inguinale *(Donovania granulomatis).*

Treponemal diseases other than syphilis which are transmitted by nonvenereal contact are:

Yaws *(Treponema pertenue).*
Pinta *(T. carateum).*
Bejel (nonvenereal syphilis: *T. pallidum).*

The viral ocular infections, trachoma and epidemic keratoconjunctivitis, are possibly transmitted by direct contact.

The primarily cutaneous infections of ringworm of the scalp *Microsporum audouini* and impetigo (staphylococcal or streptococcal) are also considered to arise from contact infection.

Syphilis

Syphilis is a disease in which the social and moral implications are so closely interwoven with its medical and public health aspects that it is difficult to discuss this infection without becoming involved in matters that have little bearing upon the epidemiology and the control of the infection.

Epidemiology. Syphilis is caused by *Treponema pallidum* and is transmitted, in practically every instance, by direct venereal contact with an active superficial lesion of the skin or mucous membrane.

203

In rare instances the disease may be transmitted through objects soiled with the patient's discharges. Occasionally, transmissions through blood transfusion have occurred. Also, infants may be infected in utero through the placenta of the infected mother.

The incubation period is usually three to four weeks but may vary from ten days to six weeks.

The infected individual is highly dangerous as long as the lesions of the mucous membrane or skin are open, because the serum of the lesion is swarming with treponemata.

Formerly, all stages of the disease were considered communicable, but it is now clear that, even without treatment, the infected person is not dangerous to others after about two years, with the exception of congenital transmission. The acute case can be rendered non-infectious by proper treatment in a very short space of time.

Prevalence of Syphilis. The exact prevalence of syphilis is not known. There has been a tendency to exaggerate the importance and overestimate the prevalence of this disease in the enthusiastic development of control methods. The data that have been collected on prevalence have not always been correctly interpreted. In general, syphilis is not common among intelligent people of the higher social ranks. Young men and women enrolled in colleges and universities seldom have a positive Wassermann reaction. It is truly a social disease—a disease of ignorance, poverty, carelessness, and negligence—an associate of crime, social maladjustment, war,* and other disturbed social conditions. It has been estimated that one adult in ten in the United States has had syphilis; that over 400,000 persons in the nation become infected with syphilis each year, that 20 per cent of deaths from organic heart disease are due to syphilis; and that syphilis is one of the four major causes of death. It is also claimed that there are almost as many recent cases of syphilis in the community as all other reportable diseases combined.

All these statements have some foundation of fact but are probably an overestimation. If one considers the types of persons that show evidence of infection, it becomes clear that the disease is quite selective in its prevalence. The data in Table 16 are taken from serologic surveys of various groups of people.

These surveys illustrate the great variation in syphilis prevalence in different economic, occupational, racial, and social groups.

---

*There is strong evidence that World War I resulted in a generally unrecognized, but nevertheless extensive, epidemic of syphilis. The epidemic prevalence of both syphilis and gonorrhea during World War II was clearly recognized.

The results of the serologic blood tests for syphilis that were secured from the first 2,000,000 reports(1) of selectees for army service in 1940-1942 provided an excellent cross section of the prevalence of syphilis in the United States and changed many of our preconceived ideas concerning the epidemiology of the disease in this country.

Syphilis has been called an urban disease, a disease of large cities and seaports, but this is not true in the United States. The urban rate in these men was 4.6 per cent while the rural rate was 4.4 per cent.

Furthermore, syphilis is not a disease of seaports, nor does it have an unduly high prevalence in large cities. The largest cities,

TABLE 16

**Positive Wassermann Tests Encountered in Mass Surveys
of Various Social Groups**

Social Group	*No. per 1,000*
American university students, unselected series	1
Large industrial plants employing skilled labor	6
Prospective blood donors, 2,044 examined	8
Premarital examinations, all persons	12
White rural unskilled day laborers, all ages	23
Street beggars	110
Railroad employees, large series	117
Negroes, all ages, southern United States	190
Convicts, large series	240
Prostitutes, large series	300-700

such as New York, Chicago, Boston, and San Francisco, all had rates of less than 2.5 per cent, whereas the rate for the nation as a whole was 4.5 per cent. Industrial areas do not suffer to an unusual degree. Rhode Island and Connecticut, the two most completely industrialized states in the Union, had rates of 1.1 and 1.2 per cent, respectively.

The extraordinary fact brought out by these data was the high prevalence of syphilis in the Negro. This rate permeated overwhelmingly all the other data. In all parts of the United States the rate in Negro men was at least ten times higher than that in white men.

Gonorrhea

Gonorrhea is an acute infectious venereal disease attributable to *Neisseria gonorrhoeae*. The incubation period of the disease is short—three to six days—and the period of communicability continues as long as the organisms are present in the discharges. Relapses are not uncommon, and female patients may be infectious for a long period. Communicability of the disease may be determined very satisfactorily by cultural methods, and to a less satisfactory degree by direct microscopic examination of the discharges.

Gonorrhea is transmitted by intimate personal contact, usually sexual, with the infected person. Newborn babies may acquire a very serious conjunctival infection, ophthalmia neonatorum, from the mother at the time of birth. Children, particularly little girls, may acquire the infection occasionally from contact with materials that have been freshly soiled with the discharges of the patient. The organism survives for only a short time in an unfavorable environment; thus practically all infection occurs by direct contact. All individuals are susceptible to infection, and a single attack does not confer immunity.

In many countries in recent years the numbers of reported cases of gonorrhoea have remained virtually static or have increased—in some countries substantially. Comparative data were presented to the Committee of the number of gonorrhoea cases reported in 22 countries and territories. In no less than 15 there has been a rise in numbers, and in four the situation appears static. The annual incidence ranges from 10 to 50 per 10,000 inhabitants. The magnitude of the reservoir of infection was also demonstrated by the morbidity statistics of gonorrhoea published in a recent ten-year review by WHO(2).

The limitations of figures of reported cases are well known, as many unreported cases of gonorrhoea are treated by private practitioners. For example, in the USA it is estimated that the incidence of gonorrhoea is five to ten times higher than is actually reported.

Available information indicates that gonorrhoea is widespread, remains uncontrolled, and is one of the most challenging health problems in many parts of the world(3).

It is a discouraging fact that syphilis and gonorrhea are far from being under control, despite the susceptibility of both infections to penicillin therapy. Indeed, after a dramatic decline in the incidence of acute cases after the general introduction of penicillin in 1946, a recent recrudescence of both diseases has been noted in several countries. This increase in syphilis has occurred in both "developed and developing" countries (to use the WHO euphemism for econom-

ically advanced and impoverished areas). A new danger is the possibility that in Africa syphilis might now move into areas in which yaws
(with its accompanying antisyphilitic immunity) has been extirpated.

In the United States, reported infectious syphilis has been on the
increase since 1957. The reservoir of untreated syphilitics is estimated at 1,200,000 cases and the true annual incidence at 60,000
cases(4). Syphilis in all its stages ranks fourth in the United States
among notifiable diseases. Other countries which have noted recru-
descences in recent years are Finland, France, Italy, and parts of
Africa.

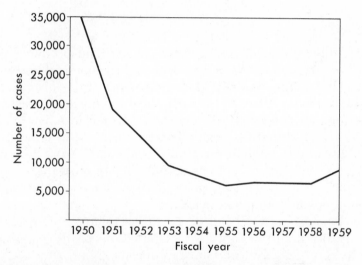

Figure 27. Primary and secondary syphilis cases reported in the United
States, 1950-1959. (Brown, W. J.: *Pub. Health Rep.*, 1960, 75:991.)

Despite these difficulties in control, the overwhelming trend since
the advent of penicillin has been downward, as is graphically shown
in Figure 27.

An important epidemiologic fact has been a shift in the age
incidence of both gonorrhea and syphilis since 1950 so that they have
been facetiously termed "childhood diseases," because a significant proportion of cases now occurs in 15- to 19-year-old age groups.

The decline in gonorrhea has not paralleled that for syphilis,
being less precipitous and less sustained.

Factors thought to contribute to the persistence of gonorrhea and
syphilis are:

1. More cases are being treated by private physicians; hence they are less adequately reported and followed up by finding and sustained treatment of contacts.

2. Increase in moral laxity and sexual promiscuity in the post-World War II era.

3. Paradoxically, the availability of antibiotics and contraceptives and the efficiency of health education campaigns in their use may foster promiscuity.

The development of penicillin-resistant gonococci has been greatly feared and watched for, but has not yet become a problem.

Chancroid

Chancroid is due to *Hemophilus ducreyi* and produces a deep, painful, ulcerated pustule, often with enlargement of the inguinal glands. The incubation period is from three to twelve days after exposure, and the disease is almost always acquired by sexual contact. It remains infectious as long as the open lesions contain the organisms. The disease is highly communicable, but is not so prevalent as the other venereal infections. In the U.S. Army, for example, it constitutes only about 5 per cent of all the venereal infections. One reason for this is that the lesions are so obvious that exposure to infection does not often take place.

The diagnosis is easily made by direct microscopic examination of smears, but multiple dark-field examinations of the lesions should be made to rule out concomitant syphilis.

Preventive measures are the same as for other venereal infections. Direct prophylaxis does not protect as well against chancroid as is the case in gonorrhea and syphilis. Greenwald(5) reports that 38 per cent of the Army personnel with chancroid had followed proper prophylaxis, whereas only 1 per cent of the syphilis cases had carried out this regimen.

Sulfonamides, streptomycin, and the broad-spectrum antibiotics are effective in treatment. Sulfonamides are preferred because the other agents are effective in syphilis and might confound interpretation of response.

Granuloma Inguinale

The etiologic agent of this disease is *Donovania granulomatis*. It is a venereal disease with a long incubation period: three to six weeks after exposure. It is rarely encountered in the United States. The chronic indolent ulcerative lesion is spread by direct contact, and the prevention is that of the other venereal diseases. Treatment is similar to that used in chancroid.

Lymphogranuloma Venereum

This disease is due to a virus that can be cultured in the yolk sac of the chick embryo.

The development of the Frei test has made us aware of the importance of this disease. The antigen for the test is prepared by growing the infecting agent in the yolk sac of the chick embryo. This antigen is suspended in saline, inactivated by heat, and a minute amount is injected intracutaneously. The skin reaction is clear-cut in positive cases and is quite specific. Complement fixation with the same antigen is also a valuable diagnostic procedure.

The disease is almost always acquired by sexual contact, though laboratory workers have contracted the disease in the handling of heavy concentrations of the virus under cultivation. It is very widespread. Lymphogranuloma has been described more frequently in Negroes, but all races and all ages are susceptible. It is more common in men than in women. Those groups having a high prevalence of gonorrhea and syphilis are also found to have a high prevalence of lymphogranuloma venereum. Surveys of prostitutes have shown the existence of positive Frei tests in 10 to 45 per cent of the individuals tested. Shaffer and his associates have also shown that persons with syphilis and gonorrhea show a prevalence of 50 to 60 per cent positive Frei tests(6).

The incubation period of the disease is from 14 to 21 days. The infection is communicable as long as the open lesion contains the virus. Since the disease is a chronic suppurative lesion, the period of communicability may be rather long. Virus has been isolated from asymptomatic individuals.

The infection responds rather indolently to the prolonged administration of sulfonamides or tetracyclines.

The preventive measures in lymphogranuloma venereum are exactly the same as those employed in the prevention of other venereal diseases. Since the condition is so difficult to recognize clinically and so frequently confused with syphilis, and since persons with syphilis so frequently have this disease also, it has been suggested that each person with recently acquired syphilis should also have a Frei test or a complement-fixation test with the Frei antigen.

The Nonvenereal Treponematoses

A number of clinically distinct nonvenereal contact infections are caused by spirochetes very similar if not identical with *Treponema pallidum*. These infections appear to be geographically restricted to certain tropical or subtropical areas and to involve family groups or communities of low socioeconomic level. In contrast to venereal syphilis, childhood infection is most common.

Transmission is by direct or indirect contact from man to man. Congenital transmission is rare. The incubation period approximates six weeks. The period of communicability is highly variable but depends upon the presence of moist dermal lesions.

Yaws occurs in Equatorial Africa, the Philippines, Burma, Thailand, throughout the South Pacific, and in scattered areas in the West Indies and Central and South America.

Bejel (nonvenereal syphilis) involves arid regions in Africa, Turkey, and the Balkans.

Pinta, which differs from the other infections in its vitiligoid lesions, occurs among dark-skinned people of Mexico, Colombia, Venezuela, and Ecuador. It is also sporadically observed in Africa and Asia. The incubation period is from one to three weeks.

With all these infections, some cross immunity and cross serologic reactions with syphilis exist.

Trachoma

Trachoma is a progressive, destructive infection of the conjunctiva which is estimated to involve 400 millions of the world's population. Some 10 millions of these victims will eventually become blind if untreated. It is now well established that the disease is caused by a virus of the psittacosis-lymphogranuloma group, which is propagable in the chick embryo and is susceptible to the action of sulfonamides and most antibiotics.

Trachoma is associated with filth, poverty, poor personal sanitation, and usually, but not invariably, with hot, arid, dusty environments. The incidence is notably high in North Africa and India. It is present among the Indians of the American Southwest but appears to be rapidly declining in that area.

Control of the disease is theoretically feasible with mass campaigns of antibiotics or sulfonamide administration, but education in personal sanitation together with economic improvements among the involved population may be equally important.

REFERENCES

1. VONDERLEHR, R. H., and USILTON, L. J.: *J.A.M.A.*, 1942, **120**: 1369.

2. *Epidem. Vital Statist. Rep.*, 1959, **12**:301.

3. Expert Committee on Venereal Infections and Treponematoses, 5th Report, *WHO Technical Report Series*, No. 190, 1960.

4. BROWN, W. J.: *Pub. Health Rep.*, 1960, **75**:990.

5. GREENWALD, E.: *J.A.M.A.*, 1943, **121**:9.

6. SHAFFER, M. L., *et al.*: *Am. J. Syph., Gonor., and Ven. Dis.*, 1941, **25**:669.

15. INFECTIONS THAT CAN BE ARTIFICALLY TRANSMITTED BY INOCULATION

A derivative of the modern practice of medicine is the growing problem of infections transmitted inadvertently from man to man by man. These infections are transmitted by hypodermic injection and are of two principal types:

1. Those transmitted by inadequately sterilized needles or syringes or other skin-piercing instruments which are contaminated with human blood.

2. Those transmitted by the injection of human blood or blood products that contain the infectious agent.

Infections in the first category include serum hepatitis, infectious hepatitis, malaria, and syphilis. Certain of these infections may be transmitted outside of medical practice through the badly contaminated needles of narcotic addicts. Outbreaks of hepatitis have also been traced to tattooing parlors.

In addition to the obligate human parasites which may be transmitted by needle, tetanus bacilli and other bacteria resident in the environment may be inoculated by grossly contaminated instruments. Such gross contamination usually involves the hastily cleaned equipment of drug addicts.

Serum Hepatitis

Serum hepatitis may be truly a disease of modern times. It appears to be unique among infections in that it is not known to be transmitted by any other means than by artificial parenteral inoculation. However, study of this disease has been curtailed by the lack of laboratory techniques to identify and propagate the infective agent. Limited studies in human volunteers have established that the causative agent is a virus of small size (hepatitis virus B) that is demonstrable in the blood of certain subjects at intervals as long as five years apart. Presumably, blood from such individuals contains virus continually and represents a constant threat to others if used for transfusion or in the preparation of plasma, albumin, or other blood products. Such carriers of virus—who are discovered after they have donated blood and transmitted the disease—are usually asymptomatic and often give no history of jaundice or liver disease. Even chemical tests of liver function may not disclose abnormalities at the time of demonstrable viremia. It is therefore almost impossible to screen out carriers in blood donor centers. The problem is complicated by the fact that the virus of infectious hepatitis (virus A) may also be transmitted by blood or blood-contaminated instruments. In this case, history taking or liver function tests may be of value in excluding potential transmitters of infection. The virus of infectious hepatitis has been demonstrated in the feces of those infected, and the disease is clearly "infectious" by personal contact or through food or water (see page 146).

The two forms of hepatitis are distinguished not only by their epidemiology but by differences in incubation period and immunity. Indeed, it is on the basis of these differences that the two viruses A and B have been provisionally identified. The 60- to 160-day incubation period of serum hepatitis contrasts with the shorter 15- to 40-day period of infectious hepatitis. However, (see page 148) intermediate periods up to 60 days have been recognized in epidemics of infectious hepatitis.

The clear-cut immunity which follows infectious hepatitis is not characteristic of serum hepatitis, as judged by the very inadequate information from human volunteer experiments. Some studies seem to demonstrate a protective effect of large doses of human gamma globulin, but others do not. Individuals of any age are subject to infection, implying that infection may not be widespread or that effective immunity may not develop. On the other hand, not all who are accidentally or deliberately inoculated with virus contract the disease. Havens and Paul(1) have proposed that such variations in apparent immunity to virus B may be due to:

1. Insufficient exposure to virus because of the artificial way of transmission.

2. The failure to develop or maintain adequate immunity following exposure.

3. The existence of multiple strains of virus that are immunologically unrelated or have a limited geographic distribution.

The increasing use of blood products and of subcutaneous injections in general has increased the relative importance of serum hepatitis as a cause of both morbidity and mortality. In the civilian population, infection rates as high as 11.9 per cent have resulted from the use of large pools of plasma(2). During military campaigns rates have been much higher. Basic research on the disease and search for effective methods of inactivating the virus in blood are confounded by the present lack of methods for cultivating the virus, which can only be detected by inoculation of human volunteers.

The origin of serum hepatitis is obscure, but it is suspected that the jaundice which followed smallpox vaccination at the end of the last century was caused by the virus. In the 1920's and 1930's, it was suspected by several investigators that the "toxic hepatitis" which followed arsenical treatment of syphilis was caused by an infectious agent.

There is no more intriguing or dramatic illustration of the insidious and potentially devastating nature of serum hepatitis than the story of yellow fever vaccination in World War II. This story is also a fine example of epidemiologic research and of cooperative investigation by military and civilian groups.

In March 1942, an unusual incidence of jaundice was noted in troops stationed in California. At this same time, outbreaks of jaundice were noted in American troops in other areas, including overseas stations, but the relatedness of these epidemics was not then apparent. The West Coast epidemic was investigated in enormous detail by an investigating team of the Commission on Tropical Diseases of the Board for the Investigation and Control of Influenza and Other Epidemic Diseases in the Army (now known as the Armed Forces Epidemiological Board). The report of these consultants to the Surgeon General of the United States Army is a masterpiece of comprehensiveness which cannot be adequately represented by the brief summary presented here (3).

Three preliminary hypotheses for the etiology of the outbreak were entertained:

"1. That a toxic agent employed by soldiers but not by civilians might be the icterogenic agent.

2. That a rapidly spreading infective agent might have been introduced into military stations from nearby civilian communities.

3. That an "icterogenic agent, like the unknown cause of infective hepatitis, had found its way into the serum — containing yellow fever vaccine from the blood of the donors in spite of the precautions taken in manufacture."

The third (and correct) hypothesis was favored by the investigators from the start, but was cautiously introduced in their report as "fantastic." Nevertheless, it was felt that earlier studies in England by Findlay and MacCallum (4) and in Brazil by Fox *et al.*(5) pointed in this direction. These same earlier studies had also excluded rather definitely the possibility that yellow fever virus itself was the icterogenic agent (this quite reasonable possibility had been considered earlier in the California outbreak, and mosquito netting had actually been used to isolate patients from potential mosquito vectors).

The first hypothesis was rapidly excluded when it was found that no common exposure of jaundiced troops to hepatotoxic agents had occurred, and that the occurrence of jaundice was not related to occupation or type of duty performed.

The possibility of an infective agent directly transmissible from man to man was also ruled out rapidly but with greater difficulty. Inevitably, some infectious hepatitis was discovered in communities adjoining army camps, and such cases were also encountered in troops. But whereas the bulk of cases of jaundice in California camps were in two peaks, in late March and early June, cases of jaundice in unvaccinated men were scattered throughout the year with a mean occurring early in July.

The relationship of jaundice to the administration of yellow fever vaccine was established on the basis of historical data from case card surveys with a reference to the time of inoculation of the vaccine and the time of occurrence of jaundice. Fortunately, records had been kept of vaccine lot numbers, and it was also determined that certain lots were icterogenic and others were not.

A review of the vaccine manufacturing procedure was then painstakingly undertaken. It was established that human serum (then thought to be necessary for the optimal growth of yellow fever virus) had been used in the tissue culture medium. Although most of the serum was heated at 56° C for one hour before use, it is now known that this temperature is quite inadequate to destroy the virus of serum hepatitis.

Thus, the efforts to prevent an old disease—yellow fever—in American troops resulted in the extensive artificial dissemination of a "new" disease, which ironically enough also produced yellowing of the skin.

Human serum is no longer used in the manufacture of yellow fever vaccine, and hepatitis has not been reported since this change in manufacturing procedure.

In addition to the major problem of serum hepatitis, a number of other infections have been inadvertantly transmitted from man to man by needle; these include syphilis, malaria, and measles. It is evident that any infection with a stage of blood stream invasion could in theory be so transmitted. Prevention of such transmission depends upon:

1. Careful screening of blood donors for evidence of past or present infection—especially of syphilis, hepatitis, or malaria. It is also unwise to use blood from those who have received blood dona-

tions themselves within the previous six months period. Donation of blood by those who have been in contact with patients with infectious hepatitis in the recent past should also be prohibited.

2. Restricting the number of donors to plasma pools to minimize the chance of contamination of any one lot.

3. Treatment of plasma by irradiation or heat for reduction or elimination of serum hepatitis virus.

4. Use of adequate sterilization for needles and syringes and surgical instruments. (Boiling in water for 30 minutes, autoclaving at 121° C at 15-lb pressure for 20 minutes, or with dry heat 180° C for 1 hour[1]).

5. Elimination of illegal clandestine self-administration of narcotics by addicts by the establishment of rehabilitation and treatment centers where drugs may be administered by qualified medical personnel.

Potential Hazards of the Future

It has already been suggested that a human virus (hepatitis virus B) may be inadvertently inoculated with the living virus vaccines for smallpox and yellow fever. Preliminary field trials of live poliovirus vaccines have resulted in infection of large numbers of people with retrospectively recognized monkey viruses present in the tissue in which the vaccine had been produced. It may be anticipated that the newer live vaccines which will be produced for other diseases will have similar potential hazards that may be difficult to recognize and to eliminate. The present requirements of the Division of Biologic Standards of the National Institutes of Health forbid the release of vaccines which contain extraneous viruses. It is to be hoped that the presence of such viruses may be detected by methods other than inoculation of man.

The Intrauterine Transmission of Infection (Congenital Infections)

Another way in which man-to-man transmission of infection occurs is *in utero* by transplacental transmission. In general, most infections severe enough to induce bacterial septicemia in the mother result in spontaneous abortion, with or without actual infection of the fetus. However, a variety of infectious agents (from protozoa to viruses) are able to traverse the placental barrier and to infect the fetus yet allow its survival into the postpartum period. Most infections that permit survival of the infant are acquired late in pregnancy (toxoplasmosis, syphilis, tuberculosis, poliomyelitis), but the virus of rubella may induce nonfatal but teratogenic infection of the fetus in the first trimester (see page 200). It is not yet clear whether other viruses may cause congenital defects.

The prevention of this sort of disease transmission must obviously be directed at prevention of the specific infections in the mother prior to or early in pregnancy. There is some evidence that vaccinia may compromise the outcome of pregnancy if inoculated in the first trimester. If live virus vaccines of other types are developed in the future, their use in pregnant women must be undertaken with caution.

REFERENCES

1. HAVENS, W. P., JR., and PAUL, J. R.: in *Viral and Rickettsial Infections of Man*, 3rd ed., ed. T. M. RIVERS, and F. L. HORSFALL, JR.: Lippincott, Philadelphia, 1959.

2. MURPHY, W. P., JR., and WORKMAN, W. G.: *J.A.M.A.*, 1953, **152**: 1421.

3. SAWYER, W. A., *et al.*, *Am. J. Hyg.*, 1944, **39**:377 **40**:35.

4. FINDLAY, G. M., and MacCALLUM, F. O.: *Tr. Roy. Soc. Trop. Med. and Hyg.*, 1937, **31**:297.

5. FOX, J. P., *et al.*: *Am. J. Hyg.*, 1942, **36**:117.

SECTION IV

The Control of Infections Directly Transmissible From Man to Man

There is surprisingly little direct evidence concerning the mechanisms by which most infectious agents are transmitted from man to man. Certain widely held assumptions have been made about mechanisms of transmission which are based on:

1. Epidemiologic (circumstantial) evidence.
2. Knowledge of the site of multiplication of the parasite in the host.
3. Studies in experimental animals.
4. Limited experiments in human volunteers.

On the basis of these methods of study, it has generally been concluded that the enteric infections (Table 13) are transmitted by ingestion of fecally contaminated material and that the infections resulting from primary invasion of the respiratory tract (Table 14) are "air borne," i.e., are caused by inhalation of microorganisms suspended in the air. It is possible—even probable—that such assumptions are correct, but it should be remembered that the only established *sine qua non* for the transmission of both enteric and respiratory infections seems to be close contact, proximity, and association between the donor and recipient of the infection. Earlier impressions that measles and other respiratory viruses were more communicable than, for example, poliomyelitis have been changed following recent recognition of the high communicability of poliomyelitis when suitable methods for the detection of cases *and the recognition of subclinical instances of infection* are utilized.

Also, the inefficacy of attempts at air sterilization or decontamination indirectly stress the need for close physical proximity in transmission of even the "air-borne" infections. On the other hand, with such enteric infections as poliomyelitis, virus is detectable and apparently multiplies in the pharynx, where it is at least potentially a source of contagion.

The studies of the Commission on Respiratory Diseases have suggested that the spread of streptococcal infections may require direct contact with nasopharyngeal discharges rather than aerosol dissemination of streptococci. This point and the others mentioned above have obvious importance with respect to control measures.

With the few exceptions listed in Table 8, it is unlikely that the environment is an important source of infective agents transmissible from man to man. These exceptions include bacteria which may actually multiply in the environment, such as staphylococci, strepto-cocci, and *Salmonella typhosa*, as well as the stable enteroviruses and the virus of infectious hepatitis. In general, the pathogens of the respiratory tract are extremely unstable and cannot survive long in the external environment.

Even more unstable in the environment are the microorganisms responsible for direct contact infections, especially those involved in venereal diseases. It is therefore understandable that transmission of such infections occurs largely across mucous membranes or at mucocutaneous junctions and rarely through the intact skin, because a moist, warm, nutritionally favorable milieu must be found quickly by such organisms. Even so, the acquisition of venereal infection can be prevented by prompt washing of even these highly susceptible sites.

The Inevitability of Certain Infections

In those special situations in which infections are transmitted from man to man by artificial means (e.g., through the hypodermic needle by physicians or drug addicts), there is an obvious opportunity for destruction of the parasite during its trip from one man to another. With the vast majority of infections transmitted from man to man, however, other methods of control are needed. It will be seen in the subsequent discussion that the most effective of these methods of control accept the inevitability of transmission, or indeed, sometimes, of infection, and it is their purpose to create a last line of defense within man himself, by the administration of specific drugs or the mobilization of specific immune mechanisms in the potential victim.

Even if it were possible by ultraviolet irradiation or other means to insulate the child from contact with the causative agents of the "diseases of childhood," *such a procedure would put the child in*

undue jeopardy if infection were postponed until his adult years.
Almost without exception, primary infections result in more severe
disease in the adult than in the child. Therefore, methods of disease
control which merely postpone the infection without inducing
specific resistance are not only unrealistic, but dangerous.

Some General Considerations in the Control of Infections Transmissible from Man to Man

It is obvious that realistic methods of disease control depend on
definition of the source of the infectious agent and identification of
the susceptible host. These problems should be considered:

1. Is the chief source of infection the clinically diagnosed case?
2. Do subclinically infected carriers contribute to the spread of
infection?
3. If subclinically infected carriers do not spread the infection,
which groups are most susceptible: young, old, male, female?

The answers to these questions will vary with each individual
disease, and the natural history of each disease must be defined
before the appropriate methods of control, based on knowledge of
transmission, can be implemented. If the clinical case (as in tuberculosis) is a major source of infection, then case-finding methods will
be of value in control. On the other hand, case finding will offer little
in the control of poliomyelitis, in which most infections are subclinical or inapparent and where specific methods of therapy for the
identified case are nonexistent.

Not too long ago, it was the general assumption of public health
practice that the clinical case was the important source of contagion
in almost all childhood infections. This attitude led to the formulation of legislation (much of it now scientifically obsolete) which required the isolation of patients with "communicable" diseases at
home or in "pest houses," the placarding of homes, and often the
quarantine of contacts. Increasing awareness of the equal or greater
importance of the nondiseased carrier as well as the development of
antimicrobial drugs which rapidly suppress pathogenic bacteria in
the patient have led to recognition of the need for revision of much
of this legislation.

16. CASE DETECTION, ANTIMICROBIAL THERAPY, AND CHEMOPROPHYLAXIS IN THE CONTROL OF CONTAGIOUS DISEASES*

Infections Controllable by Case Finding of Clinically Apparent Infections (Disease)

Infections in this category include those with high clinical attack rates (in which inapparent infections are therefore not important) and certain chronic infections in which contagiousness and exposure may be protracted. Infections in which case finding is useful include:

Pulmonary tuberculosis (adult or nonprimary type).
Leprosy.
Infantile diarrhea.
Typhoid.
Serum hepatitis (by screening of blood donors by history).
Measles (high clinical attack rate).
Venereal infections (in the male, and indirectly, in the female named as his contact).
Smallpox.

Tuberculosis is the prototype of infections in which case finding is of great importance in the control of the disease, despite the fact that most tuberculous infections are not manifest by disease. Such infections, which are of the primary type and noncavitary, do not contribute to the dissemination of *Mycobacterium tuberculosis*. In recent years, case finding has become even more important as specific antituberculous drugs have been developed; now the result of case finding is not only the isolation and public health education of

---

*There are a number of points of attack in the control of contagious diseases. It is obvious that in the classification of diseases in accord with their vulnerability to one or another method of control, the same disease could be considered in several categories. Thus, in the several categories in this chapter, tuberculosis appears in each, although the best method of control depends on specific circumstances.

the patient, as carried out in the past, but also the administration of specific therapy to aid the patient and to serve as prophylaxis for the dissemination of infection in the community. The hopeful and aggressive approach of contemporary tuberculosis experts culminated in the Arden House Conference on Tuberculosis in 1959 with the drawing up of the recommendations that follow.

Arden House Conference Recommendation

The major recommendation of the conference is a program for the widespread application of chemotherapy as a public health measure for the elimination of tuberculosis in the United States.

Goal. To sterilize that important part of the reservoir of tubercle bacilli that presently exists throughout the country in persons currently suffering from active tuberculous disease, whether presently known or unknown to public health authorities, and in selected persons who previously have had active disease and were inadequately treated.

Technique. Mobilize all resources for a widespread application of the scientifically demonstrated and medically accepted procedures of adequate chemotherapy. These include the proper dosage of appropriate drugs or combination of drugs given continuously over an adequate period of time — procedures that are known to destroy tubercle bacilli in the human body, render the patient's disease noncommunicable to others, and minimize the possibility of reactivation.

Infections Controllable by Specific Treatment of Clinical Cases

The availability of highly effective chemotherapy in the form of such orally administered drugs as isoniazid has partially resolved the need for legal restraint and hospital confinement of "open" or infectious cases of pulmonary tuberculosis. Not only may the period of hospitalization be reduced, but the contagiousness of patients who "sign out" or refuse hospitalization may be demonstrably lessened. This has been shown by a study of the occurrence of secondary cases among contacts of treated and untreated cases.

There are other infections that are not considered in the foregoing section in which the clinical case is *not* the most important method of transmission, yet certain of these infections are amenable to specific antimicrobial treatment, and such treatment will contribute to the curtailment of transmission in the community. These infections are listed below in addition to tuberculosis in which treatment of the case is a major method of prevention of spread.

Tuberculosis.
Leprosy.

Streptococcal infections.
Staphylococcal infections.
Typhoid fever.
Bacillary dysentery.
Venereal infections (chiefly male).
Malaria (not transmissible man to man but reduction in parasitemia may interfere with mosquito transmission).
Ringworm of the scalp (now treatable with griseofulvin).

Infections Controllable by Case Finding of Clinically Inapparent Infections by Laboratory Procedures

Certain infections can be controlled in part by the detection of nondiseased carriers. Infections in this category are few in number because (a) the detection of such infections is dependent upon the availability of easily implemented laboratory procedures, and (b) this method of control is only important in certain limited epidemic situations. Appreciable numbers of the population may carry pathogenic organisms in the absence of epidemics. However, the presence of this reservoir of undiseased carriers is usually suspected on the basis that sporadic manifest disease has occurred. This group of infections includes:

Typhoid fever (detection of carrier by stool culture).
Meningococcal infections (nasopharyngeal culture).
Staphylococcal infections (nasopharyngeal or lesion culture).
Streptococcal infections (nasopharyngeal or lesion culture).
Tuberculosis (chest X-ray revealing cavitary but asymptomatic infection).
Gonorrhea in the female (by culture or fluorescent antibody techniques).

The prospects for terminating the typhoid carrier state are good if the carrier is subjected to cholecystectomy. Penicillin in large dosage may also be effective, otherwise prevention of infection depends upon the education of the carrier and his supervision with respect to food handling. In the case of the other infections, potentially effective antimicrobial therapy is available; with staphylococcal infections in particular, carriers among hospital personnel can be restricted to prevent their contact with the unduly susceptible, such as the newborn infant or the surgical patient.

The amount and duration of antimicrobial therapy used for significant reduction in secondary disease transmission may be much less than that needed for therapy of active disease. Such chemoprophylaxis will not usually eliminate the organism carried except in the case of the exquisitely sensitive meningococci and gonococci. However, the number of bacteria can be so reduced that transmission of infection is similarly diminished. It should be noted that this type of infectious disease control is useful only in certain epidemic situations and sometimes only at particular times of the year. The epidemic prevalence of meningococcal meningitis is associated with an increase in carriers of type I meningococci. This increase may last for several years. *However, the seasonal fluctuation in the occurrence of*

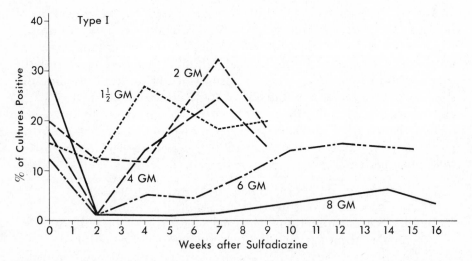

Figure 28. Type I menigococcus carriers before and after graded doses of sulfadiazine. (Aycock, W. L., and Mueller, J. H.: *Bact. Rev.*, 1950, *14*:115.)

meningitis during this period cannot be related to the carrier rate per se. Still another determinant of meningitis in the military is its predilection for the young recruit. However, the carriage of meningococci (and hence the risk of meningitis in future contacts) can be dramatically reduced by the administration of relatively small doses of sulfadiazine quite inadequate for the treatment of the established disease. As indicated in Figure 28 the effect of a single dose of 8 gm is sufficient to eliminate the detectable carriage of type I meningococci for as long as 16 weeks after its administration.

The development of immunofluorescent techniques for the detection of bacterial antigens offers promise for better detection of the female carrier of gonococci who is (usually) asymptomatic. Penicillin treatment of sexually promiscuous individuals so detected will materially reduce the spread of the disease and might eventually lead to its elimination. Therapy of the male in whom sexual activity is restricted by his acute and painful symptoms contributes to the reduction of gonorrhea only insofar as such therapy prevents evolution of the infection to a chronic state which results in protracted carriage of gonococci.

However, the prophylatic use of antigonococcal drugs is so effective as to be actually conducive to promiscuity. This fact together with evidence that the acquisition of syphilis may not be prevented by penicillin doses that are adequate to prevent gonorrhea is already posing new public health problems. A special danger is the fact that penicillin may prevent the primary chancre from appearing as well as other manifestations of the infectious state, yet the individual may later develop the more serious sequelae of syphilitic infection.

Prophylaxis with Specific Antimicrobial Drugs (Chemoprophylaxis) to Prevent or Postpone Infection in Susceptible Contacts

It would seem to be a reasonable and obvious procedure to reduce the spread of infections treatable with drugs by administration of the appropriate antimicrobial drugs to contacts exposed to such infections. As a matter of fact, this measure contributes very little to the control of infectious diseases and is employed only in certain limited circumstances. These circumstances are related to:

1. The biology of the etiological parasite.
2. The nature of the infection which it causes.
3. The mechanism of its transmission.
4. The availability of a specific antimicrobial drug.

Thus, antimicrobial prophylaxis is most effective in infections in which:

1. The parasite is highly drug susceptible (to low, briefly maintained concentrations of drug). Such parasites are usually incapable of establishing persistent or latent infection after antimicrobial treatment.
2. Infection is manifested by easily recognizable disease in the primary case.
3. The time of contact can be sharply defined.

4. Antimicrobial drugs of low toxicity are available that may be conveniently administered.

Of all the infectious diseases only gonorrhea meets these "ideal" requirements for contact chemoprophylaxis, and then only with the reservation that the male contact must anticipate the probability of infection in his partner, because her symptoms may not be evident.

Infections caused by the biologically similar meningococcus are similarly amenable to prophylaxis with antimicrobial drugs, but the recognized case of meningococcal disease is not an important factor in spread of infections.

In World War II, the incidence of bacillary dysentery was reportedly reduced by mass sulfonamide prophylaxis. However, the rapid evolution of sulfonamide-resistant shigella limited the value of this approach to controlling the disease. As with other enteric infections, environmental sanitation remains the most important factor in dysentery control.

The administration of the antituberculosis drug, isoniazid, to children who are family contacts of sputum-positive adults is now under study as a method of tuberculosis prevention. The Expert Committee on Tuberculosis of the World Health Organization has recognized the use of two types of chemoprophylaxis, each directed at a different stage in the infectious process. In the terminology of the Committee(1),

Primary chemoprophylaxis—the use of anti-tuberculosis drugs in those not infected, i.e., non-reactors to tuberculin; secondary chemoprophylaxis— the use of anti-tuberculosis drugs in those who are infected as demonstrated by a significant reaction to the tuberculin test, but who have no pathognomonic signs or symptoms of tuberculous disease.

Primary chemoprophylaxis has not been widely endorsed because of the greater usefulness of BCG vaccination in the tuberculin-negative person who is heavily exposed to infection. On the other hand, secondary chemoprophylaxis, which is essentially the prevention of disease in those recently and already infected, offers great promise in controlling childhood tuberculosis in areas of high tuberculosis prevalence.

It should be pointed out that it is not clear with respect to other infections whether chemoprophylaxis actually prevents the acquisition of infection or merely its sequel of disease, even if drug is given prior to contact with the parasite. It is probable that for any given disease either primary or secondary chemoprophylaxis may be operative, depending upon whether or not circumstances of host-parasite contact permit the establishment of the parasite in the tissues of the host. The effectiveness of antigonococcal and anti-meningococcal prophylaxis may reflect the inability of these organisms to "get started" and initiate infection in the presence of antimicrobial drugs. It is clear, however, with the arthropod-borne diseases, malaria and scrub typhus, that administration of specific drugs such as quinacrine (Atabrine) or tetracycline, even for long periods of time, does not prevent infection but only postpones the eventual advent of disease.

Chemoprophylaxis in Persons Peculiarly Vulnerable to Infections or Their Sequelae

Probably the greatest value of chemoprophylaxis at present is in the control of the late sequelae of Group A streptococcal infections, rheumatic fever, and nephritis, and definitively, the chronic residual of rheumatic heart disease. During World War II and in military and civilian studies since, it has clearly been shown that the mass administration of penicillin can reduce the streptococcal carrier rate, lower the incidence of streptococcal pharyngitis and scarlet fever and, most importantly, reduce the incidence of rheumatic fever and other late manifestations of streptococcal infection. It is also true that antistreptococcal therapy for developed streptococcal pharyngitis may still reduce the expected rate of subsequent rheumatic fever.

Only a minority of hypersensitive individuals are vulnerable to rheumatic fever following a streptococcal infection. Once this vulnerability is recognized by the occurrence of the initial attack, the protracted administration of penicillin may prevent both future streptococcal infections and their threatening sequelae in the vulnerable (rheumatic) subject. This type of chemoprophylaxis has received wide acceptance and is a good example of preventive medicine and public health directly administered by the individual medical practitioner.

The prophylactic use of antibiotics to prevent bacterial infection in other potentially vulnerable patients is less clear-cut and generalizations cannot be made. It is popular in academic circles to view with horror the "promiscuous" use of antibiotics in the absence of a specific therapeutic indication. This commendable caution can be carried too far sometimes, because of unwarranted extrapolations among basically differing problems. For example, the prophylactic use of penicillin to prevent the pneumococcal pneumonia which may follow influenza in an elderly or cardiac patient is quite different from the administration of a tetracycline drug to prevent recurrent urinary tract infections in a patient with a congenital anomaly of the urinary tract.

In the first case, it is reasonable to anticipate that pneumonia may occur within a certain brief period of time; that if pneumonia does occur, it will probably be pneumococcal and the pneumococcus will be susceptible to the action of penicillin.

In the second case, eventual infection is almost inevitable, but the time of infection and the nature of the bacterial pathogen are unpredictable. Chemoprophylaxis in this case may indeed tend to select a bacterial invader which is resistant to the drug being employed chemoprophylactically.

Another type of chemoprophylaxis which appears to hold promise is the protracted daily use of broad-spectrum antibiotics in chronic pulmonary disease to prevent the recurrent acute infections accompanying such disease which may be life threatening.

The whole concept of antimicrobial prophylaxis or chemoprophylaxis deserves re-evaluation at the present time.

REFERENCE

1. Expert Committee on Tuberculosis: *WHO Tech. Rep. Series,* No. 195, 1960.

17. SPECIFIC ARTIFICIAL IMMUNIZATION AND THE CONTROL OF INFECTIOUS DISEASES

The Prevention, Modification and Treatment of Infectious Diseases with Preformed Antibody or Gamma Globulin (passive immunization)

It would seem that the use of specific antibody would be a logical method for the prevention and therapy of infectious diseases. Yet this approach has limited applicability.

1. Antibody, whether in the form of specific immune serum or the purified serum fraction, gamma globulin, is costly to produce and limited in supply.

2. Antibody must be administered parenterally and in relatively large amounts.

3. Whether the antibody is of human or animal origin, it is rapidly eliminated from the recipient who is "passively immunized" with it, so that effective immunity rarely persists beyond two to three months.

4. If nonhuman in origin (heterospecific), the antibody, with accompanying or contaminating serum proteins, will induce the formation of other antibodies, which 7 to 14 days after injection may be associated with "serum sickness" in the recipient. Repeated or booster injections of antibodies may cause immediate and occasionally fatal anaphylactic reactions.

In the decade prior to the introduction of antibacterial chemotherapy, antibody was used with fair success in the treatment of several acute pyogenic infections including pneumococcal pneumonia and meningococcal and *Hemophilus influenzae* meningitis. Specific antibody has not been of any importance in the prevention of bacterial infections except in rare individuals with abnormally small amounts of serum gamma globulin (agammaglobulinemia or hypogammaglobulinemia).

231

In the case of diphtheria and tetanus in which disease is dependent on *in vivo* production and absorption of microbial toxins produced during infection, the administration of antitoxin antibody in large amounts may be therapeutically useful in binding unabsorbed toxins. The injection of smaller amounts of antitoxin provides effective immunity for two to three weeks after exposure. The increasing use of active immunization with toxoid is gradually superceding antitoxin (which is usually of horse serum origin) in the prevention of diphtheria and tetanus (see p. 250).

The most important use of preformed antibody is with human gamma globulin for the prevention of those diseases in which:

1. The pathogenesis of the disease is dependent upon a stage of blood stream invasion (viremia), during which time the parasite is accessible to humoral antibody.

2. The contact period may be precisely defined.

3. The infection is sufficiently common so that high titer antibody may be found in the gamma globulin fraction of serum pools.

Among the diseases that may be prevented or modified by the injection of gamma globulin during the early incubation period are measles, rubella, mumps, poliomyelitis, and infectious hepatitis (see Table 17). Of these diseases, only measles consistently meets the criterion of a readily definable contact period because clinically mild or inapparent infection may characterize the other diseases. However, there are circumstances, as in institutional or household epidemics of hepatitis, when the period of contact is similarly definable.

Gamma globulin is of little use in poliomyelitis because of rapid spread of infection (often inapparent) within households, so that by the time the paralytic "index" case is recognized, all members of the household are infected (p. 176).

The relative mildness of rubella and varicella and the apparent variability of protection of different lots of gamma globulin have not led to widespread use of gamma globulin prophylaxis in these infections.

The control of those viral diseases listed in Table 17 will ultimately depend on active immunization with vaccines not yet available (except for poliomyelitis). Passive immunization with preformed antibody (gamma globulin) is an extravagant and cumbersome stopgap procedure, but nevertheless it is of real value in special circumstances—especially in the prevention of disease in children with pre-existing disability.

Active Immunization by Vaccination. The Prevention of Disease by the Artificial Induction of Specific Immunity

The induction of disease-specific immunity by artificial active immunization (vaccination) is a major triumph of preventive medicine. Ideally the effective vaccine induces protracted immunity by presenting the recipient with antigen identical with the disease-producing agent, yet so modified that it is not injurious to the subject or his associates. Although no such perfect vaccine exists, several, such as the 17D yellow fever vaccine, are virtually free of toxicity yet highly effective in producing lasting immunity.

TABLE 17

The Prevention or Modification of Disease with Specific Preformed Antibody

"PASSIVE" IMMUNIZATION

Antitoxic Antibody	Usual Antibody Source
Tetanus*	Equine
Diphtheria	Equine
Antiviral Antibody	
Measles	Human (gamma globulin)
Infectious hepatitis	Human (gamma globulin)
Poliomyelitis†	Human (gamma globulin)
Mumps†	Human (gamma globulin)
Rubella†	Human (gamma globulin)
Rabies*	Equine

*Not acquired by human-to-human contact.
†Rarely of practical value.

Because the ultimate producer of vaccine-induced immunity is the host himself, the reagents used in the activation of this immunity may be (and often are) relatively crude preparations. The final reagent (antibody) which is manufactured in the host is pure and specific. Furthermore, the initial or primary immunization of the subject induces a state of altered reactivity to the antigen so that its re-injection subsequently as a "booster" is followed by a secondary immune response which is more rapid and of greater degree than before (see Fig. 29).

Because all infective agents of human disease (since they contain protein or polysaccharide) are potentially antigenic, vaccines could, in theory, be developed to stimulate antibody production against any of them. In fact, effective vaccines have been produced using living bacteria (BCG)*, nonviable bacterial cells (typhoid), modified exotoxins (diphtheria), type-specific polysaccharides (pneumococcal pneumonia), and living and inactivated viral particles. Even so the universal application of artificial active immunization to the control of infectious diseases would be completely unwarranted.

For example, there would be little point to injecting the population at large with the undeniably potent vaccines which have been used experimentally for pneumococcal pneumonia. Even if only the more important lower-numbered types were included in such a vaccine, the incidence of primary pneumococcal or lobar pneumonia is small and unpredictable in its distribution. When the disease does occur, it can be contained readily in most cases by the use of powerful chemotherapeutic agents such as penicillin.

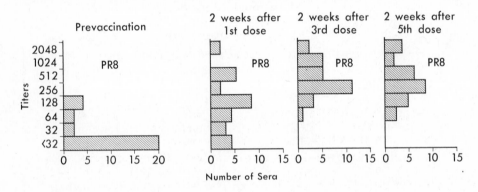

Figure 29. Booster response to immunization with influenza A (PR8) vaccine. (Quilligan, J. J., et al.: J. Clin. Investigation, 1948, 27:572.)

Somewhat different examples are the vaccines for typhoid and tuberculosis. In the United States, these vaccines contribute relatively little to the control of their respective diseases, but they are of value in certain populations at high risk of infection.

The special importance of vaccination in the general population is in the control of the intrinsically human contagious diseases which are perpetuated by human-human contact (see Tables 13 and 14). These infections are as world-wide in their distribution as man himself. They know neither geographic nor absolute seasonal limitation for they are not dependent upon the nuances of the environment or the life cycles of vectors but only upon the vagaries of human-to-

---

*Vaccine prepared from Bacillus Calmette-Guérin.

human contact and human susceptibility. Thus, contact of man with these agents is almost certain and is not subject to environmental control.

Because many of these contagious agents may infect and be transmitted without producing manifest disease in all cases, the time at which contact occurs is unpredictable and cannot be defined for any given human being. Therefore, the inevitability of recurrent contact with the obligate human parasites must be accepted as a fact of life, for the finest of sanitary engineering cannot block the measles virus in its brief journey between two wrestling four-year-olds. Instead, the four-year-old must himself be so modified that contact, or even infection, with the virus does not result in disease.

It is particularly important at the present time, with new viruses identified every year, to consider carefully not only the indications for vaccination against these agents in the individual patient, but also the contraindications, i.e., whether the contribution of the virus to human morbidity warrants the production of a vaccine. With the great plagues eradicated, we are now entering a period with the leisure and the methods to examine the public health aspects of morbidity from minor diseases as well as those with directly fatal issue. Thus, while there was no real cause for debate about the need for vaccination against smallpox and its devastating mortality, the place of adenovirus vaccine in the medical scheme of things still awaits definition.

The Nature of the Vaccines Currently in Common Use

Although many vaccines can be commercially produced, only those with the characteristics summarized in Table 18 are currently in common use. These vaccines include two bacterial toxoids, three vaccines containing living or inactivated bacterial cells, and living and inactivated vaccines made from six viruses.

Of these vaccines, only those for diphtheria, pertussis, tetanus, and smallpox are used widely in the general population. The first three (DPT) are usually administered in combination in infancy and early childhood. Smallpox immunization is also carried out routinely in the United States before admission to public schools and before foreign travel. In recent years, the Salk (inactivated) poliomyelitis vaccine has been recommended for wide-scale use in members of the population less than forty years of age. One commercial preparation of DPT also includes the Salk vaccine antigen. Response to this quadruple vaccine is apparently as good as to the original diphtheria-pertussis-tetanus preparations.

The other vaccines listed in Table 18 as being in common use are not utilized in mass immunization; however, they are valuable in certain special circumstances, considered later in this book.

Vaccines Less Commonly Used

Other vaccines in less common use or of less established efficacy include:

1. Vaccines now largely superseded by the availability of anti-microbial drugs (the rickettsial vaccines for spotted fever, typhus, scrub typhus, and Q fever). These vaccines are still useful for the prevention of disease in special groups at high risk, such as laboratory or field workers.

2. Vaccines which may be only temporarily effective but which may postpone infection to a time more dangerous for the host. This is the case with the inactivated mumps virus vaccine. This vaccine has not yet received sufficient study to determine the duration of induced immunity. Because such complications of the disease as orchitis are more common and more severe after puberty, it would be unwise to postpone the disease to that time.

3. Vaccines still in the experimental stage and of limited effectiveness (vaccines for arbor virus infections, especially Japanese B encephalitis).

4. Vaccines of questionable effectiveness for which it seems unreasonable to anticipate success. (The vaccines for cholera and bacillary dysentery — essentially focal diseases of the bowel without systemic invasion.)

The Evaluation of Response to Vaccination

Vaccines are designed to induce specific immunity to disease. The ultimate measure of their effectiveness is their capacity to reduce the incidence of disease (morbidity) or mortality in human beings exposed to infection under natural conditions. A "protection ratio" may be derived from controlled studies by comparing the attack rates in vaccinated and unvaccinated members of the exposed populations:

$$\text{Protection ratio} = \frac{\text{(incidence in vaccinated)}}{\text{(incidence in unvaccinated)}}.$$

TABLE 18

Vaccines in Common Use

Vaccine	Source	Constituents
Toxoid		
Diphtheria	Culture	Formalin-modified toxin (filtrate of broth culture)
Tetanus	Culture	Formalin-modified toxin (filtrate of broth culture)
Bacterial (noninfective)		
Pertussis*	Culture	Formalin-modified toxin (filtrate of bacterial cells)
Typhoid, paratyphoid	Culture	Heat-killed bacterial cells
Bacterial (infective)		
BCG†	Culture	Viable tubercle bacilli (Calmette-Guérin) of reduced virulence
Viral (noninfective)		
Influenza	Chick embryo	Formalin- or ultraviolet-inactivated A and B strains
Poliomyelitis (Salk)	Monkey kidney tissue culture	Formalin- or ultraviolet-inactivated virus types 1, 2, 3
Rabies (Semple) (Lilly)	Rabbit brain Duck embryo	Phenol- or ultraviolet-inactivated "virus fixe"
Adenovirus (3, 4, 7)	Monkey kidney tissue culture	Formalin-inactivated types 3, 4, 7
Viral (infective)		
Smallpox	Calf lymph	Vaccinia virus
Yellow fever (17D)	Chick embryo	Tissue culture-adapted yellow fever virus
(Dakar)	Mouse brain	Mouse brain-passaged yellow fever virus
Poliomyelitis	Monkey kidney tissue culture	Polioviruses 1, 2, and 3 (reduced neurovirulence)
Rabies (Flury LEP§) (Flury HEP**)	Chick embryo brain Chick embryo	Flury strain chick embryo-passaged rabies virus

* Bacterial cell suspension; usually included with diphtheria and tetanus toxoids as DPT.

† Vaccine prepared from Bacillus Calmette-Guérin.

§ Low egg passage (less attenuated).

** High egg passage (more attenuated; less antigenic potency).

For most vaccines the arithmetic value of this ratio is less than 0.6.

Because many factors influence response to vaccination, it is desirable to have some ready indication other than challenge by the natural infection (which may never occur). Such indications of response may not necessarily be analogous to immunity, but they may serve as a guide to the antigenic potency or viability of the vaccine or the ability of the subject to respond. The same tests used in determining past or present natural infection may be used in the evaluation of vaccines directed against them. Thus, delayed cutaneous hypersensitivity to tuberculin or diphtheria toxin (Schick test) may be used as a test of successful vaccination with BCG or diphtheria toxoid.

Similarly, convenient skin tests are not available for other commonly employed vaccines. However, the cutaneous site of smallpox vaccination is easily observed, and the characteristic course of the dermal infection is an obvious indication of successful inoculation with vaccinia virus. The local lesion produced with BCG is a less exact indication of inoculation, but it is of some value in indicating vaccine viability.

The presence of humoral neutralizing antibody has been frequently and consistently correlated with specific immunity, especially in studies of influenza and poliomyelitis vaccines. However, except in experimental studies, it is hardly practicable to assess the adequacy of immunization by serologic studies.

For the most part, the potency of most vaccines is inferred from:

1. Past experience in field trials with comparable antigen doses and immunization schedules.

2. Tests of vaccine viability (measurement of infective virus) when live virus vaccines are used.

3. Antigenic potency in experimental animals. (Much work needs to be done in this direction, particularly with respect to correlating the results of animal and human immunization with identical lots of vaccine.)

Neither natural nor vaccine-induced immunity is absolute, and either may be overridden by large challenge doses of infecting organisms or by environmental or endogenous factors that impair the nonspecific resistance of the host. The relative inefficacy of typhoid vaccine may reflect the large numbers of bacilli which may be ingested in contaminated water or food in this enteric infection. In contrast, the challenge dose of respiratory-borne pathogens (which cannot multiply in the environment) is not susceptible to such wide variation.

The Duration of Artifically-induced (Vaccine) Immunity: Relation to Mechanisms of Vaccine Immunity

It cannot be stated categorically that vaccine-induced immunity will be more or less "solid" or enduring than the immunity that results from a natural infection. Neither can it be said that "live" vaccines in general induce more lasting immunity than "dead" ones. For example, immunity from tetanus toxoid (a nonviable reagent) persists for at least as long as that following inoculation with living vaccinia virus. Furthermore, the immunity from tetanus toxoid far exceeds that of the natural infection, following which immunity does not develop, whereas, the immunity following smallpox far outlasts that from vaccinia.

The foregoing comparisons are somewhat spurious, but they serve to emphasize the imprecision involved in speaking of vaccination in general rather than in terms of the particular disease.

In the first place, the route by which tetanus toxoid is given permits better dissemination of antigen to antibody-forming lymph nodes than occurs during natural tetanus infection in which toxin migrates along peripheral nerves from the local lesion. Also, the immunity from tetanus vaccine is specifically antitoxic. Infection and invasion by tetanus bacilli are not, and need not be, prevented to prevent the disease. Furthermore, the amount of toxin formed during infection is small, and may itself serve as an effective booster of pre-existing toxoid-induced immunity.

On the other hand, the cutaneous route by which smallpox vaccine (vaccinia) is given is presumably less effective in disseminating antigen than the extensive viremia of smallpox. Furthermore, the respiratory route by which the challenge virus enters is remote from the site of cutaneous vaccination so that factors of local immunity are less operative in containing infection. That local or regional immunity occurs is illustrated by the need for rotation of vaccination sites in certain repeatedly vaccinated persons in order to effect a "take." It is clear that certain inactivated vaccines (mumps and poliomyelitis) do not prevent infection, yet the sequel of infection of the gut with either wild or vaccine strains of live polioviruses is a relative immunity to enteric reinfection.

The immunity of inactivated influenza vaccine is said to be equal to the relatively brief immunity which follows the natural disease. Yet the assumption that naturally acquired immunity to influenza is brief has been derived from a few studies in military or institutional situations. In these cases, attack rates (and presumably challenge doses) were high and probably unrepresentative of exposure within the general population. Certainly, population immunity to influenza does rise and remains high following the introduction of new viral strains, but the role of continuing reinfection in such population immunity is probably important(1).

It is only reasonable to suppose that vaccination procedures most closely simulating natural infection will induce immunity comparable to that of the disease. It is suspected (but unproved) that those infectious agents which induce enduring immunity persist within the host for his lifetime, acting continually or recurrently as antigenic stimuli.

Yellow fever vaccine, a live, parenterally introduced vaccine against a parenterally introduced infection, appears thus far to have induced persisting immunity for as long as six years as judged by persistence of neutralizing antibody.

Immunization with "killed" or inactivated vaccines would appear to be less promising in inducing persisting immunity without frequent "recall" or booster injections. However, it is entirely possible that natural challenge with the infection itself may "boost" primary vaccine immunity in time to forestall its late effects, or disease(2). This postulate remains to be proved, however. In the case of diphtheria, childhood immunization with toxoid clearly does not produce enduring immunity. It is now a cause of grave concern that diphtheria may occur during epidemics among previously immunized adults who have not had recent booster injections. The problem is compounded by the hypersensitivity to toxoid which exists in immunized adults, so that low doses of toxoid must be cautiously administered.

The Anamnestic or Secondary Response to Booster Injections

The declining immunity which follows primary injection of nonliving antigens may in most instances be quickly "recalled" by later "booster" injections (Fig. 29). Even in the absence of residual detectable antibody, the latent immunity from the initial priming with antigen may be evidenced by an accelerated production of antibody in the subject. If the incubation period of the disease to be prevented is sufficiently long, or if contact has not yet occurred, booster injections in previously immunized subjects may be used effectively to supplement the less desirable passive transfer of preformed antibody (p. 245). The situations in which booster injections are most frequently used are in the prophylaxis of tetanus, diphtheria, and typhoid. It has long been recognized that the incidence and severity of unfavorable "reactions" are greater in subjects who have been previously injected with, and hence sensitized to, diphtheria toxoid. For this reason, prior skin testing with *toxin* (Schick test) to determine immunity status, or with *toxoid* (Moloney test), to determine sensitivity to toxoid has been carried out before re-immunization of adults. Recently, careful studies have shown that simple reduction of toxoid dose may obviate such tedious pretesting and yet provide an effective antigenic stimulus for both diphtheria and tetanus(3).

The waning immunity following smallpox vaccination must be periodically "boosted" by revaccination (Table 11). In this case, the secondary immune response is visibly accelerated ("vaccinoid") as evidenced by the more rapid progression of the vaccinia lesion, which reaches its peak in less than a week in contrast to 8 to 10 days in the case of the primary reaction. Immunity to smallpox is concomitantly accelerated.

The Use of Adjuvants with Inactivated Vaccines

Another method for prolonging the immunity induced by non-living vaccines is to use adjuvant materials with the antigen. Such "adjuvants" are chemically diverse, and include aluminum phosphate and mineral oils. Their mechanism of action is not fully understood, but they seem to enhance and prolong the response to primary immunization. The use of adjuvants is still experimental, and the possibility of chronic toxicity has deterred their general acceptance. This important problem deserves further study, however.

The Route of Administration

It is well established that immunizing antigen must be injected into or beneath the skin to evoke immunity. Such parenteral administration is necessary to deliver intact protein antigen to the antibody-forming cells of the reticuloendothelial system. An obvious exception to this rule is live poliovirus vaccine which must be delivered by oral (enteral) ingestion to the site where it will multiply.

Because smallpox vaccination is essentially a dermal infection, it is best inoculated into the superficial layers of the skin by multiple puncture or pressure techniques. The intradermal route is also used to forestall the systemic effects of influenza or typhoid vaccines. This route is purported to allow the establishment of immunity with smaller doses of antigen than are effective subcutaneously. However, virtually all comparative studies of the relative efficacy of the intra-

TABLE 19

The Similar Effects of Intradermal and Subcutaneous Injection of Influenza Vaccine When Similar Time-dose Schedules Are Used

COMPARATIVE FREQUENCY AND MAGNITUDE OF ANTIBODY RESPONSES IN SUBJECTS INJECTED BY SIX SCHEDULES*

Study Group	Injection Route	Dose† (ml)	No. of Subjects	Percentage	Percentage of Subjects with Antibody Titer‡ of 4 Units or More	Percentage of Subjects with Antibody Titer‡ of 8 Units or More	Mean Titer of Antibody§
Prevaccination	—	—	116	100	9.4	1.7	3.1
Schedule A	Subcutaneous	1.0	67	100	86.0	53.0	17.2
Schedule B	Intradermal	0.1 (X2)	95	100	61.0	35.0	10.6
Schedule C	Subcutaneous	0.1 (X2)	50	100	84.0	56.0	17.2
Schedule D	Subcutaneous	0.5 (X2)	41	100	91.0	66.0	28.0
Schedule E	Intradermal	0.2 (X2)	46	100	76.0	45.0	14.9
Schedule F	Subcutaneous	0.2 (X2)	39	100	84.0	30.0	13.0

* From McCarroll and Kilbourne (4).
† Dose, 200 CCA units/ml. Method periodate inactivation of inhibitor; egg-ferret-mouse-line antigen.
‡ Hemagglutination-inhibiting antibody titers—reciprocal of serum dilution at end point.
§ Geometric mean titer of all serums in group, assigning value of 2.5 to titers < 5.0 (starting dilution).

dermal and subcutaneous routes of injection have not used identical dose schedules. Because small doses intradermally may apparently induce the same response as larger subcutaneous doses, it has been frequently and erroneously concluded that intradermal inoculation is superior to subcutaneous in immunizing efficacy. Such conclusions have been derived from studies in which:

1. Immunization was not truly primary.

2. The antigenic mass used subcutaneously was larger than necessary for optimal response.

3. The efficacy of several small doses intradermally was compared with that of a single subcutaneous injection.

In 1957, when suboptimal and identical doses of Asian influenza A2 vaccine were given(4) by identical schedules to members of a population without any possible prior experience with the antigen, no significant differences were noted in response to subcutaneous or intradermal injection (see Table 19).

REFERENCES

1. KILBOURNE, E. D.: *Am. Rev. Resp. Dis.*, 1961, **83**:265.
2. SALK, J. E.: *Ann. Int. Med.*, 1959, **50**:843.
3. LEVINE, L., *et al.*: *Am. J. Hyg.*, 1961, **73**:20.
4. MCCARROLL, J. R., and KILBOURNE, E. D.: *New England J. Med.*, 1958, **259**:618.

18. THE ROLE OF ARTIFICIAL IMMUNIZA-TION IN PUBLIC HEALTH: SPECIFIC VACCINES FOR SPECIFIC PURPOSES

Vaccines for the Prevention of Mortality

The decrease of the killing infectious diseases of man (with their major impact in infancy and childhood) is due principally to environmental sanitation rather than to artificial immunization. But several vaccines — two of them the earliest known — are important methods of control for diseases with high mortality rates. Immunization against smallpox and rabies antedates the recognition of their viral etiology. The principles established over a century ago by Pasteur (with rabies) and Jenner (with cowpox) have been the basis for all subsequent vaccines. These principles include the concept of reducing virulence by "attenuation" or passing or deriving the vaccine strain in or from a different (nonhuman) host.

The diseases which contribute importantly to mortality but are preventable by vaccination include:

Smallpox.
Rabies.
Yellow fever (jungle type).
Diphtheria and pertussis (to a lesser extent)

Although usually considered as causes of general morbidity, diphtheria and pertussis may cause significant mortality in infants and young children.

Tetanus, although uncommon, can kill as many as 40 per cent of its victims, so that vaccination should be considered potentially life-saving with this disease. Similarly, the total mortality from poliomyelitis is small, but the use of vaccine, particularly in adults, has undoubtedly saved lives.

For completeness, the effective vaccine for the prevention of

244

Rocky Mountain spotted fever should be mentioned. However, the great reduction in mortality in spotted fever through the use of tetracycline antibiotics has almost eliminated the need for vaccination.

Vaccines for the Reduction of Mortality in Special Risk Groups

Certain vaccines which are not widely or routinely employed in the general population may have value for the reduction of mortality in groups at special risk of infection or severe disease.

Influenza vaccines have assumed special importance with the recognition that the disease may be fatal in certain patients with cardiac or chronic pulmonary disease or pregnancy. These persons are no more liable than others to acquire the infection but are peculiarly vulnerable to its effects. It is currently recommended by the Surgeon General of the U.S. Public Health Service that such persons receive annual boosters of polyvalent influenza vaccine following primary immunization.

The use of BCG for the prevention of tuberculosis is usually restricted to children in certain crowded, economically deprived populations in which morbidity is predictably high. In such circumstances it is obvious that mortality is also reduced through prevention of miliary and meningitic forms of the disease.

Rabies represents a unique situation in which the incubation period after exposure is so long (14 to 42 days in man) that primary active immunization can be effected in time to prevent the development of disease. The special groups in which mortality may be prevented would therefore include humans bitten by possibly rabid animals in addition to farmers, animal trainers, veterinarians, and others at special risk. Because the case fatality rate of rabies is 100 per cent, reduction of morbidity by immunization is equivalent to reduction in mortality.

None of the rabies vaccines currently available is completely satisfactory. Of the two inactivated preparations (Table 18), the traditional Semple vaccine is the most reliable antigenically. However, serious hypersensitivity reactions to brain tissue components make it undesirable for wide-scale use. A modification of this vaccine which represents duck embryo passage material is apparently less dangerous in this respect. Two live-virus vaccines have been produced by multiple serial passages of the Flury strain of virus in chick embryos. These vaccines, LEP (low egg passage) and HEP (high egg passage) are now used widely in the immunization of domestic animals. The HEP (less virulent but also less antigenic strain) has recently been used as "base line" immunization of those constantly exposed to animals. Because antibody measurements are not easily or reliably correlated with immunity in rabies, the immune status of individuals so vaccinated is somewhat unpredictable. In cases of actual specific exposure, booster injections of living or inactivated vaccine may be given—often supplemented by injection of specific immune serum.

In the case of dog-bite victims who have not previously received primary immunization, the live virus vaccines are not relied upon for the "emergency" induction of primary immunity.

Vaccines as Supplements to Environmental Sanitation

The basic control of yellow fever as an arthropod-borne disease and typhoid as an enteric infection depends on sanitation of the environment. In a sense, rabies also is similarly controlled in most countries by immunization and regulation of the domestic canines, which comprise the important reservoir of infection.

Nevertheless, vaccines for these three diseases together with the vaccines less commonly used for plague, the rickettsial diseases, and the arthropod-borne encephalitides are valuable adjuncts for disease control. Although control of the urban-dwelling mosquito vector is the key to control of urban yellow fever (p. 164), similar environmental control of jungle mosquitoes and animal reservoirs is a virtual impossibility with the jungle form of the disease (p. 109). In the latter case, specific immunization of residents and visitors of the endemic areas is the only feasible control method.

Although the efficacy of typhoid vaccination still remains in dispute, several carefully controlled studies, including one in Yugoslavia (1), suggest its value for those who have not acquired natural immunity from childhood exposure in an endemic area. Certainly, the severity of the disease is less in those who have received specific immunization(2).

Vaccination as a Quarantine Procedure

It is paradoxical that the countries of Asia in which yellow fever has never occurred nevertheless require proof of vaccination for yellow fever from foreign travelers. This measure is obviously not for the protection of the traveler but for the protection of the countries visited, especially if the traveler has recently gone through an area (South America or Africa) in which yellow fever is endemic. In such a case, specific immunization is in effect a quarantine procedure to prevent the importation of the infection into areas in which there are potential vectors for the transmission of disease to the susceptible population. Without this precaution, in these days of swift air travel, persons incubating yellow fever could easily pass from yellow fever zones to any part of Asia in considerably less time than the three- to six-day incubation period of the disease and thus disembark as unrecognized reservoirs of infection. This possibility is forestalled by the requirement that a traveler carry a certificate as evidence of anti-yellow fever vaccination at least ten days before. Such certificates are valid for six years.

The United States and many other countries require smallpox vaccination within a three-year period before citizens are permitted to leave the country. Again, in this case the vaccine is not primarily for the protection of the individual traveler, but for the protection of the country to which he will return — by preventing his acquisition of the disease abroad. The following brief note published in the "Morbidity and Mortality Report" of the U.S. Public Health Service(3) epitomizes the problem involved in the air age:

> The Division of Foreign Quarantine has informed us that recently smallpox was imported to Madrid, Spain by a child who flew from Bombay to Rome on TWA flight #809, January 26 and from Rome to Madrid on Alitalia #346, January 27. Diagnosis was made on February 6 and death occurred on February 14.
>
> A secondary case in Madrid was confirmed on February 23, and 13 additional cases were reported for the week ending March 4.

The infections other than yellow fever and smallpox that are susceptible to international quarantine regulations are cholera, plague, louse-borne relapsing fever, and louse-borne typhus. For none of these are vaccines important as quarantine measures, although certain Asian countries require cholera vaccination of travelers prior to their entry into the country.

Vaccines for the Reduction of Morbidity in Certain Groups at High Risk

Young adults when crowded together in schools or military camps seem to be particularly susceptible to epidemic infection with respiratory viruses. Vaccines are available for the control of certain of these infections, namely those caused by influenza and adenoviruses. Both the influenza and adenovirus vaccines are polyvalent and contain the viral strains most commonly encountered in epidemic form: influenza A and B and adenoviruses 3, 4, and 7. Extensive studies by the Commission on Influenza of the Armed Forces Epidemiological Board have proved the efficacy of these vaccines under field conditions.

In times of widespread prevalence of influenza when all members of the population are at risk, the general use of vaccine may be considered with special reference to such key personnel as policemen, firemen, physicians, and nurses, in whom simultaneous illness (no matter how benign) may jeopardize the public safety.

In contrast, the use of currently available adenovirus vaccines for other than the special military or school situations seems completely unwarranted because there is no evidence that the virus types in the vaccine cause epidemic disease in the general population. In this sense, the adenovirus vaccine is a highly effective prophylactic for which there is no disease!

The Case of Live vs. Inactivated Viral Vaccines: A Consideration of the Poliovirus Vaccines as a Prototype of the Problem

As we pointed out in Chapter 12, poliomyelitis is a relatively new disease. Its emergence has paralleled improvements in public sanitation, which have postponed infection to later childhood and adulthood. In infants the infection is rarely paralytic but, unfortunately, the threat of crippling or death increases with the age of the victim. Thus, public consternation virtually demanded the production of vaccines against this "statistically unimportant disease."

Poliomyelitis, of course, is not unimportant. It is one of the few viral infections directly transmissible from man to man that can cause permanent disability or death. This disability, which usually involves the young, is not only tragic but puts a great economic burden on the family and the community if optimal care and rehabilitation are employed.

In countries with inadequate sanitation, poliomyelitis is relatively unimportant because:

1. Most infections occur very early in life and hence are more apt to be asymptomatic.

2. The primary burden of disease—the fatal enteric infections such as typhoid and bacillary dysentery—eclipses the rare fatalities from poliomyelitis.

Inactivated Poliovirus Vaccine (Salk). To date (1962), only one poliovirus vaccine—the inactivated Salk vaccine—has been commercially and widely used in the United States.* The encouraging results of the rigidly controlled field trials in 1955 have since been abundantly confirmed. Careful supervision of production by both industry and government† eliminated the early difficulties with antigenically poor lots which contained residual live virus. At least four injections of the Salk vaccine at appropriate intervals (Table 20) are necessary to produce optimal immunity. The duration of this immunity is still unknown. Until this problem is solved, annual or biannual boosters are advisable for those at risk.

By June, 1960, more than 400 million doses of Salk vaccine had been released in the United States. Although 70 million doses were exported, most of the remainder was used in vaccination programs within the United States. At that time, surveys indicated a complicated picture of the distribution of vaccinated subjects in the population, varying not only with age but with socioeconomic group. Ninety per cent of 5- to 14-year-olds in the upper socioeconomic group and only 25 per cent of the 15- to 39-year-olds in the lower socioeconomic group had been vaccinated(4). Since 1955 the poor acceptance of polio vaccine by lower economic groups coupled with the more extensive vaccination of school-age children has produced a significant shift in the paralytic disease away from the well-to-do child and back to the preschool child of the slum area. This experience re-emphasizes the gap that public health education must close between scientific accomplishment and its implementation. As reported by the World Health Organization(5):

It has been possible during 1959 to arrive at what is considered to be a firmer estimate of the effectiveness of inactivated vaccine as used in the U.S.A. The main sources of the data were (a) the case reports submitted to the Poliomyelitis Surveillance Unit, (b) the Census Bureau random sampling, and (c) an intensive study of a local epidemic in Des Moines, Iowa. From these data, the effectiveness ratios by age group and vaccination status for triple vaccinated persons were estimated to be over 90 per cent in the age group 0-14 and 82 per cent for the age group 15-39; for persons vaccinated 4 times the ratios were 96 per cent and 86 per cent respectively.

Reduction of the severity of disease acquired despite vaccination is another indication of the efficacy of vaccination, albeit seldom ap-

[*Text continued on p. 251.*]

*The background of this accomplishment has been reported in Chapter 12.

†The standards for vaccines and other biological reagents are now set and supervised by the Division of Biologic Standards of the National Institutes of Health.

TABLE 20

Recommendations for Immunization of the General Population*

I. SUGGESTED SCHEDULE OF IMMUNIZATION IN AREAS WITH ADEQUATE PUBLIC HEALTH MEDICAL SERVICES: TO BE MODIFIED AS REQUIRED TO SUIT LOCAL CONDITIONS†

Age	Proposed Schedule
2-6 months	Diphtheria-pertussis-tetanus triple vaccine: 3 doses with 1 month's interval between each dose
6-7 months	Smallpox vaccination
7-10 months	Poliomyelitis vaccine (inactivated): 2 doses with 1 month's interval
15-18 months	Booster dose of triple vaccine; simultaneously, third dose of poliomyelitis vaccine
2-4 years	Fourth dose of poliomyelitis vaccine
5-6 years	Booster dose of diphtheria-tetanus vaccine; simultaneously, smallpox re-vaccination
10-15 years	Booster dose of diphtheria-tetanus vaccine if Schick test positive: no injection of diphtheria prophylactic in Schick pseudo-reactors

*WHO Technical Report Series No. 198.

†*Tetanus:* An individual who has been effectively immunized with a primary course of tetanus toxoid followed by 1 or 2 booster doses should be given a further dose of tetanus toxoid if exposed to the risk of tetanus. If the injury is extensive, a dose of tetanus antitoxin should also be given. If tetanus antitoxin is given to a non-immunized individual, active immunization with tetanus toxoid should be begun 4 to 6 weeks later.

Poliomyelitis: The use of live attenuated polio virus vaccine is not included in this schedule because of the still limited knowledge about its efficacy when given orally to infants. This procedure may become the method of choice in countries where there is a high incidence of clinical disease in early infancy. In these countries immunization with inactivated vaccine may have to be begun earlier than suggested in the schedule, but in such circumstances the antibody response will be negligible in a considerable proportion of infants because of the presence of maternal antibody.

It is suggested that the fourth dose of polio virus vaccine be given within 1 to 2 years after the third dose of the primary course since (a) antibody titers may have fallen to low levels by that time and (b) clinical disease has occurred in children after 3 doses. If the polio antigens, particularly types I and III, are improved, it may be possible to postpone the fourth dose until school entry.

Quadruple vaccine (DPT and polio) is not recommended at present.

TABLE 20 (*Continued*)

II. Suggested Schedule of Immunization in Areas with Inadequate Medical Services: To Be Modified as Required To Suit Local Conditions‡

3-6 months	Smallpox vaccination and simultaneously first dose of triple vaccine *with alum*
	Second dose of triple vaccine 1 to 3 months after first dose
5-6 years	Booster dose of diphtheria-tetanus vaccine; simultaneously smallpox revaccination

‡ It is envisaged that this schedule will be used in countries with a low incidence of clinical poliomyelitis. In such areas poliomyelitis vaccine should not be employed routinely, but should be available to those at special risk of clinical disease.

Smallpox and triple vaccine should not be given simultaneously either to infants with a history of convulsions or other evidence of central nervous system disease or to those convalescent from an acute infection.

The injection of an alum-containing mixed vaccine carries a slight risk of provocation poliomyelitis in young children. It is recommended that the content of aluminium hydroxide or phosphate should not exceed 2 mg/ml and that the mixture should not be given to infants over 6 months of age.

---

preciated. A study of 424 children with poliomyelitis showed that while 50 per cent of the unvaccinated patients suffered moderate or severe paralysis, only 11 per cent of the vaccinated patients were so affected(6). The incidence of nonparalytic poliomyelitis is also reduced by vaccination.

Live Poliovirus Vaccines. Even prior to field testing Salk vaccine, the first experiments on humans with a "live" poliovirus vaccine were undertaken in 1952(7). In the past decade, an enormous amount of money and energy has been expended by several groups of American investigators in efforts to perfect living infectious vaccines for the prevention of poliomyelitis. The proponents of live virus vaccine have not questioned the efficacy of the Salk vaccine. They have believed, however, that more enduring immunity could result from ingestion of an attenuated living virus which would simulate the experience of natural infection. Three types of vaccine have now been produced—the Sabin, Koprowski, and Lederle (Cox) vaccines—and more than 65 millions of people, most of them under 15 years of age, have been inoculated in field trials of varying number and nature. Although interpretation of several of these trials is difficult because many of the subjects may have been previously immunized by natural infection or by Salk vaccine, it can be concluded that:

1. Live virus vaccines stimulate antibody production and immunity in a variable number of subjects, depending on:
   a. The strain of virus used.
   b. Whether single or multiple strains are given.
   c. Whether single or multiple dose regimens are employed.
   d. The prevalence of other interfering enteroviruses in the population.
2. Serious reactions or disease from live virus vaccines have not been detected.

In spite of these observations, the caution shown by public health authorities in delaying licensing* of the vaccine for commercial production is both understandable and commendable in view of certain other facts. The use of live poliovirus vaccines raises problems unprecedented in the history of public health.

The oral ingestion of live poliovirus vaccines perfectly *simulates natural infection* in contrast to the live virus vaccines used for smallpox and yellow fever. Like natural infection (and unlike Salk vaccination), live poliovirus vaccines stimulate the development of local immunity in the gut, which reduces the possibility of reinfection. Most importantly, *the vaccine viruses may spread from the vaccinee to household contacts and others.* Thus, since the vaccination procedure is a contagious one, the potential effects of vaccine viruses upon the community as well as upon the vaccinated subject must be considered. (To a very limited extent this is true of vaccinia, which rarely infects contacts with pre-existing dermatoses.)

"Contagious immunity" is an exciting prospect which has suggested to some investigators that the avirulent vaccine viruses might spread and eventually replace all existing virulent wild strains of poliomyelitis virus. A sobering alternative is that multiple serial human passages might increase the risk of mutant vaccine strains with increased virulence, resulting in paralytic disease.

Although the viral strains of the vaccines have been carefully selected from laboratory strains with reduced virulence for the monkey, the correlation of this property with reduced virulence for the human is still not clear; nor have any other biologic or physical prop-

---

*At this writing (April, 1962), at least two pharmaceutical companies in the United States have been licensed to produce and market oral live poliovirus vaccine containing the "Sabin" strains of virus.

erties of the virus been linked unequivocally with virulence or avirulence. The potential for mutation always exists, and studies with earlier, less attenuated strains showed that neurovirulence for the monkey could be regained during two successive human transfers.

The past experience with the 17D yellow fever vaccine should not be forgotten. In that case, human transfer was not involved: instead, mutation occurred during tissue culture passage so that one lot had increased neurovirulence for man(8).

Another unprecedented danger is the possibility that live poliovirus vaccines, made in monkey kidney tissue culture, may contain simian viruses which had been latent in the tissue. This danger is more than hypothetical. It has been recognized retrospectively that many of the vaccine lots used in field trials have not only contained simian virus but have infected the recipients, as shown by antibody response. The fact that no acute reaction or disease accompanied such infections is not entirely reassuring, because the ultimate or chronic disease potential of the monkey viruses is not known.

Live vs. Dead Poliovirus Vaccines: A Summary of Considerations Pro and Con

The advantages of immunization with inactivated poliovirus vaccine are:

1. A finite (measured) mass of antigen is administered.

2. There is no danger of virulent virus mutation with the non-multiplying antigen.

3. Vaccination is limited to the vaccinee.

4. The efficacy of the vaccine in preventing paralytic poliomyelitis is now well established in closely controlled trials and general field experience.

Potential disadvantages of the "dead" virus vaccine are the possibilities that:

1. The potency of the antigen may be impaired by the procedures which kill (inactivate) the viruses.

2. If residual live virus survives the inactivation procedure, it is potentially virulent for man in vaccines presently available.

3. The duration of immunity is unknown — revaccination may be necessary throughout adult life.

Whether the fact that inactivated vaccine does not prevent poliovirus infection is an advantage or disadvantage is debatable. Obviously the Salk vaccine does not curtail the circulation and persistence of wild viruses but neither does it prevent natural infection of the subject, which may occur in the Salk vaccinated subject without inducing disease but boosting immunity.

On the other hand, advantages of the live poliovirus vaccines are:

1. They simulate natural infection; therefore may produce lasting immunity to disease and at least partial immunity to reinfection.

2. Mass immunization is far simpler and safer with a vaccine which may be given by mouth.

3. Immunization may be "contagious" if vaccine viruses spread to contacts.

4. Ultimately, wild virulent viruses may be displaced by the vaccine strains.

However: .

1. Mutation to neurovirulence for man may occur in the laboratory, in the primary vaccinee, or in the community. Such mutation might particularly jeopardize nonimmune adult contacts of vaccinated children.

2. Immunization might be blocked by interference from unrecognized enterovirus infections.

3. The importance of contaminating simian viruses from the tissue cultures in which vaccine is produced has not yet been determined.

A choice between the two vaccines, however, may not be necessary. The initial administration of inactivated Salk vaccine prevents paralytic disease but not infection of the gut. It may be logical to follow such primary immunization with live virus vaccines which will boost humoral immunity and induce local enteric immunity to poliovirus infection.

REFERENCES

1. CVJETANOVIC, B. B.: *Am. J. Pub. Health*, 1957, **47**:578.

2. TURNER, R.: *South African Med. J.*, 1959, **33**:639.

3. *Morbidity and Mortality Report of the United States Public Health Service,* March 10, 1961. Government Printing Office, Washington, D.C.

4. *Poliomyelitis Surveillance Report, No. 191,* U.S. Pub. Health Service, Government Printing Office, Washington, D.C.

5. Expert Committee on Poliomyelitis, *Third Report, WHO Tech. Rep. Series,* No. 203, 1960.

6. WYMAN, M. G., *et al.: California Med.,* 1957, **87**:1.

7. KOPROWSKI, H., *et al.: Am. J. Hyg.,* 1952, **55**:108.

8. FOX, J. P., *et al.: Am. J. Hyg.,* 1942, **36**:117.

SECTION V

New Hazards to Man and New Problems of Environmental Sanitation

Although it may well be questioned whether the problems discussed in this section are basically new, their increasing magnitude and recent emergence to general attention are certainly new phenomena.

The lower atmosphere in which man has lived exclusively prior to the space age has never been free of natural pollutants, and the earliest efforts at food preservation involved the use of additives, but in our technologically advanced and industrialized society the threats to human health from air pollution and the use of chemical food additives have aroused grave concern. At least some of this concern appears to be justified, but much of the speculation concerning the etiologic role of environmental chemical pollutants in human disease is indeed only speculation and is reminiscent of the early days of medical bacteriology.

In the following pages, an effort is made to summarize the positive evidence linking chemicals in the environment with illness in the general population and to emphasize the problems involved in securing such evidence. The more obvious relations of certain industrial hazards to occupational diseases are considered in Chapter 30.

19. AIR POLLUTION

The air man breathes is rarely free of contaminating gases, liquids, or solid particles. The composition of unpolluted air of the lower atmosphere is summarized in Table 21. Contamination of this atmosphere may occur from natural sources or from the activities of man. Such contamination is usually termed "pollution" if it is potentially deleterious to living plants, animals, or human beings. A broad definition of air pollution covering both natural and man-made contamination, without implication concerning health, states that "air pollution is any air-borne substance which is neither water in any of its phases nor a component of dry air"(1). This type of definition is obviously useless for legal purposes; therefore, the implication that the pollutant is harmful in some way is present in most legislation.*

The Nature of Air Pollutants

In physical terms, there are two principal categories of air pollutants:

1. Substances which exist in the gaseous state at less than 200° C.
2. Aerosols of liquids or solids (particles dispersed in an air or gaseous medium).

It is of interest that air-borne particles may indirectly influence the state and composition of the atmosphere.

Dust or aerosol particles may show greatly enhanced surface activity by virtue of increased surface area, adsorption of gas molecules or other properties that facilitate chemical reactions. Many substances that oxidize only

*There has been no consistency or uniformity in the use of the terms "pollutant" and "contaminant" in publications relating to air pollution. It is proposed here that the distinction between these terms which has been observed in the case of water pollution is useful and should — for the sake of uniformity — be observed in the newer field of air pollution. In this usage, a *pollutant* is any unwanted or undesirable substance, and a *contaminant* is a pollutant with the capacity to induce human disease.

slowly in their massive state will oxidize with extreme rapidity or explode when dispersed as fine dust in air. Adsorption and catalytic phenomena are influenced particularly by the state of dispersion of the solid or liquid phases in the gas dispersion medium of heterogeneous systems. Thermal radiation effects become much more pronounced if suspended solid or liquid particles are present in the air. Such particles absorb radiation and conduct heat rapidly to the surrounding gas molecules, which may be quite transparent to the radiant energy. Aerosol particles may act as condensation nuclei to facilitate the condensation of water vapour upon them and thus promote the formation of fog or ground mists(2).

TABLE 21

Average Composition of the Atmosphere °

Gas Component †	Composition (p.p.m. by volume)	Composition (p.p.m. by weight)
Nitrogen	780,900	755,100
Oxygen	209,500	231,500
Argon	9,300	12,800
Carbon dioxide	300	460
Neon	18	12.5
Helium	5.2	0.72
Methane	2.2	1.2
Krypton	1	2.9
Nitrous oxide	1	1.5
Hydrogen	0.5	0.03
Xenon	0.08	0.36

° From M. Katz (2).
† Water vapor is also present in variable amounts.

The interaction of atmospheric contaminants is of more than academic interest. It now seems probable that the eye-irritating toxicants of Los Angeles smog are formed from the interaction of certain hydrocarbons and oxides of nitrogen as induced by ultraviolet irradiation in the air(3).

Natural Air Pollutants

The air pollutants not artificially produced by man include:

1. Water vapor of fine-particle water aerosols (fog).
2. Dust (minerals, soil, or particles of animal and vegetable matter, including pollen).
3. Bacteria and their spores and fungi.
4. Salts (derived from ocean spray).
5. Aromatic compounds resulting from animal or vegetable fermentations which may produce noxious odors.
6. Products of combustion of natural origin (forest fires, volcanic eruptions, etc.).
7. Radioactive materials. Natural or background radiation varies from 0.0003 to 0.0006 roentgen per day. (These amounts are far below the 2 to 10 r daily dose which may induce acute illness within weeks.)

TABLE 22

Air Pollutants[*]

Group	*Examples*
Solids	Carbon fly ash, ZnO, $PbCl_2$
Sulfur compounds	SO_2, SO_3, H_2S, mercaptans
Organic compounds	Aldehydes, hydrocarbons, tars
Nitrogen compounds	NO, NO_2, NH_3
Oxygen compounds	O_3, CO, CO_2
Halogen compounds	HF, HCl
Radioactive compounds	Radioactive gases, aerosols, etc.

[*]From L. C. McCabe[1].

It is probable that such natural or background sources of atmospheric pollution play little role in human disease. However, atmospheric dissemination of microbial pathogens has probably occurred (p. 123), and an increase in incidence of positive skin reactions to histoplasmin was observed after a tornado in the Middle West[3].

It is also possible that levels of natural radioactivity will increase as the surface of the earth is disturbed by the encroachments of man.

If the proportion of the population exhibiting allergy to pollen continues to increase, then air pollution from vegetable sources will also become increasingly important.

Man-made Pollutants

The most common and important air pollutants are the products of combustion. It is predictable that the concentrations of such pollutants will continue to increase in industrialized urban societies until revolutionary improvements take place in the efficiency of combustion processes.

More than 100 combustion products have been identified in the atmosphere, but they may be classified into the relatively few general types indicated in Table 22.

The Principal Sources of Man-made Pollutants. Particular types of combustion are usually associated with the production and release of characteristic pollutants. The most thorough investigations have been made on those pollutants that: (a) result from the combustion of coal (the fuel in greatest industrial use), and (b) are most amenable to detection and measurement by simple techniques. Such pollutants are not necessarily related to human disease.

Perhaps the best studied of the pollutants derived from coal combustion is sulfur dioxide. The concentration of this gas has been measured in British industrial and urban areas for many years. Sulfur dioxide has undeniable economic effects related to its corrosive actions on buildings and its injurious effects on vegetation. Its role in human disease is less clear, as is discussed further in this chapter.

Fluorides may be introduced into the atmosphere through the manufacture or processing of phosphate fertilizers, aluminum, pottery, or bricks. An indirect result of even small amounts in the air (0.001 part per million) is the production of fluorosis in animals which feed upon the fluorine-contaminated vegetation of the region.

Nitrogen Oxides. Katz(2) has described nitrous oxides as the:

> Second most abundant atmospheric contaminant in many communities, ranking next to sulfur dioxide. These oxides are important by-products of the chemical industry in the manufacture of nitric acid, sulfuric acid by the chamber process, nitration of organic compounds, and the manufacture of nylon intermediates, and are formed in varying quantities in internal combustion engines from the air supplied to the fuel. Significant amounts are liberated in the exhaust gases of trucks and passenger automobiles.

Carbon Monoxide. Concentrations of carbon monoxide vary considerably in urban areas and directly reflect the patterns of automobile traffic.

The importance of the automobile as a source of air contamination has only recently been appreciated. In addition to carbon monoxide, aldehydes and potentially carcinogenic hydrocarbons (including benzpyrine) are emitted from automobile exhaust. Indeed, the major contributor to the smog of Los Angeles appears to be the automobile.

It is the particulate matter in the atmosphere which usually attracts public attention to air pollution, because it comprises the smoke which reduces visibility and results in gritty fallout which soils clothes and lowers public morale. These particles are usually more than 200μ. When pollution stems from industrial sources and the combustion of coal, measurement of dustfall is a useful index of air pollution and its control. Particles smaller than 1μ remain suspended for these do not spontaneously settle out but must be removed by filtration or precipitation. The concentration of particulates has shown a direct correlation with the number of persons contributing to community pollution.

The Influence of Climatic and Meteorologic Conditions

The production and perpetuation of a polluted atmosphere are dependent not only upon sources of combustion but also upon climatic and meteorologic conditions which prevent the dilution and dispersion of pollutants. Conditions of weather and terrain that hinder the free circulation of air may result from many circumstances. The most notable air pollution disasters, however, have occurred in lowland valleys or river plains during periods of fog and temperature inversion.

The mechanism of temperature inversion is illustrated in Figure 30. The warm cap of air produced by radiation from the ground prevents normal upward displacement of air and contaminants; therefore those contaminants are retained and accumulate in the lower stratum. When such meteorologic conditions are sustained, immediate and acute effects upon human health are noted. The topographic advantages for transportation and water supply offered by river valleys, however, not only attract but foster industrial development of their environs.

The notorious smog of Los Angeles results not only from the combustion products of millions of automobiles but also from the unusual topographic features of the area. The city is located on a narrow coastal plain which is bounded by the Pacific Ocean on the west and by mountains on the east, north, and south. Thus, sea breeze and terrain lead to the accumulation of a large air pocket over the city, especially in summer and early fall when temperature inversions are more likely to occur.

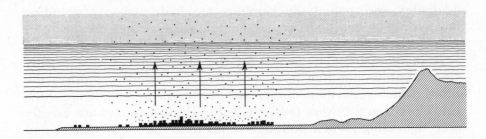

Thermal inversion, common in Los Angeles, is the main meteorological factor in smog formation. Except in an inversion, air temperature decreases with height; the warm surface air rises, carrying pollutants away.

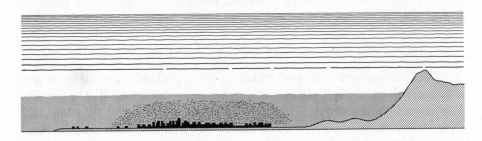

Inversion sets in when cool sea air moves in under warm desert air and is trapped. The normal temperature gradient is reversed in the inversion layer, the base of which (at the surface in this drawing) forms a lid over the city, concentrating pollutants.

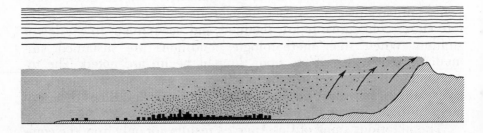

Inversion persists until the weather changes, as when the warm air is high enough to permit the cool sea air to escape and carry away the accumulated smog. Thermal inversions occur in Los Angeles about 100 days a year, but they are also common elsewhere.

Figure 30. The effects of a temperature inversion on the development of smog. (McDermott, W.: *Scientific American*, Oct., 1961.)

Acute Epidemic Disease Associated with Air Pollution

Even the most cautious investigators of air pollution acknowledge that acute disease may occur in association with air pollution — usually in association with unusual and exacting meteorologic conditions. Three such episodes that have been thoroughly studied occurred in:

1. The Meuse Valley of Belgium in 1930.
2. Donora, Pennsylvania, in 1948.
3. London in 1952.

As indicated in Table 23, the Meuse Valley and Donora episodes were remarkably similar, occurring in similar topographic settings and weather conditions, in association with similar industries, and resulting in similar illnesses. The London episode differed principally in having a different probable source of pollution and a more precipitous onset of illness. In none of these epidemics has the responsible pollutant been conclusively identified.

The Donora experience is worth recounting as a particularly well-studied example of the effect of acute air pollution on a community. An extensive report of the disaster has been published by members of the U.S. Public Health Service team which investigated the problem in retrospect two months after its occurrence(3). One of the authors of the original report has summarized the story as follows:

During the last week of October 1948, a temperature inversion and an anticyclonic weather condition characterized by little or no air movement occurred over a wide area of the north-eastern portion of the USA. The unusually prolonged stable atmospheric condition, associated with fog, resulted in the accumulation of atmospheric contaminants to abnormal levels of concentration, particularly in highly industrialized areas. The city of Donora was one such area.

Donora is located on the inside of a sharp horseshoe bend of the meandering Monongahela River some 30 miles south of Pittsburgh. The narrow plain immediately adjacent to the river is occupied on the Donora side of the river by a large steel and a large zinc reduction plant. Just beyond this narrow plain, as well as the one in the town of Webster on the opposite bank, the terrain rises sharply. On the Donora side the hills rapidly reach a height of 400 feet (1150 feet above sea level) in a 10% grade.

On the morning of 27 October 1948, the atmosphere of Donora became very still, there was a marked weather inversion and fog enveloped the city. This weather phenomenon was associated with an accumulation of atmospheric contaminants. The condition continued until 31 October, when an afternoon rain occurred and the change of weather was associated with clarification of the air. In that interval of four days there was a great deal

TABLE 23*

Comparison of Three Major Air Pollution Crises

	Meuse Valley, 1930	Donora, 1948	London, 1952
Weather	Anticyclonic, inversion, and fog	Anticyclonic, inversion, and fog	Anticyclonic, inversion, and fog
Topography	River valley	River valley	River plain
Most probable source of pollutants	Industry (including steel and zinc plants)	Industry (including steel and zinc plants)	Household coal-burning
Nature of the illnesses	Chemical irritation of exposed membranous surfaces	Chemical irritation of exposed membranous surfaces	Chemical irritation of exposed membranous surfaces
Deaths among those with pre-existing cardio-respiratory disease	Yes	Yes	Yes
Time of deaths	Began after second day of episode	Began after second day of episode	Began on first day of episode
Ratio of illnesses to deaths	Not available	75:1 to 300:1	Illness rates not in expected proportion to that of deaths
Autopsy findings	Inflammatory lesions in lungs included parenchyma	Inflammatory lesions in lungs did not include parenchyma	Inflammatory lesions in lungs included parenchyma
Suspected proximate cause of irritation	Sulfur oxides with particulates	Sulfur oxides with particulates	Sulfur oxides with particulates

*From H. Heimann(3).

of respiratory tract illness among the residents. During the same period there were 17 deaths in the community, which normally experienced an average of two deaths in an equivalent period of time.*

The U.S. Public Health Service was asked to assist the state health authorities to make an epidemiological study of the episode, with the ultimate object of avoiding such occurrences in the future. The study was begun early in December of the same year, about two months after the episode. The investigation was planned to determine the following: (a) the health effects that occurred among the people and domestic animals; (b) the qualitative and quantitative nature of the contaminants that had accumulated in the air and (c) the meteorological conditions that existed at the time of the episode.

The primary method used to study the human effects was the household canvass by questionnaire to obtain data on descriptions of the sicknesses that had occurred and of their prevalence. This canvass was carried out by public health nurses in a statistically valid sample of the population. (One third of the total population constituted the sample.) For a selected portion of those who were said to have been ill, physicians obtained more detailed clinical information by interview. Further medical data were obtained from a review of the medical records of patients who had been hospitalized during the episode and from autopsies. Blood studies were made for three purposes: (a) to determine the blood content of influenza antibodies, since the outbreak of illnesses in the Donora episode resembled in some respects that of an epidemic of influenza; (b) to enumerate the percentage of polymorphonuclear eosinophilic leukocytes in the blood, to be used as an indicator of the part that allergy may have played in the clinical manifestations and (c) to evaluate the presence in the blood of abnormal chemical elements, either in kind or in amount. Chest roentgenograms were made of a limited number of persons. Teeth, bone and urine samples were chemically examined for fluoride content to provide auxiliary evidence in regard to the relationship that fluorides may have had to the acute clinical manifestations. A veterinary physician investigated the occurrence of sickness among both farm animals and pets during the episode. Finally, records of general morbidity and morality of the community were studied for varying periods of time before the episode.

The aerometric and other engineering studies were also done after the episode was over. The engineers attempted to determine the nature and amounts of the materials which were present in the ambient air during the episode. Their studies included a period of time when the local factories were operating fully during a later short weather inversion. The meteorologists made a study of local weather conditions, reviewing whatever past weather records were available.

It was found that during the episode almost half (42.7 per cent) of the population had suffered some symptom referable to irritation of

---

*During the days immediately following the episode three more deaths occurred among persons who became ill during the episode.

the respiratory tract. Cough was the most common symptom. In most, symptoms were described as "mild" or "moderate," but 10 per cent of the population had illness which was termed "severe." Seventeen deaths occurred among the 13,839 persons in the Donora area.

Both the frequency and severity of illness were found to be related to increasing age and to pre-existing disease of the heart or lungs but not to other factors, such as sex and occupation. In all but four of the fatal cases, there had been acute or chronic pre-existing disease.

The original report concluded that the etiologic factor may have been a combination of sulfur dioxide with its oxidation products and nonspecific particulate matter. A more recent suggestion(3) is that "metal ammonium sulfates" may have been responsible(4).

An interesting "follow-up of Donora ten years after" has been published(5). It was the purpose of that study to learn whether long-term effects of the acute episode were detectable and whether persons who had suffered acute illness in 1948 differed from those who had not. Regrettably, the findings were not clear-cut, but it was shown that "persons who reported acute illness at the time of the smog episode have demonstrated subsequently higher mortality and prevalence of illness than other persons living in the community at the time." It is not clear from the study whether the air pollution episode caused the subsequent increased disability in those who had been acutely ill or whether the acute illness observed in these subjects occurred because they had pre-existing or underlying disease which continued to progress. Most evidence—particularly that from British studies of "bronchitis"—would suggest that pre-existing disease is worsened rather than primarily engendered by acute episodes of pollution.

THE CHRONIC EFFECTS OF AIR POLLUTION
ON HUMAN HEALTH

Although 33 states have introduced legislation for the control of air pollution, it must be admitted that direct evidence for the etiologic role of atmospheric contaminants in human disease is almost totally lacking. With the exception of the acute Donora-like episodes which have affected mainly the chronically ill, few clues are apparent. The difficulties in making such an etiologic association are many:

1. It is basically more difficult to assess the etiology of chronic disease than acute disease—and it is the relation of chronic pulmo-

nary disease to air pollution that is chiefly under study. For example, it is possible that the continued inhalation of concentrations of pollutants which are not acutely toxic might produce disease by their cumulative effects.

2. The number of atmospheric pollutants is many, and "air pollution" differs quantitatively and qualitatively from city to city. The markedly differing incidence of "bronchitis" in the United States and in the British Isles might be an effect of the differences in the fuels used (and therefore combustion products)—principally petroleum in the United States and coal in the United Kingdom. It is obviously pointless to equate "air pollution" in Los Angeles and London as similar etiologic agents of disease.

3. The diseases of air pollution are as undefined as their etiologic agents. There is little agreement among American and British physicians concerning the diagnosis of bronchitis, asthma, and pulmonary emphysema. The 34-fold higher mortality rate from "bronchitis" in Great Britain may reflect the fact that "bronchitis" is rarely indicated as a primary cause of death on an American death certificate. Even pulmonary emphysema, which is the more common American diagnosis, is more often listed as a secondary than as a primary cause of death in America(6). Even if differing terminologies for obstructive ventilatory disease are reconciled, it is still not clear if this category of disease is the most important sequel of air pollution. In addition to the other diseases of the respiratory tract such as lung cancer, it is possible that certain air pollutants absorbed via the respiratory route may exert their effects elsewhere within the body. Certainly this is true of certain occupational exposures to industrial air pollutants (e.g., beryllium and radium).

4. A practical and immediate problem for the practitioner of public health and for the legislature to decide is the arbitrary point at which a "nuisance" or a source of "minor discomfort" or "irritation" constitutes a threat to public health. Must the community await evidence that an air contaminant threatens life before acting to eliminate it? The improvement in public morale and civic pride which followed reduction of the grime of Pittsburgh attests to the value of positive action.

It is obvious from the foregoing factors that the relation of air pollution to human disease is indeed a formidable problem. Its resolution will require the application of the most advanced and critical methods of epidemiology and toxicology, pathology and clinical medicine. It seems probable that the etiology of disease will prove to be multifactorial and variable from one environment to another. In the meantime, it is pertinent to review briefly the available evidence that air pollution may have long-term effects on human health.

It has been a logical approach to assess the long-term effects of air pollution in relation to diseases of the respiratory tract. Most studies have compared the mortality rates from chronic pulmonary diseases in urban (polluted) areas with those of rural areas. More recently, door-to-door surveys by the National Health Survey of the United States and measurements of pulmonary function have been made to assess differences in morbidity from chronic respiratory disease. From the different types of studies, evidence has accrued that the incidence of chronic respiratory disease (bronchitis, asthma, pulmonary emphysema, carcinoma of the lung) is higher in urban dwellers (especially those in heavily industrialized areas) than in rural residents. It is not clear, however, whether the increased risk of living in an urban area is necessarily related to atmospheric pollution or to other concomitants of city living. For example, the higher rate of lung cancer in city dwellers has been ascribed by some to the increased consumption of tobacco (personal air pollution), although other studies have claimed a ninefold higher incidence in nonsmoking urban residents than in nonsmoking country dwellers(7). Furthermore, the air of many cities contains substances, e.g., benzpyrine, which are known to be carcinogenic in experimental animals. A variety of noncarcinogenic pollutants, including sulfur dioxide, ozone, and nitrogen dioxide, may induce airway resistance and pathologic changes in the lungs of laboratory animals.

Radioactive Air Pollutants

The influence of radioactive atmospheric pollutants on human health is equally equivocal, although there is considerable evidence that intense occupational and industrial exposures have resulted in serious late effects, usually neoplastic. Workers in the pitchblende mines in Czechoslovakia developed a relatively high incidence of lung cancer that seemed related to exposure to radon gas. The increased risk of leukemia in radiologists also seems well established. The promiscuous use of X-ray for diagnostic purposes is under careful scrutiny because of evidence that X-irradiation of infants in the thymus region may be followed by an increased rate of thyroid cancer or leukemia.

Now that man is befouling the general atmosphere with products of nuclear fusion and fission, the importance of such pollutants is being carefully studied. The wide study carried out by the Atomic Bomb Casualty Commission in Hiroshima and Nagasaki has provided some valuable preliminary information about the hazards of direct whole-body irradiation, but the effects of fallout (radioactive dust) remain to be determined. In this connection, the interrelation of preventive medicine and geopolitics is nowhere better stated than by the following(8):

When considering latent effects of contaminating the atmosphere with ionizing radiation, it becomes necessary to recognize that fall-out from a single explosion will persist for decades and its effects will extend over generations. Geneticists agree that the number of mutations—and most of these are harmful—is strictly proportional to the amount of radiation received. There is no "safe" or harmless dose. Some evidence also implies that even small doses of radiation may cause leukemia and bone cancer in a small proportion of exposed persons, but this small proportion must be applied to the entire world population. Thus, nuclear explosions of the past twelve years may indeed be causing an unknown number of cases. Taking into account the exposure of the entire world population this number may not be inconsiderable.

The Effect of Air Pollution on Pre-existing Disease

Although a primary role of air pollution in the initiation of chronic disease remains in doubt, its adverse effects on certain members of the population with pre-existing cardiac or pulmonary disease has been established in such acute disasters as the Donora episode.

Less direct evidence suggests that chronic exposure to air pollutants may affect the health and longevity of persons with cardiopulmonary disease; e.g., in the British Isles, the mortality from chronic bronchitis is higher in the cities with greater amounts of air pollution(9). This occurrence of increased mortality from bronchitis might, of course, be related to urban factors other than air pollution. However, mortality rates charted in relation to increase in atmospheric pollution have shown suggestive associations in several cities.

Acute morbidity from chronic pulmonary disease has similarly been linked to air contamination—using such indices as rates of hospitalization of asthmatics or reduction in pulmonary function in pulmonary disease patients.

Air Pollution and Preventive Medicine

It must be obvious that until more precise relationships between air pollution and human disease have been observed, preventive measures must be general, empirical, and imprecise. Nevertheless, it makes little sense to permit combustion products of proved noxious potential to continue fouling the atmosphere because of a lack of definitive proof of their role as incitants of disease. On the other hand, it is equally true that actions which are too hasty may do more harm than good. For example, elimination of one contaminant from the atmosphere may actually interfere with its interactions with and removal of another contaminant of greater pathogenic potential(3). In spite of the ambiguous nature of the problem, there are several reasonable steps which may be taken by the community for the reduction of air pollution and the prevention of its possible sequels.

A fundamental problem of air pollution control is the fact that air pollution parallels the progress of an industrialized society. Therefore, to attack the problem of atmospheric contaminants as a categorical evil is a procedure which cannot win widespread support because industry itself contributes so much to the public health. It has been pointed out that the problems of environmental sanitation in the nineteenth century were less difficult because "the malaria mosquito and the typhoid bacillus . . . had no friends"(10). Quite properly, the automobile industry and those supplying food, light, and heat to homes and hospitals have many advocates who must be convinced of the value of costly methods for pollution control. The simple fact is that *no single atmospheric pollutant or combination of pollutants has been conclusively linked to the induction of serious disease in the general population.*

Nevertheless, as the earlier parts of this chapter have indicated, there are strong indications that air pollution is deleterious to physical and mental health so that an aggressive approach to its control seems mandatory. As with no other problem in public health, control will depend upon the participation of nonmedical specialists for both the conduct of research and the design of preventive methods. Medical and industrial collaboration has already resulted in the enactment of legislation in 33 states of the union. In addition, the need for interstate cooperation in topographically related areas (as in New York City and Northern New Jersey) has been recognized.

Since more than public health is involved, a comprehensive program for the control of air pollution should consider also the protection of plants, animals, and buildings and the furtherance of continued economic growth.

In summary, the progressive community will ensure:

1. *Reduction in fly ash and smoke, which comprise the obvious and esthetically obnoxious "dirt" of the environment and which reduce visibility and ultraviolet irradiation.*

In effect, the smoke and ash problem is easily solved by conversion from coal to petroleum products as a fuel source. The results of a wholesale conversion of this nature are dramatically exemplified in the story of Pittsburgh—once known as the "smoky city." When the majority of residents switched from coal to "smokeless fuels" within a thirteen-year period, and all railroads and riverboats were converted to diesel engines, the reduction in dustfall was so great that the face of the city changed—and concomitantly the morale of its inhabitants.

2. *Preliminary studies and regulation of industrial plant design to prevent local atmospheric pollution.*

A special laboratory of New York University College of Engineering conducts "mock-up" studies of proposed factories and their stacks under conditions simulating the topography and wind conditions of the proposed building sites. Such studies have saved industry thousands of dollars by preventing improper design which might be in conflict with existing air pollution legislation. It is significant that industry is sufficiently concerned with public relations to avail itself of such research in preventive design.

3. *Reduction in the combustion products of gasoline engines: chiefly those of automobiles and trucks.*

The state of California has already enacted legislation requiring that cars purchased in the state possess "blow-by" devices which reduce the amount of unburned hydrocarbons released into the atmosphere.

Urban planners are also considering new methods of public transportation which will permit abolition of automobiles from cities.

4. *Research on the etiologic role of atmospheric pollutants in human disease.*

This last measure is not only the most important but also the most difficult to effect, being perhaps more related to basic physiologic research than to the air pollution problem per se.

REFERENCES

1. McCabe, L. C.: in *Air Pollution*, 1961, p. 39, WHO Monograph Series No. 46.

2. Katz, M.: *ibid.*, p. 142.

3. Heimann, H.: *ibid.*, p. 177.

4. Hemeon, W. L.: *A.M.A. Arch. Industr. Health.*, 1955, 11:397.

5. Ciocco, A., and Thompson, D. J.: *Am. J. Pub. Health*, 1961, 51:155.

6. Landau, E., and Morton, J.: *Am. Rev. Resp. Dis.*, 1961, 83:405.

7. Stocks, P., and Campbell, J. M.: *Brit. Med. J.*, 1955, 2:4945.

8. Breslow, L.: *Am. J. Pub. Health*, 1958, 48:913.

9. Stocks, P.: General Register Studies on Medical and Population Subjects No. 1, London, England, Her Majesty's Stationery Office, 1947.

10. Prindle, R.: *Am. Rev. Resp. Dis.*, 1961, 83:403.

20. OTHER CHEMICAL HAZARDS OF THE ENVIRONMENT: POISONS, DRUGS, AND FOOD ADDITIVES

The environment of the industrialized society is not only beclouded by products from the combustion of fuel, but it is also increasingly burdened by vast numbers of new chemicals of ambiguous potential used in medicine, agriculture, food processing, the cosmetic industry, and in vermin control. In addition, other products such as detergents, bleaches, and cleaning fluids — some highly toxic — are an essential part of the contemporary human environment.

The benefits of the modern chemical environment are easily discerned. The selective toxicity of certain chemicals has been of great use to agriculture for the destruction of weeds and predatory insects. Other chemicals fertilize poor soil; the use of antibiotics and medicated feeds has produced a revolution in the growing of food animals. In part because of these advances in industrial chemistry in the United States, 13 per cent of the population is able to produce food for the remaining 87 per cent(1). The contributions of the cosmetic industry may be less practical and more controversial, but life is certainly more pleasant in this day of the lipstick and the deodorant. Public health and medicine are obviously indebted to the manufacturing chemists for the development and production of the powerful new therapeutic and prophylactic agents, including antibiotics, steroids, and pesticides.

The hazards of the chemical environment are not easily recognized unless they are acutely manifest as accidental poisonings or occupational diseases. Yet the sheer volume of chemicals manufactured (10,000 new compounds in 1960 [2]) has aroused concern because of the difficulties in accurate assessment of their toxic potential.

The Ways in Which Chemicals Create Environmental Hazards

Toxic chemicals may affect man's health in a variety of ways. Atmospheric (air) pollution has been considered in some detail (Chap. 19). Industrial wastes are also discharged into streams and waterways where they may influence the public health indirectly through their deleterious effects on fish, game, and recreational facilities.

More directly, chemicals threaten the general public as:

1. Poisons not intended for ingestion which are accidentally inhaled or ingested.

2. Medicines and drugs, many of them nonprescription preparations.

3. Cosmetics, most of them topically applied.

4. Constituents inadvertently introduced into food, such as penicillin or pesticides in milk.

5. Chemicals that are deliberately added to foods for any of several reasons—the so-called "food additives."

The problems involved in the control of these environmental hazards are quite different from one another and will be considered separately.

Accidental Poisoning. The ingestion or inhalation of readily available household products or gases causes more than 2,500 accidental and almost 4,000 self-induced deaths a year in the United States. One third of the accidental deaths from ingestion occur in children less than five years of age. It is estimated that approximately 600,000 children swallow toxic chemicals every year(2).

Both the prevention and the treatment of this steadily growing health menace have been beyond the scope of the practicing physician, often because:

1. The toxic compounds in many products, such as cleaning fluids, polishes, and bleaches, are not identified upon the product label.

2. Even when identified, the compounds may be so new that there is little if any toxicologic information available concerning them, since such products are not intended for oral consumption.

In addition to the important educational campaigns of the pediatricians and the National Safety Council, two promising approaches have been made toward the control of accidental poisoning. First, the Congress of the United States has enacted legislation (Federal Hazardous Substances Labeling Act) requiring an additional number of household products to list their ingredients on their labels. Formerly, such labeling had been mandatory only for drugs, pesticides, and products containing strong alkalis.

Secondly, the American Academy of Pediatrics has collaborated with regional and local public health services in the establishment of poison control centers. These centers act as repositories of up-to-date information on the identification of probable poisons in various proprietary products as well as their antidotes. They also function as fact-gathering agencies which record and tabulate information on individual cases reported by the physician.

The poison control center has met a real public health need. Since the establishment of the first center in Chicago in 1953, the number of centers has multiplied so that by March, 1960, there were more than 364 centers throughout the United States(3). In 1957, the participation of the federal government was secured by the establishment of the National Clearinghouse for Poison Control Centers in Washington, D.C., as an activity of the Public Health Service.

The typical poison control center is staffed day and night for the purpose of answering telephone inquiries. Most centers are located in hospitals which have resident physicians available at all times. Details on toxic products as well as information on therapy are available for the physician. Since the setting up of the National Clearinghouse, these centers are in a position to undertake epidemiologic research on poisoning and to assist local health departments in poisoning outbreaks.

The Toxic Hazard of Medicines and Drugs. The rapid succession of new drugs produced by the pharmaceutical industries has presented the Food and Drug Administration (FDA) with an increasingly difficult job of safety evaluation. It has long been recognized that the manufacturers' protocols of toxicity tests in animals and preliminary trials in human beings have not always been adequate guarantees of safety. Toxicity may be revealed sometimes only after widespread use of a drug. Unless the scattered instances of toxicity from general use are recognized, described, and collated promptly, needless morbidity or death may occur. The haphazard methods of the past have included publication of case reports, warnings from manufacturers, or casual verbal communication among physicians. The physician has been hampered in his task as sentinel of the public health by:

1. The widespread pharmaceutical practice of using special proprietary names instead of generic designations for drugs. This

makes it difficult to recognize that four or five different names may indicate a single antibiotic and, thus, reactions to these drugs may have a common cause.

2. The fact that, conversely, drugs with similar generic names which differ only with respect to one chemical grouping may have widely different toxicogenic potentials. For example, demethoxy-tetracycline may induce cutaneous hypersensitivity to sunlight in some patients, although the parent compound does not.

3. Aggressive promotion of new drugs with little or no reference to their toxic potential.

To aid the individual physician and the FDA in the prompt evaluation of toxicity hazards of new drugs, an Adverse Reaction Reporting program has been instituted under the direction of the FDA. This program has enlisted the participation of a number of hospitals which provide a representative sample of the medical specialties. If toxic effects are noted, either by this means of evaluation or any other, the FDA is authorized to ask the manufacturers to relabel the drug, warn physicians, or even to withdraw it from the market.

The physician himself bears a responsibility in avoiding the indiscriminate or promiscuous use of drugs—especially the antibiotics. This problem can only be avoided through better basic education of the medical student and physician.

Allergic or hypersensitivity reactions may occur even with compounds such as aspirin which are considered nontoxic in usual dosage.

Cosmetics. Despite the fact that cosmetics need not be tested for safety prior to their public sale, the constant introduction of new products of increasing complexity has not created a major public health problem. The toxic effects of cosmetics are chiefly local and consist of skin irritation or hypersensitivity reactions.

Because they must be capable of altering the physical state of proteins in the hair shaft, hair-waving preparations are potentially toxic to the skin and may cause a chemical burn—particularly the thioglycolic acid derivatives which comprise the majority of such preparations(4).

The most effective hair dyes are paradiaminobenzenes and aminophenols. These compounds have such high sensitizing capacities that cutaneous patch tests are required before their use.

Hair-waving preparations as well as hair dyes may be irritating or damaging to the eye.

Most antiperspirants are salts of aluminum and zinc. They may produce irritation secondary to their astringent effects. Zirconium salts are apparently capable of inducing axillary granulomata.

Potentially Toxic Chemicals Introduced into Foods Inadvertently. It has been pointed out that the productivity of modern agriculture is very much dependent on the use of chemicals employed as pesticides, fungicides, herpicides, and medicated feeds. For the most part these compounds have been introduced cautiously and with due regard for the consequences. However, the accidental ingestion of certain compounds, such as the chlorinated hydrocarbon insecticides dieldrin and DDT, by food animals may result in their deposition in animal fat or their secretion in milk.

More than fifty different drugs are incorporated into the feeds for food animals either as prophylaxis against infection or as hormonal regulators of weight gain. These drugs include almost all the antibiotics employed in human medicine, estrogenic hormones, sulfonamides, and miscellaneous parasiticides. The FDA is concerned with the possibility that these drugs—intended for animals—may eventually be ingested by the human beings who eat the animals. Indeed, the progeny of animals that eat medicated feeds may become sources of chemical toxicity, the coccidiostatic compound nicarbazine may be found in the eggs of chickens that have taken this medication with their feed(3).

Because of the hazard to human health presented by the medicated feeds and by drugs used therapeutically in animals, certain arbitrary "withdrawal times" have been established to allow excretion or metabolic destruction of drugs prior to the slaughter of animals.

The hazard of residual antibiotics in food following therapy for infection is more than theoretical. Serious hypersensitivity reactions have resulted from the ingestion of milk which contained residual penicillin from therapy for bovine mastitis. It has been estimated that 75 tons of antibiotics are used as intramammary infusions each year for the prevention and treatment of this disease(3).

The Food Additives. In modern industrialized society, the principles of saving labor and time have reached into the kitchen of the housewife so that more and more food is prepared or processed in some way before it reaches the consumer. Improvements in methods of preservation, including refrigeration, have made it possible to serve strawberries when snow is on the ground or to import lobster tails from South Africa.

Refinements in packaging often permit the buyer to view the product before purchase, thus placing a premium on its visual appeal or attractiveness (green vegetables should continue to look green, etc.). The demands of preserving foods for longer periods of time in attractive condition have resulted in a steady increase in the number and variety of substances with no intrinsic nutritive value that are added to foods. These substances may be:

1. Preservatives, which have bacteriostatic or bactericidal action.
2. Antioxidants (chiefly to prevent color change).
3. Stabilizers and thickeners.
4. Bleaches.
5. Buffers.
6. Texture modifiers.
7. Colorings.
8. Flavorings.

It has been estimated that in addition to small amounts of substances which are unintentionally added to foods, such as pesticides, the average American ingests about a pound of food additives each year. It is therefore a matter of increasing concern that the public be assured that these additives are nontoxic as determined by prolonged (instead of acute) toxicity tests in animals.

Prior to 1958, the Food and Drug Administration of the United States had to provide scientific evidence that a chemical was toxic before its use in foods could be prohibited. The emphasis has now been reversed so that the Food Additives Amendment to the Pure Food and Drug Law has decreed it to be the responsibility of industry to show a chemical is safe before it can be added to food(3). This amendment covers not only chemicals deliberately incorporated in foods but also dyes or other chemicals in the food package which may enter the food. The manufacturer must present evidence that the chemical either does not enter the packaged food or that it is not toxic in the concentration used.

The determination of toxicity depends arbitrarily on two-year feeding experiments in at least two animal species, preferably the rat and the dog. A range of dosage levels must be employed, and a completely "no effect" level determined. The data from the animal testing form the basis for setting the allowable concentration permitted in food. In setting this tolerance, the probable quantity of food consumed must be estimated as well as the possible additive or synergistic effect of the chemical with any similar chemical also in the diet.

A controversial clause of the Food Additives Amendment states that no chemical which produces cancer in animals may be used in any food in any amount. The clause led to the condemnation of large quantities of cranberries in 1959 at holiday time because they were contaminated with aminotriazole as a residual from spraying. Aminotriazole in large doses had been found to increase the incidence of cancer in rats. This episode and the great economic loss it entailed have caused misgivings about the stringency of this law.

Another problem created by the 1958 Food Additives Amendment has been the fact that it defines as "additives" all substances, whether newly proposed or already in use, which are not generally recognized as safe by competent authorities. The FDA has had to determine through consultation with qualified scientists which chemicals already used in foods are "generally recognized as safe"—a somewhat arbitrary but necessary decision.

Addition of Antibiotics to Foods. The addition of antibiotics to foods is a relatively recent practice which poses special problems. In contrast to most other food preservatives or bacteriostatic agents, antibiotic drugs are widely used therapeutically in man and may be specifically required in certain illnesses. It is therefore categorically undesirable to increase the risk of sensitization to these valuable drugs or to risk the evocation of an allergic reaction when they are not required therapeutically. Nevertheless, the United States Food and Drug Administration has approved the use of the tetracycline antibiotics in the preservation of eviscerated poultry. In Canada these antibiotics may be used for both poultry and fish.

However, the manner of use is carefully regulated, and problems of allergic reactions will probably be circumvented because (a) only small amounts of antibiotics may be employed, and (b) cooking temperatures destroy residual drug.

REFERENCES

1. Osborn, F.: *Population: An International Dilemma.* New York. Population Council, 1958.
2. Cannan, R. K.: *Fed. Proc.*, 1960, **19**:1 (No. 3, Part II).
3. Geiling, E. M. K., and D'Aguanno, W.: *Fed. Proc.*, 1960, **19**:3.
4. Lehman, A. J.: *Fed. Proc.*, 1960, **19**:15.

21. HUMAN HEREDITY AND GENETIC DETERMINANTS OF DISEASE

Although even an elementary presentation of the principles of human genetics is beyond the scope of this text, failure to consider the important role of host heredity in the incidence and expression of disease would be unwise. It is hoped that a brief review of some current concepts in human heredity and an examination of certain specific examples of genetic determination of disease will introduce the student of public health to recent and exciting contributions of genetics to the understanding of disease in human populations.

Too often the epidemiologist, although aware of the vagaries both of the environment and of the specific agents of disease, assumes a sameness or identity of members of the affected population which is unjustified. True, he recognizes the influence of age, sex, and (occasionally) race, on morbidity and mortality, but the wide variation in attack rate and severity which may occur with an infectious disease, for example, is usually attributed to the variation in the parasite or in the host environment. This orientation is entirely understandable, because the simpler chemical and genetic nature of the parasite is far easier to define than that of the randomly bred human being, and evidence has been meager that the course of disease is modified by genetic background in the human.

Biochemical methods have made it possible to begin valid and significant studies of heritable human traits other than those expressed as obvious morphologic differences (such as eye color, albinism, curly hair, and the presence of supernumerary digits). Indeed, a reliance on such crude and striking differences for the ascertainment of heritable influence has led to the common assumption that hereditary defects or disease are rare and not a matter of general concern. This attitude has been somewhat modified by the threat of mutations from atomic radiations, but only recently have the subtler contributions of genotype to disease resistance and susceptibility become widely appreciated. It is now clear that resistance to disease may be significantly modified by change in a single gene expressed as a single amino acid difference in a blood protein molecule (see discussion on malaria which follows in this chapter).

The Basis of Human Heredity

The dependence of true understanding upon minor refinements of scientific methodology is nowhere better exemplified than by the fact that the true number of human chromosomes was not determined until 1956. Until that time studies of human genetics were based on a diploid chromosome count of 48 — an erroneous count perpetuated through the years by a large number of cytologists using less than optimal techniques. The introduction of a method by Tjio and Levan (1), which separated the chromosomes within the cell, permitted a clear definition of 46, not 48 chromosomes. Since 1956 this count has been confirmed in other laboratories.

Through the process of *meiosis* or reduction division, the 46 chromosomes of the immature germ cells of man and woman are halved in number. Thus each *gamete* (mature germ cell: i.e., sperm or egg) which will fuse in conception to form the new individual (*zygote*) is *haploid* and bears 23 chromosomes. The act of fertilization then restores to the zygote the full diploid complement of 46 chromosomes, which will subsequently characterize all its somatic cells. During the growth and development of the embryo, this full complement is maintained by *mitosis* — cellular division which does not (normally) reduce the chromosome number. The mechanics of meiosis, which is actually a two-stage divisional process, result in a reshuffling and a recombination of the genetic material of the *parents* of the possessor of the gamete. According to C. Stern(2):

The recombining of genes in meiosis explains why each child of a couple, excepting identical twins, has many genetic characters that other brothers and sisters do not have. Even if individuals lived for geologic periods and had a litter of children each year, the chance of forming two identical gametes would be so small as to make it practically certain that no two children would have the same genotype.

Any deviation in the fundamental processes of meiosis and mitosis may lead to recognizable and characteristic abnormalities of the zygote produced, and the anomaly so produced may be heritable. It is now known that "nondisjunction" or failure of chromosome separation in the meiotic formation of the egg may result after conception in *trisomy* for one chromosome in the resulting zygote; thus, the chromosome count is 47 rather than the normal diploid count of 46. This condition is associated with mongolism, a relatively common syndrome characterized by idiocy, which occurs in about 0.15 per cent of the births in white populations. The greatly increased incidence of the disorder in the children of older mothers (especially after 35 years of age) is in accord with the theory that it is defective

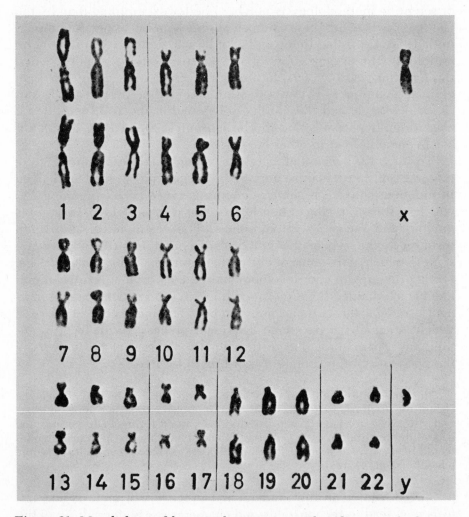

Figure 31. Morphology of human chromosomes. The idiogram of a human male. The chromosomes are from an enlarged photomicrographic print (original enlargement, 4,000 X) cut singly, paired, and arranged in rows and groups for easier identification of the different types. (Tjio, J. H., and Puck, T. T.: *Proc. National Acad. Sci.*, 1958, *44*:1229.)

division in the formation of the female gamete which is responsible for the anomaly. Other accidents of chromosomal distribution leading to atypical numbers of the X and Y sex chromosomes may be associated with abnormalities in sexual and skeletal development (e.g., Klinefelter's syndrome). It should be pointed out that an abnormal chromosome count may be compatible with survival, as in mongolism. It is also possible that studies of large numbers of apparently normal people may reveal some persons with atypical counts and no other stigmata.

The 23 sets of chromosomes which an individual possesses (one set of 23 from each parent) differ significantly in morphology (Fig. 31) and may be distinguished from one another by careful study. The *genes*, which are the basic units of heredity, are arranged in linear fashion on the chromosomes. It has been estimated that there are some 10,000 genes in the human chromosome set—or a total of 10,000 pairs—one set from each parent (2). The corresponding genes from each parent, located on corresponding chromosomes are termed *alleles* or *allelomorphs* and control the same hereditary characteristic or trait.

The chemical basis of heredity has been defined as DNA (deoxyribonucleic acid), although it is not yet clear whether each gene corresponds to a single DNA molecule.

Because genes influence embryonic and later development in complex and interrelated fashion, it is usually extremely difficult in human genetics to equate an abnormal (or arbitrarily defined) characteristic with a single gene. Thus, an apparently simple characteristic such as skin color is probably polygenic in origin. Yet, conversely, a single defective gene may have a *pleiotropic* effect and produce a disease syndrome characterized by multiple manifestations, as in phenylketonuria. In this "inborn error of metabolism," a number of effects are apparent, depending on the level of observation. Individuals with this trait:

1. Excrete large amounts of phenylpyruvic acid, which can be determined colorimetrically by the addition of ferric chloride to the urine.

2. Have severe mental impairment.

3. Have pigmentary disturbance which results in light-colored hair.

Basically, these three gross defects are related to an impairment in the metabolism of phenylalanine.

The Mechanism of Inheritance

A simple understanding of *dominance, recessiveness,* and *homozygous* and *heterozygous* inheritance is necessary for an appreciation of genetics in relation to public health.

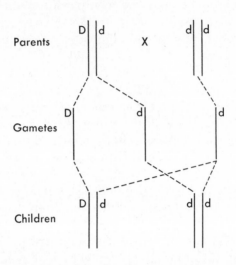

Figure 32. Marriage *Dd x dd*. Transmission of alleles from parents to children. (Stern, C.: *Principles of Human Genetics*, 2nd ed., 1960, W. H. Freeman and Co., San Francisco.)

The trait carried by a dominant allele (one of the gene pair) is always manifest in its possessor. In Figure 32 such an allele is indicated by *D* and its recessive counterpart as *d*. In this case the *Dd* parent is said to be heterozygous for either *D* or *d*, and the parent *dd* is homozygous for the abnormal allele. The transmission of the gene from parent to children is shown by the broken lines. The child with the *Dd* inheritance would exhibit the trait that is also manifest in the *Dd* parent; the *dd* child would not.

If *d* as a recessive allele carried an identifiable trait, this trait would be apparent only in the homozygous *dd* individuals; it would not be manifest in the heterozygous individual with a single recessive *d* allele. It is therefore obvious that both parents must carry a recessive trait either latently (heterozygously) or manifestly (homozygously) if any of their children are to manifest the trait.

Sex-linked inheritance involves a transmission of traits by genes located on the two sex chromosomes *XX* (female) and *XY* (male).

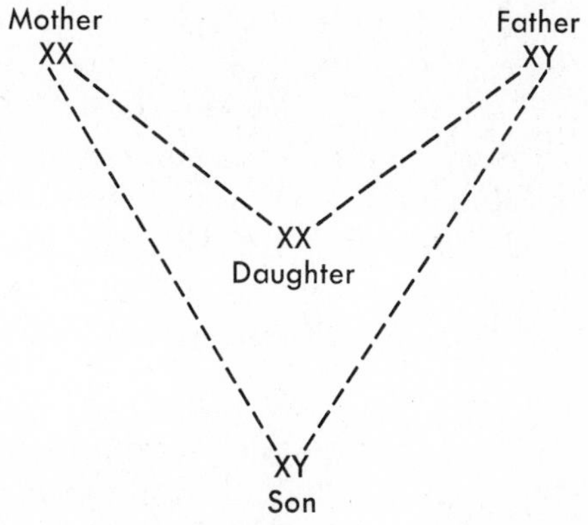

Mother
XX

Father
XY

XX
Daughter

XY
Son

Figure 33. Transmission
of the sex chromosomes.

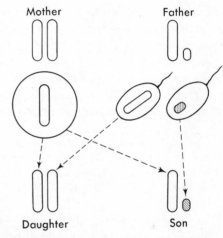

Figure 34. Transmission of the X
chromosomes from one generation
to the next. (Stern, C.: *Principles
of Human Genetics*, 2nd ed., 1960,
W. H. Freeman and Co., San
Francisco.)

Mother

Father

Daughter

Son

Inheritance from the other 44 chromosomes is termed *autosomal.*

The transmission of the sex chromosomes is illustrated simply in Figure 33. The Y chromosome is carried only by the male and transmitted only from father to son. X chromosomes are carried by both male and female and go to offspring of either sex. Few traits have been related to Y-linked genes; most so-called sex-linked traits are transmitted by the X chromosomes and are also known as "X-linked." The inheritance of the X chromosomes is diagramed in Figure 34.

X-linked recessive traits are more frequently manifest in the male because he is the recipient of only one X chromosome which is not "counterbalanced" by the normal allele of another X chromosome — as in the heterozygous female. Only the female who is homozygous in her inheritance of the recessive trait and who acquires abnormal recessive genes from both parents may be affected. The affected male, who bears only one X chromosome, is said to be *hemizygous.*

Colorblindness and hemophilia are classic examples of X-linked recessive traits. The extreme rarity of hemophilia in the woman is evidently related to the statistical improbability of marriages between carriers of this unusual trait so that a homozygous female is rarely produced.

Dominant X-linked traits are rare and not medically important.

Heredity and Environment

"Which is more important—heredity or environment?" Scientists have been unduly concerned with this pointless question in the past. The question has meaning only with reference to effects on a given trait. The differential effects of heredity and environment on the whole organism are incalculable. It must be obvious that man cannot exceed the limitations of his hereditary endowment. The extent to which he can express or manifest this endowment, however, may be greatly modified by his environment. The differing attainments of genetically identical (single ovum or monozygotic) twins reared in different environments have been noted in several studies.

Dobzhansky(3) has emphasized that the distinction between hereditary and environmental diseases is not meaningless.

But to be meaningful, the problem must be stated correctly. What we must ask is: What part of the observed variance in a given characteristic is due to the variety of genotypes existing in the individuals under study and what part to the variety of environments to which these individuals are exposed?

These factors are important to those concerned with the public health, because environmental contributions to disease are more susceptible to manipulation than the genetic endowment of the population.

The environment includes not only the world in which the infant is born, but also the womb in which he develops as well as all factors that can influence intrauterine existence. The intrauterine environment apparently differs from pregnancy to pregnancy in the same mother as is evidenced by the fact that nonidentical (fraternal or dizygotic) twins differ from each other in birth weight less than do siblings who are not twins and hence have had differing intrauterine experience.

Of great importance is the fact that environment can influence the *expression* or *penetrance* of a genetic defect or characteristic. Thus the genetically determined short stature of Oriental races may be modified by American diet, and the occurrence of diabetes in families may also be influenced by diet. Maternal age in certain experimental animals may influence the incidence of polydactylism in their progeny. Whether a gene has "high penetrance" is not necessarily an intrinsic property of the gene, but is influenced by interplay with other genes and the external environment. Of course, the expression of some traits is still not subject to environmental modification.

It is an intriguing thought that there might be many diseases that are basically genetic but which are not easily recognizable as such because they are rarely expressed or manifest. In genetic terms, the *genotype* is rarely expressed *phenotypically*. The following is a case in point(4):

About 15 years ago, a number of reports appeared from England describing infants who failed to thrive, who were found to have elevations of their serum calcium levels. Careful investigations of these cases showed that both the milk and cereals provided by the National Health Service were overfortified with vitamin D so that these infants were receiving between 1500 and 2500 I.U. daily instead of the recommended 400 to 800 I.U. The excess vitamin D was removed, and this syndrome is now almost extinct. The important question to raise here is: Why did 200 to 300 babies show mild signs of vitamin D intoxication when millions of others fed on the same diet were free from such signs? It would appear that the level of intake, which is perfectly satisfactory for most infants, was too much for specific babies, suggesting that they have some constitutional or genetic factor that makes them more susceptible to vitamin D.

Genetic Determination of Resistance and Susceptibility to Disease

Perhaps more important than the problems of diseases apparently genetic in origin is the possible influence of genetic constitution on resistance to those diseases which may affect all mankind. Because, in general, man mates randomly and is rarely inbred to any degree, it is difficult to assess the influence of his genetic background on disease incidence and mortality. Apparent racial differences in susceptibility have been seized upon by investigators because racially homogeneous groups tend to share genetic endowment to a greater extent than the population at large. Newer studies of blood groups and serum proteins have provided better methods than previously had been available for such racial categorizations.

Because the races of man are often distributed in different environments, the old question recurs: "Are differences in the incidence or severity of disease related to hereditary or environmental influence?" The notorious severity of such infections as measles in aboriginal populations in isolated communities is more probably related to absence of prior immune experience and to secondary bacterial infection than to genetically determined lack of resistance.

The high incidence of syphilis and tuberculosis in the American Negro might not be racially (genetically) determined but possibly is related to the socioeconomic environment in which most Negroes live. Nevertheless, there are persistent suggestions that non-Caucasions are subject to a more severe form of tuberculosis and that Jews are relatively resistant, perhaps through long exposure to the disease and selection through the ages. The only strong suggestion of a genetic influence on susceptibility to tuberculosis comes from the classical studies of Kallman and Reisner(5) which showed that if one identical twin had tuberculosis the chances were three out of four that the other would be affected. In the case of nonidentical twins, the chances were one in three that both would be affected if one was.

Other infectious diseases suspected of having genetic determinants include rheumatic fever and paralytic poliomyelitis. Although evidence of genetic determinants is suggestive in the case of rheumatic fever, it is less so for poliomyelitis(6). Only in the case of falciparum malaria is it strongly indicated that human genetic endowment may influence resistance to an infectious disease. This story has been put together lucidly and succinctly by Allison(7) who has contributed much to the investigation of the problem. Regardless of the resolution of this specific problem, the example is cited in this chapter in some detail because of its implications for the future study of both infectious and other diseases apparently caused by external agents.

The Sickle Cell Gene and Resistance to Malaria

In certain southern European, Asian, and African populations, an abnormal hemoglobin is detectable in certain individuals by the tendency of their erythrocytes to assume a sickle shape in vitro. In those who are homozygous for this trait, sickling can occur at physiologic partial pressures of oxygen, whereas sickling in heterozygotes occurs only at considerably reduced oxygen tension. Chemical analysis proves that all hemoglobin in homozygotes is abnormal (hemoglobin S), but that in heterozygotes there is both abnormal and normal hemoglobin present. Homozygotes are afflicted with sickle cell anemia and its attendant complications, but heterozygotes are usually free of the disease.

It is remarkable that the geographic distribution of indigenous populations possessing the sickle cell gene corresponds closely with areas in which falciparum malaria is hyperendemic or holo-endemic (transmitted throughout the year). In such areas infants and children are intensely infected, and many die before they can grad-ually develop specific immunity to the parasite. In children one to five years old, development of immunity is manifested by a decrease in parasitemia and a decrease in illness in the presence of any re-maining parasites. The state of hyperimmunity which is attained by school age is maintained throughout life in those who continue to dwell in the endemic area.

In the newborn in whom parasitemia is very high and in in-dividuals more than five years of age in whom specific immunity has developed, the parasite counts in sickle cell heterozygotes do not differ significantly from persons with normal hemoglobin. How-ever, in the critical age range between one and four years, children heterozygous for the sickle cell gene have significantly fewer *Plas-modium falciparum* in their blood. Because fatality in falciparum infections is closely associated with high parasite counts, it has been inferred that the reduction in parasitemia associated with the sickle cell trait is protective and has definite survival advantage for the host. Sickle cell trait carriers are also known to incur the potentially fatal complication of cerebral involvement less frequently. Sickle cell hemoglobin (hemoglobin S) and normal hemoglobin differ only in the substitution of a valine for a glutamic acid residue in each half molecule(7). If, as indirect evidence suggests, this minor chemical modification is sufficiently inimical to the parasite to influence the survival of man, it is a dramatic illustration of the effects on a human population of a biochemically expressed genetic mutation.

In summary, it seems probable that under the influence of malaria favorable selection of children bearing the protective sickle cell trait has occurred; a heterozygous child has a greater chance than the nonsickler or the intrinsically diseased homozygote to reach repro-ductive age and thus perpetuate the trait. This expectation is actually borne out by surveys of the ratios of normal homozygote and hetero-zygote in infancy and at the reproductive age. In the presence of malaria, the increasing frequency of the sickle cell gene through increased survival of heterozygotes tends to be limited by the dele-terious effects in homozygous individuals who are subject to actual sickle cell disease before the beginning of their reproductive lives.

When malaria no longer exerts its influence on populations carry-ing the sickle cell gene, it seems probable that the trait—no longer possessing survival value—will eventually disappear. One also wonders whether the heterozygote bearers of the sickling trait might actually be at a disadvantage in the new environments of the forthcoming air and space age in which exposure to reduced oxygen tension can be anticipated. It is ironic that the bearers of another biochemical trait thought to be protective against malaria (a deficiency in activity in the red cell of the enzyme glucose-6-phosphate dehydrogenase) are peculiarly vulnerable to toxicity effects from certain antimalarial drugs. Thus, in the modern environment with its new drugs, the cure might be worse than the disease — in those persons selected by previous environmental pressures.

The General Problem of Selection

Just as malaria has apparently favored the emergence of particular rare genetic traits, so it might be anticipated that the incidence of other diseases with genetic determinants will be influenced by both favorable and unfavorable environmental factors in contemporary industrialized societies. Hormones and antibiotics are part of our modern environment which enable the diabetic to live normally and to resist the pyogenic infections that formerly threatened his life. Accordingly, more diabetics reach the reproductive age and marry, and the incidence of this genetically based disease is increasing. Thus, protection by modern medicine can mask or counteract the influence of genes definable as "bad" or "defective" in earlier times. As long as the costly and technologically advanced environment is maintained, the diabetic or the individual with the compensated blood dyscrasia can function. As medical prophylaxis and therapy inevitably improve, it is likely that still more individuals with genetically determined disease-producing traits will survive to perpetuate such traits.

On the other hand, it is probable that the automobile, the pollutants of the environment, and the new drugs can exert selective pressure on human populations so that man may "adapt" to these newer threats as he has to the parasitic hazards of the past.

The Prevention and Therapy of Hereditary Diseases

The ancient social and religious taboos against marriage between those closely related by blood have received legislative endorsement in our society. In the United States, marriage of parent and child and between siblings is prohibited. Marriage between niece and uncle or between nephew and aunt is also illegal in most of the states(2). Irrespective of their moral implications, these laws are a step toward eugenic control of the population and the prevention of hereditary diseases. These laws also serve to lessen the chance that matings of heterozygotes will produce children who are homozygous for recessive traits. Conversely, there is a greater probability that consanguineous (blood-related) individuals carry the same recessive gene than do unrelated members of the population.

Other laws for the control of hereditary disease — especially mental deficiency — are controversial and not generally accepted. These include incarceration and even sterilization and abortion of those who are deemed unfit.

A less drastic approach has been the development of eugenic counseling as a medical or paramedical specialty. As more and more information is obtained on the incidence of genetic defects and upon their mechanism of inheritance, the prospective parent can be intelligently advised concerning the probability of his transmitting an hereditary disease, and may alter his personal plans accordingly. The further definition of new blood groups will aid in exclusion of paternity and in other problems of forensic medicine. Relationships between easily ascertained biochemical abnormalities and disease-inducing recessive genes might also be established. It is already known that individuals who are heterozygote for the gene associated with galactosemia exhibit lessened activity of an enzyme which is totally absent in the diseased homozygote and present and fully active in unaffected homozygotes. There are several other known instances in which the heterozygous individual who bears a recessive trait may be recognized by some physiologic or biochemical abnormality which is not expressed as disease, as in the homozygote.

The mutagenic effects of ionizing radiation are a constant external threat to the children of tomorrow. Safeguards must be constantly sought. The indiscriminate use of roentgenographic equipment by nonmedical persons (as for the fitting of shoes) is to be deplored, and the physician also must be educated both to protect himself and to restrict diagnostic roentgenography in his patients. The hazards of radioactive fallout have been mentioned in Chapter 19.

In a sense, the therapy of hereditary diseases has been undertaken ever since the discovery of insulin. The hemophiliac can now be maintained by products extracted from human blood; the child with pyloric stenosis can be saved by surgery. Even the potentially feeble-minded child with phenylketonuria can be spared by preventive regulation of dietary phenylalanine(8). These repairs of inborn defects are dramatic and encouraging. They are also extremely costly, less than completely adequate, and a poor substitute for the prevention of the disorders.

REFERENCES

1. TJIO, J. L., and LEVAN, A.: *Hereditas*, 1956, **42**:218.

2. STERN, C.: *Principles of Human Genetics*, 2nd ed. 1960, W. H. Freeman and Co., San Francisco and London, p. 78.

3. DOBZHANSKY, TH.: *Ann. N. Y. Acad. Sci.*, 1961, **91**(3):634.

4. HSIA, D. Y.: *ibid*, 674.

5. KALLMANN, F. J., and REISNER, D.: *Am. Rev. Tuberc.*, 1943, **47**:549.

6. SCHWEITZER, M. D.: *Ann. N. Y. Acad. Sci.*, 1961, **91**(3):730.

7. ALLISON, A. C.: *ibid.*, 710.

8. HSAI, D. Y.: *New Eng. J. Med.*, 1960, **262**:1318.

PREVENTION,

in

Book Two

PROTECTION, AND CONSERVATION
public health

SECTION I

Child Health Protection

22. CHILD HEALTH PROTECTION

INTRODUCTION

The most effective and the most important part of the community plan for promotion of the health of the individual is the child health program.

The reasons for its importance are obvious: There is so much to be done; and the results of the work have been, and will continue to be, so fruitful. In general, the younger the age group with which one works, the more effective will be the results. The material is much more pliable and responds readily to the improvements in the technique of care that is provided.

Many of the results that may be obtained in promotion of the health of children can be secured by the "mass" or group method of procedure. Thus simple techniques of limited scope may be of wide utility in protection of the whole community. For example, the sanitary supervision and control of food, and particularly pasteurization of milk, will serve to protect all the children against many forms of infection. Simple vaccination of every infant against smallpox will give protection of the whole state against future invasion by smallpox. Many other examples may be given of the application of mass techniques in child health promotion. This is in striking contrast to promotion of adult health which is, by and large, an individual and personal affair, and cannot be promoted effectively by mass methods.

Health education is much easier to promote in the younger age groups. Parents are unwilling to change their personal habits and to apply newer knowledge of preventive medicine to their own lives, but they are quite willing to utilize this information for the care of their children. One of the best illustrations of this principle is the application of newer knowledge in the field of nutrition.

301

Furthermore, children of school age are plastic and teachable. They are quite willing to accept new theories and new modes of life. Thus, in our work in promotion of sanitation in certain rural areas in the southern states, we found it necessary to wait for the emergence of a whole new generation of children to adulthood before a complete new sanitary program could be installed.

Another great advantage which accrues in working with the younger age groups is that the results are much more lasting. If a single child's life is saved, it represents the saving of many years of productivity. It has the disadvantage, of course, that the program may conserve the lives of certain individuals who will be of little value to the community and may, in fact, become permanent community liabilities, but, as we have pointed out in the chapter on population trends, the disadvantage of preservation of a certain proportion of the unfit by public health measures is not a serious defect of the over-all plan.

The preservation and promotion of the health of the individual child are much more than a matter of community interest. It is also of deep concern to parents and to physicians in private practice. Pediatrics is one division of medical science that has adopted preventive medicine as a practical policy. The pediatrician, by the very demands of his professional work, must make it his major interest to keep his patients well. The great proportion of calls in a well-conducted practice in pediatrics relates to matters concerning well babies, rather than the care of sick children.

Most textbooks of pediatrics deal extensively with such topics as: normal growth and development of children; nutrition of childhood, and especially problems of infant feeding; the prevention of communicable disease in childhood; habit training; and many other matters that are related to health promotion in childhood. For this reason, we have not given comprehensive consideration to these matters in this text, since authoritative and detailed discussion of these topics is readily found elsewhere.

In this chapter we present the community point of view in relation to child health protection under the following headings: prenatal and maternal care; neonatal care; infant hygiene; the preschool child; the crippled child; oral hygiene; and school health services. Conservation of vision is included as a child health service. The role of the practitioner of medicine in a comprehensive, coordinated plan of community-wide protection and promotion of child health is given special emphasis.

PRENATAL AND MATERNAL CARE

Infant Mortality

The infant mortality rate declined steadily for many years in the United States. This improvement was due chiefly to a reduction in mortality from infectious diseases. A leveling off in the decline in the infant death rate occurred about 1950. The curve then flattened out completely and has stabilized in most areas. It is true that there is still a wide variation geographically, with the extreme of 20.9 deaths

TABLE 24

Infant Mortality in Pennsylvania
1954 to 1958

DEATH RATE PER 1,000 LIVE BIRTHS

Age	White	Nonwhite	Total
Under 1 day	9.3	19.4	10.3
Under 1 month	17.6	33.5	19.0
Under 1 year	22.7	44.5	24.8

per 1,000 live births in Iowa, as compared with 39.4 in New Mexico (in 1957). The rural rate in the United States is slightly higher than in metropolitan areas, but it is now obvious that the infant mortality rate has stabilized throughout the nation in the general area of 25 infant deaths per 1,000 live births. In New York City, for example, the lowest rate of 23.7 was obtained in 1954. During the next six years it rose very gradually to about 26.

This over-all picture of infant mortality is influenced chiefly by the pattern of the neonatal death rate. The big gain has been made in infants who have passed 28 days of life. Actually there are now eight neonatal deaths, i.e., occurring during the first four weeks after birth, for every three deaths that occur during the following eleven months. Most of these neonatal deaths occur during the first three or four days after birth.

Moriyama[1] believes that no substantial progress will be made in further reduction of the infant mortality rate until there is "some break-through" in dealing with congenital malformations, and such diseases of infancy as prematurity, birth injury, and postnatal asphyxia.

Vinyard[2], in a study of infant mortality in Pennsylvania, has emphasized that the control of early death of infants is an unsolved problem. He also points out that the rate in nonwhites is double that of whites in every age group (see Table 24).

Perinatal Mortality

In the past, our chief concern has been with infant mortality. As neonatal deaths began to assume greater importance, it was realized that the whole span of pregnancy must be considered, and the term "perinatal mortality" was coined. Two different perinatal periods are used.

Period 1. Perinatal deaths include all deaths that occur from the time span of the first viable period of pregnancy (which is twenty weeks of gestation, with a fetal weight of 500 gm) to the twenty-eighth day of life.

Period 2. Perinatal deaths from 28 weeks of gestation and a fetal birth weight of about 1,000 gm, to the seventh day of life.

Perinatal deaths can be greatly diminished if premature labor can be prevented or postponed. Experience has shown that when mothers place themselves under expert prenatal care by the twelfth week of pregnancy, the hazard of premature birth is greatly diminished.

Environmental factors which predispose to premature childbirth should be carefully avoided(3).

Factors in Perinatal Mortality

Nearly 150,000 perinatal deaths occur in the United States each year: one half of these are fetal deaths of twenty or more weeks gestation, the other half occurs in babies dying during the first week of life. The perinatal death rate is declining, but improvement has lagged far behind the gains in the maternal mortality rate.

A major factor is failure of pregnant women to seek prenatal care in the early stages of pregnancy.

Shapiro, Weiner, and Densen(4) studied perinatal mortality in a large population under a prepaid group-practice program. A higher proportion of pregnant women in the prepayment plans began prenatal care in the first trimester of pregnancy than did the control group in the general population. The women who had early prenatal care had a much more favorable pregnancy experience.

A high perinatal mortality occurs in diabetic mothers. Puerperal toxemia is also associated with a high perinatal loss. Infectious disease in the mother, even when mild, may play a role in perinatal mortality (see Chap. 6). Other unknown factors undoubtedly influence perinatal morbidity and mortality. Most authorities now believe that if early and continuous medical supervision is applied effectively during pregnancy, at least one third of perinatal deaths can be prevented.

The protection of the health of pregnant women is an important community responsibility. Childbirth is a perfectly normal process which should bring joy to the family, and this happiness should extend to the whole community, for each new baby is an additional community asset. There is no gainsaying the fact, however, that the process of childbirth is accompanied by suffering, with a certain risk of serious illness and even death to the mother. It also represents a hazard to the newborn child. Well-planned prenatal care is the best insurance that a child has against being "ill-born."

Maternal Health

One of the significant achievements of modern medicine has been the elimination of the hazards associated with pregnancy. From 1915 to 1925, the mean mortality rate per 10,000 live births was 60 to 70. At the present time in many areas of the United States, the mean rate is 4 or less. This reduction represents 1 maternal death due to childbirth for each 2,500 live babies born.

There is good reason to believe that further improvement can be achieved.

The maternal mortality rate in the United States is higher in rural areas than in metropolitan areas; the ratio is about 5 to 3. Regional differences are striking. In Vermont, the maternal mortality rate is less than 2, and the whole group of New England states has a rate well below 3, whereas in the East South Central area, the maternal mortality rate is consistently three times higher than in New England. Maternal mortality is much higher in Negroes than in whites. The age of the mother plays a role – the older the mother, the higher the rate. Pregnant women who seek prenatal advice early in their pregnancy and who remain under supervision have a lower risk of fatality than mothers who did not receive prenatal care.

The major cause of maternal mortality is toxemia of pregnancy. Syphilis and hemorrhage, as causes of maternal deaths, have been largely brought under control.

The reduction of maternal mortality has been secured chiefly through the increased availability and improved quality of prenatal care as well as the development of almost universal hospitalization for mothers at the period of childbirth.

The methods that should be utilized to improve still further the adequate medical care of mothers before, during, and after childbirth are quite obvious and clear-cut. We know now how it should be done, but in some areas we do not apply these procedures effectively.

The purpose of the community program in prenatal and maternal care is to minimize the risks of childbirth, and to give to each baby that is born the best possible chance for survival, with optimum opportunity for a normal birth and subsequent satisfactory development.

The most important factor in good prenatal and maternal care is the alert, well-trained physician; second in importance is the well-equipped hospital, with proper facilities for delivery of the baby. The most important factor in postnatal care is the home nursing service.

The purpose of good prenatal care is twofold: first, protection of the mother, and second, insurance for the baby.

Prenatal Program

A good prenatal program requires early consultation by each expectant mother with her family physician. Not later than the third month of pregnancy, the mother should visit her physician for the purpose of securing an obstetric examination, which includes pelvic measurements. The mother then comes under the constant supervision of her doctor, enabling him to watch the development of the baby and to observe all signs and symptoms that relate to the physical and mental condition of the mother. This prenatal program includes:

1. A serologic test for syphilis.
2. Frequent supervision of blood pressure and urine.
3. Provision for proper nutrition of the mother.
4. Regular visits to the dentist during pregnancy.
5. Instruction of the mother concerning preparation for the baby and for proper care of the baby after arrival.
6. A roentgenogram of the chest, taken early in the prenatal period, is also desirable.
7. Rh testing.

Many of these activities can be carried out by a well-trained nurse.

Some obstetricians employ their own nurses for this purpose. In many communities, a district nurse is available on an hourly service basis. People unable to pay for prenatal care should receive it in clinics conducted under health department auspices, or by voluntary agencies.

Delivery of the Baby

Formerly, most babies were delivered in the home, but in cities and industrial areas in the United States more than 95 per cent of all babies are born in the hospital. The essential requirement in childbirth is that facilities be made available to each mother for an aseptic delivery, with a physician and a nurse in attendance.

In certain rural areas in the United States, particularly among the Negroes, the midwife delivers the baby. These women are, in some instances, untrained and unqualified. This type of delivery service is being eliminated as rapidly as possible. The qualified midwife, so commonly employed in Europe, has never been widely accepted in the United States. Less than 2 per cent of babies born in this nation are delivered by midwives, and the great proportion of these are born in the rural areas of the southern states.

Some communities have solved the problem of the high cost of hospital delivery service by providing a *three-day* hospital delivery plan for all normal deliveries. The mother and baby return home on the third day after childbirth, and continue the ten-day postpartum rest period at home. This is a somewhat makeshift arrangement with many defects, but it does give aseptic and inexpensive delivery service and provides for emergencies and difficult situations.

Postpartum Care

Postpartum care should provide for a period of bed rest for the mother following the birth of the baby.

Nursing care and household aid service should be given during this postpartum period. The district nursing plan of seven properly spaced one-hour visits to each newly delivered mother over a 21-day postpartum period is a satisfactory nursing arrangement. The physician should also make a final postpartum examination of the mother, usually about one month to six weeks after delivery.

Provision for Prenatal Care

Ideally, provision should be made for continuous medical care during the entire period of pregnancy by a physician of the patient's own choosing. This physician should make all arrangements, including pre- and postpartum nursing care, laboratory service, and hospitalization; he may be paid a flat fee for these services. Many persons, unable to pay for the complete service, enroll in a publicly supported prenatal clinic. This service is free. Nursing care is furnished to these mothers on a part-pay or on a free basis, and hospitalization, with medical care, may also be given free by the community or paid for on a part-cost basis. A more satisfactory plan is prepayment insurance. This furnishes a complete full-coverage arrangement which provides for all the costs of standard prenatal care, delivery, and postnatal obstetric service.

The difficulty with existing plans for care of pregnant mothers in the lower economic groups is that often there is little correlation between the various services. The nursing service may be given by a voluntary district nursing association; delivery service may be furnished by a municipal hospital or by a private philanthropic institution. The prenatal clinic is often conducted by the health department, but may be supported by private agencies.

The prenatal clinic which is conducted by a private or public agency may be quite efficient, but it tends to be impersonal. The home nursing care is excellent, but is not under the direct supervision of the physician who has the responsibility of the delivery.

Obviously, we are in a stage of evolution, where we know perfectly well *what to do,* but have not yet solved *how it should best be done.* The science of obstetrics is well advanced, but a system to provide these benefits to all mothers at a moderate cost has not been devised.

Prenatal care, delivery, and postnatal care represent a *unit of service* which is a joint family and community responsibility. It is not unreasonable to hope that a simple, easily administered procedure can be worked out in the near future to fit the needs of each mother and the economic structure of each family and each community.

NEONATAL CARE

Prematurity

Prematurity has become the most important cause of death during the neonatal period. Many of these deaths can be prevented. Two chief modes of attack are: (a) prevention of prematurity, and (b) provision for adequate care of babies prematurely born so that they might have the opportunity for survival.

What is prematurity? It has been defined as a termination of pregnancy during the twenty-eighth to the thirty-seventh week of gestation. For all practical purposes, any baby weighing less than 2,500 gm at birth should be handled as a premature baby. Thus, in a plural birth, the twin babies may have reached 10 full lunar months of gestation but at birth may weigh less than 2,500 gm each. They should be treated as prematures.

Prevalence of Prematurity. There are no exact data on prevalence of prematurity in the United States. The rate varies in different parts of the country, in different races, and in different social and economic conditions. Approximately 5 per cent of all babies born alive weigh less than 2,500 gm. Over 70 per cent of these babies weigh over 2,000 gm, and with reasonable care each of these babies should survive. The smaller the baby, the less the chance of survival. About 5 per cent of premature babies weigh less than 1,000 gm at birth. Even with most expert care almost all of these babies will die. If they survive they are often physically or mentally handicapped.

Under highly advantageous conditions the survival rate of premature babies is as presented in Table 25.

TABLE 25
Survival Rates of Premature Babies

Weight at Birth	Number of Babies	Number Survived 28 Days	Per Cent Survived
Under 1,000 gm (2.2 lb)	104	4	3.8
1,001 to 1,500 gm	133	77	58.0
1,501 to 2,000 gm	249	220	88.6
2,001 to 2,500 gm	784	760	96.0

These data indicate that great efforts should be expended to prolong pregnancy until the fetus weighs at least 1,500 gm (3.3 lb). The chance of survival below this stage of development is small, and the infant will have great difficulty in developing into a normal child. Most premature babies weighing 2,000 gm or more do well, with adequate care.

Prevention of Prematurity. In many instances the cause of a premature birth is not known. However, there are certain known factors tending to produce prematurity that are controllable; at least they can be influenced in some degree. Thus if suitable preventive measures are employed, a reduction in premature births may be anticipated.

Maternal syphilis is an important cause of premature birth. A community-wide plan for compulsory blood test for syphilis for all pregnant women is an excellent preventive procedure. If all pregnant women with syphilis are given early and adequate treatment, the chances are the baby will be normal and born at full term.

Other factors that may produce premature birth are the toxemias of pregnancy, placenta previa, and also premature separation of the placenta. Often the obstetrician is in a serious dilemma; if pregnancy is allowed to continue, the toxemia may result in maternal convulsions and possibly in death. If pregnancy is terminated, the premature baby will have little chance for survival.

Severe illness of the pregnant woman, particularly severe infections, were formerly an important cause of premature birth. Malaria and pneumococcus and streptococcus infections are good examples of that situation. With modern antibiotics, the skillful clinician can now handle these situations promptly and effectively. Trauma of the mother is an important cause of prematurity which can be prevented in most instances, if suitable precautions are observed.

A few simple general hygienic measures should be taught the mother by her physician, as follows:

1. Proper diet, exercise, rest, and recreation.

2. Avoidance of exposure to infections.

3. Special precautions to avoid falls, accidents, and other trauma. Sexual intercourse should be interdicted after the seventh month of pregnancy.

4. Adjustment of daily routine with avoidance of overwork, fatigue, and anxiety.

5. Secure assistance, if necessary, from the economic and social point of view.

Overwork and malnutrition are important factors in the production of prematurity and should receive special consideration. Despite the utilization of every available preventive measure, a certain number of babies will be born prematurely. The community should make adequate provision for their care.

A Community-wide Plan for the Care of Premature Babies. The hospitalization of premature babies is a very expensive procedure. The essentials of a plan are to:

1. Develop optimum facilities for hospital care of full-term babies.

2. Establish standards of optimum care of premature infants.

3. Provide for care of prematures in each hospital that has a maternity service.

4. Provide a special center for the care of the most difficult problems in premature care.

5. Plan for suitable transportation facilities for the premature babies to the special center.

6. Plan for follow-up home care of prematures by the public health nurse.

An understanding of the scope of these plans in a large community may be obtained from New York City data. In this city the above criteria have been accepted as a goal, and special centers have been provided to meet the needs of the city.

Practically all babies are born in hospitals that have facilities for care of prematures. Babies of 2,000 gm weight or more are, for the most part, cared for by the hospital in which they are born. Only a few of these babies are transferred to the special center. About a fourth of the babies sent to the special centers weigh from 1,000 to 2,000 gm, while 16 per cent of all babies sent to the special center weigh less than 1,000 gm. As we have already noted, premature babies weighing under 1,000 gm seldom survive, even to reach a special center, and are a very poor risk at best. Despite the skilled care given at the special center, 25 of the 34 babies transferred in 1946, which weighed under 1,000 gm, died.

An analysis of the experience of the New York Health Department helps us clarify planning for community-wide premature care programs. It is clear that in the average community only 4 or 5 per cent of premature babies will weigh less than 1,000 gm. Most of these babies will not live long enough to reach a special center. Even if they do, and are given ideal care, at least three out of four of them will not live.

This group, therefore, does not require major community planning. A considerable proportion of babies weighing between 1,000 and 1,500 gm will survive if given the expert care of the special center. They will not survive without this care. Although only 7 per cent of total prematures, this is a critical group requiring special consideration.

Most premature babies (89 per cent) weigh between 1,500 and 2,500 gm. A number of these will require special center care, but if the over-all plan is adequate, with development of facilities for premature care in each maternity hospital, then the majority of these babies may be cared for in the hospital in which they are born.

Obviously, therefore, the greatest benefit of the plan is the saving of the lives of premature babies through adequate though relatively simple facilities developed in the hospital in which they are born. The special center is reserved for the most difficult problems and with full realization that a considerable proportion of the babies sent there will not survive.

A necessary part of the plan is coordination of care for the premature in the hospital and in the home. Home visits should be made by the public health nurse to prepare the home for reception of the premature baby. These visits are most necessary. Frequent follow-up home visits by the nurse after the baby is discharged from the hospital will save many lives and often prevent hospital re-entry of the baby.

Birth Trauma

Injury at birth can be reduced markedly if a good prenatal program has been followed. Better training of physicians in the field of obstetrics and better preparation of the mother for delivery, with a comprehensive program for good prenatal care of the prospective mother, constitute the best insurance the baby can have against trauma at birth.

Malformations

It has always been assumed that malformation of the newborn baby was accidental, and little or nothing could be done to prevent neonatal deaths from this cause. But as we gain new knowledge of the physiology of pregnancy, evidence is now emerging that some of these conditions may be prevented. Erythroblastosis foetalis is an illustration of this point.

Erythroblastosis Foetalis. A group of related clinical conditions, of varying degrees of severity, are the result of hemolysis of the red cells in the newborn infant. These conditions are called erythroblastosis foetalis, icterus gravis neonatorum, and congenital anemia of the newborn.

These conditions are due to a specific immunization of an Rh negative mother with an Rh positive factor, which comes from the blood of the fetus in utero. The fetus inherits the Rh positive factor from the father (about 87 per cent of the population are Rh positive). The Rh factor is an inherited Mendelian dominant; thus when the reaction occurs, the father and infant are always Rh + and the mother always Rh −. The marriage of an Rh positive man with an Rh positive woman, or an Rh negative man with an Rh positive woman, produces no change in the red cells of the baby. Only when an Rh positive man is married to an Rh negative woman is there any potential danger. The first child of their marriage may be quite normal, but while in utero it may sensitize the mother so that subsequent pregnancies may result in disaster.

This fetal hereditary condition occurs in less than 1 pregnancy in every 500. Thus it is clear that factors other than heredity may play a part in incidence. Parents do not always transmit the Rh factor to their offspring; variations in placental permeability may occur, or the condition may be mild and unrecognized.

Women with repeated abortions should certainly have their Rh status determined. If it is Rh negative, then the husband's blood should be examined and further studies carried out.

Treatment of the baby with erythroblastosis may be successful if blood transfusions are given as soon as the condition is suspected. Where parents have given birth previously to infants with this disease, then transfusion should be given, as a preventive to the newborn baby as soon as possible. The donor should be Rh negative.

Prevention of Developmental Defects

The brilliant experimental studies of Ingalls[5] have changed many previous concepts concerning developmental defects of the newborn and give hope that many of these conditions may be prevented.

All congenital defects are not determined genetically at the moment of conception. Many are acquired during fetal development. They are usually a fetal manifestation of critical stress on the mother at some stage of pregnancy.

In some instances the fetus dies. The anomalous child is one who has survived the intrauterine stress. The type of deformity is directly related to the stage of development of the fetus at the time it was subjected to stress; e.g., harelip deformities occur during the sixth week of pregnancy; cleft palate during the seventh week; mongolism during the eighth week; deafness during the ninth week. The reason for this is that the critical stage of development of the particular organ affected occurs on that date. The stress may be due to rubella* or another natural infection as well as to traumatic radiation, exposure to carbon monoxide, uncontrolled diabetes, or many other factors.

*See discussion on rubella as a cause of congenital malformation on page 200.

Thus it is clear that many "congenital defects" of the newborn can be prevented if adequate prenatal care is given to the mother, particularly in the early stages of her pregnancy. Elective operations should not be performed, complex dental procedures should be avoided, diabetes should be well controlled, and anemia, systemic hypertension, and hypothyroidism should be given attention. Other factors also play a role. This is a most fertile field for clinical and epidemiologic study.

THE INFANT HYGIENE PROGRAM

The baby is well launched on life by the time he has reached one month of age. The essential health protection measures that should be provided for him are:

1. Protection from infection.
2. Provision for normal physical, mental, and emotional development.

The important infectious diseases to which the infant is most susceptible are:

1. The respiratory infections.
2. Gastrointestinal diseases.

One of the most deadly of the respiratory infections in infancy is whooping cough. Most babies are immune to measles and diphtheria until about the sixth month of life, but newborn babies are susceptible to whooping cough, and the mortality rate from this disease in infancy is very high. The common cold is also a source of trouble in infants since these small babies are particularly susceptible to secondary infections, such as a pneumococcus infection which produces otitis media and pneumonia. The most important strain of pneumococcus in the production of infant pneumonia is type 14, a relatively avirulent strain in adults. The reason for this phenomenon is unknown.

Measures that may be employed in protection of the infant from respiratory infectious diseases, including whooping cough, measles, and diphtheria, have been presented in Chapter 17. A satisfactory routing program of immunization procedures for the normal infant is given in Table 20 in the section on the communicable diseases of childhood (p. 250).

The control of infant diarrheas is often a matter of proper food. The former high death rate of babies from summer diarrhea has been almost entirely eradicated throughout the whole United States. The most important single factor that produced this effect was sanitation of the milk supply, particularly universal pasteurization of milk.

Education of the Mother

The most important part of an infant hygiene program is intelligent care of the baby by its mother. The health instruction of the mother can be carried out by her own physician, a clinic physician, or the public health nurse.

Normally, the baby should be seen by the physician once a month during its first three months of life, then every other month for the first year.

The community should provide a child health center where mothers who cannot afford private physician fees can come at regular intervals for advice concerning the care of their babies. The major problems that arise relate to:

1. Infant feeding and food habits of children.
2. Mental hygiene, particularly in relation to habit training.
3. Prevention of communicable disease.

The clinic service is supplemented by public health nursing supervision. The nurse visits the home soon after the baby is born to be certain that the mother and baby are receiving good postpartum care. From that point on, the public health nurse serves as a liaison agent between the family and the well-baby clinic or the private physician.

Hospital Service

The community has not fulfilled its obligation in infant care until provision has been made for adequate hospitalization facilities for the care of sick babies. As already noted, special provision must be made for care of premature infants. The correction of congenital defects of the newborn, such as clubfoot, cleft palate, and other types of congenital defects, also requires immediate and skilled attention. In many instances, these services must be provided from community resources.

State and Federal Government Responsibility
for Provision for Infant Care

The Children's Bureau of the federal government has been very active in stimulating nation-wide programs for infant health promotion. National funds that were provided under the Social Security Act of 1935 made possible the development of effective state divisions of child health within each of the state health departments. All state health departments were thus enabled to promote effective local child health services throughout every area in the state. These community-wide services have been instrumental in instituting programs for care of the crippled and neglected child, in broad educational programs concerning the proper care of children, and in the promotion and advancement of community responsibility for the care of the health and the welfare of children. These programs are based on the thesis that the promotion of child health is a local responsibility—a joint function of the individual, the practicing physicians, and the community.

THE PRESCHOOL CHILD

For administrative reasons, it has been convenient for state and local health departments to separate community-wide child care into certain arbitrary divisions. Under this plan, the preschool age period of health care extends from the first birthday to entrance in school at about six years of age.

From the point of view of the family and the practicing physician, this division is an artificial one. The essential thing to be remembered is that child health protection should be continuous.

It is true that the health protection measures employed for a child from age one to six years must have a different orientation than the procedures followed for infants or school-age children. These years of a child's life are the period of adjustment to life contacts.

The important problems in child health protection to be solved during this period are:

1. Prevention of communicable disease.
2. Establishment of sound nutrition and good food habits.
3. Habit training and mental adjustment to life situations.
4. Provision for correction of physical defects and for detection of incipient disease. Provision of facilities for dental care are particularly important for this age group.

The instruction of parents concerning the techniques of child health care, particularly in the principles of normal nutrition and in mental hygiene, is the most important factor in a well-rounded plan for the preschool child. The family physician or the pediatrician should provide these services to all parents in the community.

In the past it has been the custom for the physician to visit the family only when called into the home in case of illness. But a well-balanced program of child health care, as outlined here, requires that the family physician see the well child at regular intervals. The American Academy of Pediatrics has recognized this trend and has prepared an outline, giving a detailed plan of procedure to be followed in the health care of a normal child. Many pediatricians make an agreement with families in their practice whereby they supervise the health of the child according to a satisfactory schedule for an annual fee.

Well-child Stations and Well-child Conferences

Families that are unable to pay for private pediatric service may secure health supervision of their children through the health department well-baby stations. These stations not only give medical advice concerning normal growth and development of the baby but also provide free immunization against communicable disease and correction of dental defects in the younger age groups; tuberculosis testing is done, and roentgenologic service is provided if it is required; laboratory diagnostic service is furnished as well as diagnosis of defective vision. These child health stations do not correct physical defects nor, as a rule, do they remove defective tonsils and adenoids or give medical or surgical care to sick children. There are exceptions to this rule. Some stations provide dental care, others make provision of glasses for children, and others have posture classes for orthopedic defects.

Hospitalization

Each community must provide facilities for suitable hospitalization of children who suffer from the more serious communicable diseases or who require correction of physical defects. This includes convalescent care for the crippled child and for children with cardiac disease. In so far as possible, the family should pay for these services either on a fee-for-service or an insurance-plan basis. In case the family is unable to pay, it becomes a community responsibility to provide the needed hospitalization.

Public Health Nursing in the Child Health Program

The public health nurse is a very important element in child health promotion. Her work is done chiefly through home visits. Through her intimate contact with the family, she is able to carry out her educational work and to secure correction of defects. She also is able to aid in the prevention of the spread of communicable disease. The nurse serves as the connection between the physician, the clinic, the health department, the hospital, and the home. Her work in the well-baby clinic is important, for she takes the interval history and gives advice to the mothers, explaining the physician's orders and illustrating how these orders can be carried out most effectively.

Her function is to give advice and instruction rather than to provide direct nursing service. She may give nursing care to a child in the home as an instructional measure, but her duty really is to teach the mother how to care for her own child. Thus the primary function of the nurse, whether in the home nursing visit or during the visit by the mother and child to the well-baby station, is to provide instruction and not to furnish direct service (see Chap. 44)

THE CRIPPLED CHILD

Nothing has a greater appeal to the human heart than the suffering of a crippled child. In fairly recent times it was the custom (and, in fact, among primitive peoples today it is the practice) to put these children out of their misery by means of a merciful death. In the Middle Ages, before even the simplest community health and welfare programs had been formulated, cripples were given special privileges. They were allowed to solicit alms and hold certain privileged occupations. Special hospitals and institutions for the care of crippled children were among the first charitable organizations developed as a community enterprise. It is curious, therefore, that so little attention was paid by official health services during the nineteenth century to prevention and treatment of crippled children, even after many effective methods were available for this purpose. The Social Security Act of 1935 was the first nation-wide official recognition of the importance of prevention and care for the crippled child.

This act made provision for funds to be allocated by the federal government to each state "To extend and improve services for locating crippled children, and for providing medical, surgical, corrective and other services and care, and facilities for diagnosis, hospitalization and after-care for children who are crippled or who suffer from conditions leading to crippling." Each state, in order to receive the subsidy from the federal government, was required to work out an acceptable plan for the consummation of the objectives of the general plan and to match federal appropriation with state funds, on a parity basis. Part 4 of Title V of the act provided for the establishment and extension of plans for vocational rehabilitation of the physically disabled.

These authorizations gave special consideration at first to orthopedically crippled children, but as the years went by this interpretation was broadened. There is no gainsaying the fact that the Social Security Act has revolutionized community planning in the care of the crippled and has extended proper facilities for the correction of serious physical defects of children to the most remote rural areas of the land. It has also changed our concept as to what a crippled child is, and has emphasized the responsibility of the community for the transformation of these cripples from liabilities to social assets.

What is a crippled child? In a broad sense, a crippled child is a child who does not attain his normal growth and development. He does not realize, to the fullest degree, his potential physical and mental capacities. Formerly a crippled child was considered in a narrow sense as one with an orthopedic defect: with bone, joint, tendon, or muscle deformity. But the line was hard to draw. A child with defective vision from "squint eyes" had a muscular deformity which was subject to early correction. Cardiac disease is a crippling defect of one of the most important muscles of the body. Cleft palate is an important crippling defect which is remediable when operated upon early in life, yet it was not included in the category of crippling conditions of childhood. It is now customary to broaden the interpretation of the activities of the bureau of crippled children to the more inclusive functions of a bureau for the care of physically handicapped children.

A Community Program for the Care of Handicapped Children

1. **Appraisal.** A suitable scheme must first be devised for appraisal of normal growth and development. Defects must be discovered early if they are to be checked and effectively treated. Various methods have been devised, such as the grid-graph method of Wetzel, in order to obtain a normal curve of growth and development which can be applied to any given child and thus aid the physician in making an early diagnosis of incipient defect.

2. Early Recognition of Physical and Mental Defects of Childhood. The second part of the program is a corollary of the first. It is obvious that amelioration of a crippling defect can be accomplished best if the defect is recognized in its early stages.

3. Correction of Defects. Early recognition of defects is of little value unless a comprehensive plan is instituted for correction or amelioration of the physical defects that are encountered.

4. Preventive Measures. It is perhaps just as important to institute preventive measures in a crippled children's program as it is to institute corrective measures. The avoidance of crippling defects often cannot be secured by a direct approach, but many indirect methods may be employed which can, in the long run, prevent the occurrence of physical defects. One of the best examples of this principle is safety education, in the attempt to prevent accidents.

5. Rehabilitation. One of the most important and also most neglected parts of the crippled children's program is organization of community facilities so that a crippled or defective child may receive education and training to utilize his natural talents and become a useful, productive individual.

No one group can encompass all the activities that must be undertaken in order to supply the community's needs in the care of the handicapped child. The physician plays the most important part in the plan, but the school, the hospital, the convalescent home, the public health nurse, the social welfare worker, and the voluntary organizations all contribute to the program.

Administration of a Program for the Care of Handicapped Children

It is the responsibility of the whole community to organize its facilities so that the plans can be executed properly. This administration is assigned to the bureau of handicapped children of the health department. Its duties include:

1. Reporting. A system must be devised for the reporting and centralized recording of names of all handicapped children in the area.

(a) Hospitals, clinics, and private physicians are required to report to the bureau of handicapped children each case of congenital malformation and birth paralysis that is encountered at the time the baby is born.

(b) Through the department of education, crippling defects are discovered by schoolteachers, school nurses, and physicians, in preschool and school children. These are reported to the central bureau.

(c) Private physicians, clinics, and hospitals report to the central bureau those crippling and handicapping conditions encountered in their practice which may require the utilization of any of the available community facilities needed for the correction of the defect and rehabilitation of the individual.

In addition, the bureau itself should organize a case-finding program in order to search the community for those children who may have unrecognized or neglected remediable crippling defects.

2. Facilities for Correction of Defects. The early recognition and the centralized reporting of crippling defects are of no avail unless the community provides the facilities for the proper correction of these defects. The load is a heavy one since the correction of an orthopedic defect is a long and expensive process. The incidence of serious handicaps varies in any area. Facilities must be prepared to meet the need for the particular community. In the average community there are about 2.5 crippled children in each 1,000 of the total population. This represents perhaps 8 cripples per 1,000 persons under 21 years of age. The types of defects that are encountered vary considerably. In past years, bone and joint tuberculosis comprised more than 50 per cent of all crippling conditions. This ratio is now reduced to less than 5 per cent.

The Social Security Act made special provisions for community subsidies to provide for the various types of proper remedial care wherever these facilities were not available. In most cities, hospital facilities and skilled orthopedic care are available for the correction of crippling defects, but the prolonged convalescent care so often required for these children has not been provided. Most parents do not have funds to pay for the prolonged and expensive surgical and hospital care needed to correct these orthopedic defects. Under the Social Security Act, direct provision is made for payment to surgeons and to hospitals for the necessary services. The following case provides a simple example of the effectiveness of a community-wide, well-planned program in providing care for a crippled child:

J. B. is a seven-year-old white girl whose family has a low income. She is the fifth child in the family. Her mother had a normal puerperium and delivered at term after 10 hours' labor. It was a frank breech presentation; the breech was broken up, the left leg brought down, and the head delivered by forceps. The baby weighed 3,400 gm (7 1/2 lb). The child appeared normal, and the neonatal period was uneventful.

When the child was two years old, friends of the family noticed that she held her head to one side, but the mother paid no attention to the matter. The condition gradually became more noticeable, and at five years of age the mother brought the child to the well-baby clinic because her head "tipped to one side."

The girl was friendly, intelligent, alert, well developed, and well nourished. Physical examination was negative except that the occiput was drawn to the left, the chin downward and to the right. The sternomastoid muscle was prominent on the left and under constant tension. There was marked limitation of motion in abduction of the head to the right and rotation to the left. A roentgenogram of the cervical spine showed no bony abnormality.

The family was advised to have an operation performed to correct the defect, but they had no funds. Suitable hospital arrangements were made by the bureau of handicapped children, and a tenotomy was done of the sternal and clavicular attachments of the left sternomastoid muscle, and a rubberized head cap and elastic traction applied, starting from the opposite mastoid region. The child had an uncomplicated course, the deformity was completely corrected, and at the end of two years there was no limitation of motion of the head and only a small, almost invisible scar in the linear folds of the neck near the clavicle. The hospital, the surgeon, the hospital social service worker, the district nurse, and the child health station of the municipal health department all participated in planning for the welfare of this child.

3. Preventive Measures. Measures to prevent the occurrence of crippling or to prevent the gradual advance of a crippling process are difficult and discouraging, but they are an important function of the community-wide program.

Broad, general educational measures aid in the prevention of handicapping defects. Many parents do not realize the seriousness of an apparently minor physical defect in their child or the necessity for early and radical correction, so that neglect often occurs, and an appeal for assistance is not made until too late. General preventive measures, such as correction of posture and relief of foot strain can be applied by the physician to prevent physical deformity. The prevention of rickets by a proper dietary regime and the prevention of the serious bone deformities of osteomyelitis by specific therapy, will aid in the reduction of crippling defects throughout the community.

The best example of the value of general preventive measures in the reduction of crippling defects is the marked reduction in bone and joint tuberculosis in the children of the community that followed the control of tuberculosis in cattle and the pasteurization of milk, together with the reduction of human pulmonary tuberculosis.

Congenital dislocation of the hip, clubfoot, and other birth abnormalities may often be readily corrected if recognized early in life and if suitable therapeutic measures are promptly applied.

4. Special Educational Facilities. Each crippled child is entitled to an education. In many instances extensive crippling, with mechanical difficulties such as casts or splints, makes it impossible for the child to go to school. The department of education furnishes teachers for children in convalescent homes or sends teachers to the homes of individual crippled children so that each may develop according to his ability.

Wallace(6) has emphasized the necessity for community co-ordination of all facilities for handicapped children. She estimates that there are between five and six millions of handicapped children in the United States. These categories include orthopedic defects, neuromuscular and neurologic lesions, birth injuries, convulsive disorders, hearing impairments, visual defects, speech defects, malocclusion, cleft palate, the mentally retarded, the emotionally disturbed, and other categories. In some areas, chronic diseases of children such as diabetes, nephrosis, and celiac disease are considered as crippling conditions.

The care and rehabilitation of the handicapped child is a prolonged and expensive procedure. The community must be prepared to carry a considerable share of the financial outlay for these children. This may be done successfully through coordination of activities of voluntary organizations with the activities of the local, state, and federal health authorities.

Among the essential community facilities that should be established are:

1. Early case-finding procedures.
2. Referral and counseling devices.
3. Diagnostic centers for evaluation and treatment.
4. Rehabilitation facilities.

These facilities include: (a) social, (b) educational, (c) vocational, (d) recreational, (e) foster homes planning, (f) home care, and (g) institutional care.

There are many community agencies interested in specific problems of the handicapped child. Several of these agencies are organized on a national basis, with local chapters in each community. It has become quite evident that maximum results can be secured through close interrelationship and planning of all community agencies, voluntary and official, that are concerned with the diverse needs of the handicapped child. Closest coordination is required in those phases of the program related to rehabilitation.

5. Rehabilitation. The most difficult and the most frequently neglected part of the whole community plan is vocational training, vocational guidance, and industrial placement of handicapped persons. Several communities in the United States, usually on a voluntary agency basis, have attempted to meet this situation directly. If the crippled or handicapped child is to take his place in the world, he must be given special training, according to his aptitudes. Employers are not as likely to employ crippled persons, when normal, healthy laborers are readily available. Employers may, in a sense, be penalized if they employ cripples, since the workmen's compensation laws apply to crippled and to handicapped persons as well as the healthy men, and the crippled person seems a much greater occupational risk.

Vocational guidance is perhaps the most essential part of the whole plan. The crippled person must adjust his life in order to realize fully all his capabilities, yet live within his physical limitations. He always has before him the fact that much of the world's important work has been accomplished by men who labored with indomitable courage, under severe physical handicaps, to fufill difficult tasks most successfully, despite their physical incapacity.

Health Care of the Adolescent

The health needs of the adolescent have received relatively little consideration. In 1960 there were more than 13 millions of persons in the United States between the ages of 15 and 19 years. Most of their health problems are a carry-over from earlier years.

During this age period, mortality and morbidity rates are at a very low level; hospitalization rates are at a minimum. The old enemies of adolescence—tuberculosis, typhoid fever, and rheumatic fever—have been brought under more adequate control.

Accidents are the most important cause of death in this age group and are much more common with boys than with girls.

The greatest health problem in this transitional period from youth to adulthood is emotional stress and resultant maladjustment to life situations.

In some areas, *adolescent units* have been established in hospital clinic services, to give special attention to adolescent health problems.

Dr. Gallagher(7), chief of the Adolescent Unit of the Boston Children's Hospital, has pointed out that adolescents are not children and not adults. Furthermore, there is a vast difference in the health problems of the 13-year-old and the 18-year-old. The period of adolescence is characterized by rapid physical growth and greatly increased nutritional needs. Adolescents have an excessive interest in themselves and their physical development. Sexual development is often of great concern. There is a conflict in their desire for security and desire for independence. This confusion can lead to major emotional conflicts that require sympathetic guidance from parents and teachers as well as sound medical supervision.*

*An excellent adolescence reference book for teachers and parents is *Your Adolescent at Home and in School*, Frank, L. K., and Frank, Mary, Viking Press, New York, 1956.

REFERENCES

1. MORIYAMA, I. M.: *Pub. Health Rep.*, 1960, **75**:391.

2. VINYARD, J. H.: *Pub. Health Rep.*, 1960, **75**:407.

3. *A Guide to the Study of Perinatal Mortality and Morbidity, 1959*, A.M.A. Committee on Maternal and Child Care.

4. SHAPIRO, S., WEINER, L., and DENSEN, P. M.: *Am. J. Pub. Health*, 1958, **48**:171.

5. INGALLS, T. H.: *J.A.M.A.*, 1956, **161**:1047.

6. WALLACE, H. M.: *Children*, 1958, **X**:20.

7. GALLAGHER, J. R.: *Medical Care of the Adolescent.* Appleton-Century Crofts, New York, 1960.

23. DENTAL HEALTH

Dental hygiene and oral hygiene are frequently considered as synonymous terms. This is a mistake since dental hygiene is but a part of a more comprehensive subject. Furthermore, oral hygiene does not consist of the application of antiseptic mouthwashes and other topical therapeutic agents.

Many of the diseases of the mouth are local manifestations of general bodily dysfunction. Early signs of vitamin deficiency, for example, are often encountered in the mouth. This is particularly true of vitamin C deficiency, in which the early symptoms of scurvy appear predominately as swelling and tenderness of gums. In niacin deficiency, the primary signs of the disease occur on the tongue and other mucous surfaces of the buccal cavity. Vincent's angina will be found, as a rule, in necrotic tissue, and thus is a manifestation of an underlying disease, usually a nutritional deficiency. Leukoplakia and similar troublesome lesions of the mucous membrane of the mouth and tongue are also usually symptoms of underlying disease. Syphilis and cancer of the lips, mouth, and tongue are frequent etiologic factors in oral disease. Thus, oral hygiene does not consist merely of topical applications for therapeutic purposes; it involves an analysis of the underlying cause of the conditions that are encountered. Preventive measures must be directed toward the elimination of the basic causes that produce a general infection or other abnormal condition which may first manifest itself as an oral lesion.

Dental Caries

On the basis of existing knowledge, one must include dental caries, and pyorrhea as well, as belonging to the general category of a local manifestation of an underlying systemic disturbance.

Dental caries is the most important and most perplexing problem of oral hygiene. It is an almost universal defect of all mankind, and its causes have not been determined. There is no field in medicine that offers a better opportunity for effective research than dental pathology. More scientific studies should be done on the etiology, bacteriology, and epidemiology of dental caries. It should prove to be a valuable field of endeavor.

Great variation occurs in the extent and degree of severity of dental caries encountered in different parts of the world, and even in different parts of the United States. The best data that we have of the incidence of these defects have been obtained from the initial examination of young men for Selective Service in the United States Army in 1940 and 1941. Of the 2,000,000 men examined, some 900,000, or over 40 per cent, were rejected for physical or mental disabilities; 188,000, or 21 per cent, of these rejections occurred because of severe dental defects. In this initial group, dental caries was the most important reason for rejection of young men for Army services.

There is good evidence that there has been no decrease in dental caries in the population, in spite of almost 50 years of increasing knowledge in preventive medicine that has accumulated since World War I (1914-1918), and in spite of the active nation-wide organization of local health services during this period. Provision has been made in many cities and states for dental clinics for the children of the poor. Extensive promotion of child health services has occurred, with education of all the people in relation to nutrition and to personal hygiene. The toothbrush has become an important article of commerce during the past 25 years. Nevertheless, dental caries is still prevalent.

Nutrition and Dental Caries

There is strong evidence that adequate nutrition for the mother, during her pregnancy, has a beneficial effect upon the formation of a sound foundation for good teeth in the fetus. Subsequent optimal nutrition of the baby and of the growing child, with an abundance of milk, fresh fruits and vegetables, and sunshine is believed to play an important part in good dentition. Many dentists believe that once the teeth are fully formed, they are not markedly affected by changes in general nutritional status.

There is also good evidence that decay of carbohydrate food residues in the mouth, particularly carbohydrate concentrates such as candy and sugar, plays an important part in the chemistry of tooth decay. It is not true that "a sound tooth never decays" nor that "a tooth brushing a day keeps the dentist away," but there is ample evidence that proper tooth brushing at regular intervals and a clean mouth, free from food debris in the tooth interstices, do promote oral hygiene.

Dental Care

Since we have no sure method of preventing dental caries, and since we do not know its primary causes, it is obvious that the most logical preventive plan at present is to remove caries in its incipiency. This requires a plan whereby the young child visits the dentist early in life—at about the third year—and makes periodic visits to the dentist thereafter at intervals of about one visit every six to nine months. The purpose of the frequent visits is to check dental decay in its incipiency; if this check-up is followed by immediate correction of the defects found, the method becomes a true disease prevention plan.

Education and Oral Hygiene

Education of the public, particularly education of the school child, has done much to promote knowledge concerning the importance of sound teeth. This education is of little avail, however, unless facilities are readily available in the community for correction of dental defects at a cost that the individual can afford to pay.

The major purpose of the educational program is to motivate the child to secure adequate dental care. The community must be ready to provide the necessary facilities for those children who cannot secure dental care through their own family resources.

Health Department Dental Clinics

Most local health departments have developed a dental service for correction of dental defects. These clinics are intended particularly for correction of dental caries discovered in children at the school medical examination. A social service worker determines whether the child is entitled to free care. The usual plan is to furnish a service for children from 6 to 12 years of age on the theory that this is purely a preventive service; that if the child is convinced of the importance of good teeth, he will seek and pay for subsequent dental care during adolescence and adult life, maintaining the good foundation given him during his early years.

Unfortunately, this theory has not worked well in practice. Frequently the whole value of the initial care is lost because there is no community-wide plan for continuous dental supervision. Dental caries can advance rapidly during adolescence and other periods when the nutritional demands of the body are very great, e.g., during pregnancy and during the period of lactation. Thus, an ideal program should provide readily available facilities for dental care for the adolescent and the young adult. Furthermore, best results in caries prevention are secured if the child begins dental care before he enters school. The ideal time for the first visit to the dentist is not at six years but rather at the fourth or even the third birthday. No satisfactory plan has yet been worked out that will bring young children who need early dental. care to the dentist's office or to the dental clinic.

Dental Insurance

Obviously the most satisfactory arrangement for adequate dental care is a system of periodic prepayment on a group basis, which will provide for all the usual contingencies of a good personal continuous program of dental hygiene from early childhood through adult life. There are, at present, no actuarial data that make it possible to determine what this service should cost. Such a plan should be put into effect at the third year of childhood and be continued throughout adult life, with special emphasis on adolescence. It should cost much less, in the aggregate, than the present method of dental correction. Our existing policy is, in effect, to neglect the care of the teeth in adult life until caries has developed, often to such a degree that extensive, costly, and time-consuming repair work is required.

Tentative programs for prepayment toward dental care have been developed by The Dental Insurance Plan, Inc., Group Health Dental Insurance, and other organizations. By 1961, some 560,000 people were benefited by some type of dental care insurance. Nearly one half of these beneficiaries lived in New York State.

The Effect of Fluorine on Dental Caries

It has been noted for some years that if a community water supply contained one part per million of fluorine, the people enjoyed a relative freedom from dental caries both in the deciduous and permanent teeth. If the fluorine content of the water is high—over two parts per million—an undesirable condition called "mottled enamel" will prevail.

Dean's study(1) in Illinois can be taken as an example. It revealed that Monmouth, with a fluorine content of the water supply of 1.7 parts per million, showed an average of 2 D.M.F. (i.e., decayed, missing, or filled teeth) in each child examined, whereas Quincy, a nearby city with only 0.2 p.p.m. of fluorine, had a caries index of 6.3 D.M.F. per child.

These observations were widely repeated and led to several community experiments in which fluorine was added to water supplies, and the diminution of dental caries was studied. In each instance a similar community in the vicinity has been used for the control observations.

Ast(2) has reported on the results of water fluoridation in New York State. This careful and prolonged study showed clearly that addition of fluorides in the concentration of one part per million to a municipal water supply reduced caries incidence in children by at least 65 per cent and had no untoward effect on the general population.

Ast and Schlessinger(3) have reported subsequently on a ten-year follow-up of their original studies. The results are most encouraging and conclusive.

The U.S. Public Health Service(4) in 1959 made a comprehensive report on fluoridation in the United States. The conclusions were:

1. One part fluoride per million added to the water supply will prevent 65 per cent of dental caries in children. The cost is less than ten cents per person per annum.

2. This procedure is approved by every major scientific and professional organization in the United States.

3. Forty-two millions of people now enjoy this benefit: seven millions in areas where natural waters contain fluorides; the remainder have fluorides added to the municipal supply. Most of the people that are benefited live in large cities.

4. There is no evidence that fluorides in the concentration of one part per million are in any manner injurious to the population.

5. Other methods of administering fluorides to children are not suitable as mass public health measures. Fluorides in suitable amounts could be added to milk, salt, bread, or other foods consumed by children. The great difficulty is adequate dosage, since varying amounts of these foods are utilized. Fluorides in tablet form have been used widely, particularly in Europe. Intelligent cooperation on the part of parents would make this a very useful measure, but it is not suited to mass application over a long period of time.

Community Acceptance

The peak year of community acceptance of water fluoridation was 1953, when 378 municipalities instituted the procedure. Since then the program has been slowed down by the active opposition of well-organized national groups. The chief arguments are: (a) opposition to adding a "poison" to the water, (b) invasion of human rights, (c) rejection of a new discovery that conflicts with entrenched belief, (d) dental caries is a relatively mild rather than destructive disease that can be handled by individual preventive or therapeutic measures.

It now seems probable that complete acceptance of fluoridation of water will require long, patient educational efforts on the part of all the health agencies interested in the welfare of children.

Topical Application of Fluorides. Extensive studies have been made of the value of application of sodium fluoride directly to the teeth of children in an attempt to prevent dental caries. Some authors have reported a caries reduction rate of 40 to 50 per cent, but these studies have not been well controlled nor have they been analyzed on a sound statistical basis. The procedure is time consuming and relatively expensive, and there is doubt that the method is of great value as a public health procedure.

REFERENCES

1. DEAN, H. T., *et al.: Pub. Health Rep.*, 1939, **54**:862; 1942, **57**:1155; 1950, **65**:1903.

2. AST, D. B., *et al.: Am. J. Pub. Health*, 1950, **40**:716.

3. AST, D. B., SCHLESINGER, E. R.: *Am. J. Pub. Health*, 1956, **46**:265.

4. Report on Fluoridation in the United States, *Pub. Health Rep.*, 1959, **74**:513.

24. SCHOOL HEALTH SERVICES

Medical inspection of school children was inaugurated in 1894 in the public schools of Boston by Dr. Samuel Durgin, famous health officer of the city at that time. Personal hygiene had been taught in the schools for years, but the concept of a medical service for school children began with Dr. Durgin. The purpose of this health service was to prevent the spread of contagious disease, particularly scarlet fever and diphtheria, through the schools.

In 1906 Massachusetts passed a law requiring annual medical inspection of all school children, and many states copied or modified this law. The school nurse was introduced into the school health service by New York City in 1902.

The initial stages of planning for the protection of the health of the school child were pioneer efforts that served an excellent purpose at the time, but were frequently faulty in concept and in execution. There have been many changes through the years in our attitude toward the functions of a school health program, and many changes also have been made in the method of administration of the service. It seems probable that our ideas in this field will continue to change, as indeed they should. In this short section, we shall attempt to present only a brief summary of present conceptions of the aims and purposes of a school health service. Those interested in the details of school health, theory and practice, are referred to the many excellent books on this subject.

Environmental Sanitation

The school authorities should provide a healthful environment for the school child. This function is the direct responsibility of the school administrator. Provision should be made for proper lighting and ventilation of classrooms, for adequate washroom and toilet facilities, with a system for sanitary disposal of sewage. Individual drinking fountains, proper seats and desks for the children, adequate and safe recreational facilities, provision for protection against fire hazards, and provision for cleanliness of the school are essential. Provision should be made also for hot lunches in rural schools, and the cafeterias of city schools should provide well-planned menus at cost. These facilities should be provided for all schools, from the one-room country school to the municipal high school with 5,000 students. Standards for sanitation of the school and environs are promulgated and enforced by the state department of education. This is the first and most fundamental step in good school health service. The state health officials can be of real assistance in promotion of proper standards; local health department personnel should aid the community schools in meeting and maintaining proper environmental sanitation in each and every local school.

Health Instruction

The education of the children in the principles of healthful living is of paramount importance in the promotion of the public health of the nation. Those engaged in health education find it very difficult to change the health habits and to influence the point of view of adults. However, much can be done with adults who are associated with the school-age child, in the form of parent-teacher association meetings, at which speakers from the health department can give the adults information on health problems and mental hygiene. Also, at the time of the medical examination of the child in school, the school physician and nurse may do an effective amount of health education with both the parents and children. A new social concept— such as community responsibility for health promotion—requires a period of 25 to 50 years for general adoption by a nation. It is the new and enlightened generation, which is educated in the public schools, that will make a real advance possible.

Health education in the school is the function of the schoolteacher. The health officer and the public health nurse may furnish teaching materials and give advice in the teaching program, but the teacher is the key person in the presentation of the material to the children. She not only teaches the principles of public health but also guides the children so that proper health habits are inculcated in their own lives. They in turn carry this influence back into their own homes. This plan can become effective only when the teacher herself has been well trained and is sincerely interested in the welfare of her pupils. The health department can be most effective when it aids in the teaching of teachers and imbues them with an enthusiastic interest in the promotion of child health. The health department should have in-service training courses for teachers and principals concerning the health of the school child. In addition, the student teachers may be assigned in pairs to observe teacher-nurse conferences and school medical examinations.

Physical Training

Physical training in the public schools is based on sound theory and should be of great value to the children. Unfortunately, physical training has been greatly overemphasized in many schools, and in some instances the effects have been harmful. Competitive games between schools lead to community rivalry. The physical trainer becomes a "coach," whose position depends upon winning games. The young and immature students are exploited by the athletic department, and by the community, to win games, sometimes in order to pay for an expensive gymnasium or mammoth stadium. Often the director of physical training is the sole judge of whether a boy is physically fit to take part in a grueling athletic contest. In some instances, he is director of the entire school health program, including the medical and nursing services. This is bad administration and leads to great confusion. One point should be emphasized: namely, that the school or family physician, not the physical trainer, should determine whether a child may participate in competitive games or other athletic activities.

Physical training has a definite place in health promotion of the child, but it should not overwhelm all the other parts of the program. Ideally, physical training should be planned so that it will suit the talents and personal aptitudes of each student: thus he will not only learn coordination and development of physical stamina, but he will also acquire a real interest in a suitable form of physical exercise which may be carried into the postschool years and throughout his adult life.

Prevention and Control of Communicable Disease

The average school child is disabled by illness (i.e., sick for seven consecutive days) about once a year. About four out of five of these illnesses are due to communicable disease. Thus a school program for prevention of contagion should have value. There are specific measures that school authorities can take to prevent spread of contagion.

1. Smallpox Prevention. Most states require that a child be successfully vaccinated with smallpox vaccine before entering public school. This is an excellent law. The child may be vaccinated by his private physician or by the health department. A better procedure is one in which all children are vaccinated during the first year of life, and again on entering school. This should be sufficient for lifetime immunity, unless the individual has a known exposure to smallpox in some subsequent epidemic. In such instances, a precautionary third vaccination is desirable.

2. Diphtheria Immunization. All children should be immunized against diphtheria in infancy. A single "booster" dose can be given to these children when they enter school to increase their protection against diphtheria. Children who have not been immunized against diphtheria in early childhood should be immunized immediately when they enter school.

3. Immunization Against Poliomyelitis. Some school authorities have organized intensive programs for immunization of children against poliomyelitis. A much more effective plan is a community-wide program of protection of children against all the various childhood diseases during infancy and the preschool period.

4. Tuberculosis Prevention. A discussion of case-finding methods in tuberculosis is presented in Chapter 16 in the section on that disease. Skin tuberculin testing of school children, with supplementary roentgenogram or fluoroscopy of the chest of all children who manifest positive Mantoux tests, has been carried out extensively by mass methods in the schools of many communities. This method has educational value, but there is a great question as to whether the number found of cases of actual or potential tuberculosis is commensurate with the time and cost that the method involves. In areas of high tuberculosis prevalence, this method can be used effectively. The adolescent high-school student profits most by this type of service.

The major activities of the school authorities in control of common communicable diseases of childhood are:

1. To notify the department of health of suspected cases of reportable communicable disease encountered in the school.

2. To encourage parents to keep sick school children at home, and also to keep the sick child away from younger brothers and sisters.

3. To isolate and send home children who seem sick, particularly if they have a temperature of 100° F or over.

4. Daily inspection. The teacher is familiar with her students and is quick to notice any change in appearance. Each morning she should make an inspection of her class and if a child seems to be ill, she should refer the child to the school nurse. If a school nurse is not available for morning sick call, written instructions should be provided by the school physician to the teachers, giving symptoms which warrant exclusion of a child from school, and indicating the procedures to be followed if it seems necessary to send the child home.

If a child develops a communicable disease, then a certificate of return to normal health by the private physician or school doctor should be required before the child may be permitted to re-enter school.

Skin Diseases. Certain communicable skin diseases are the bane of the teacher and the school nurse. Those diseases most frequently encountered in school children are: scabies, impetigo, pediculosis capitis, and ringworm of the scalp and skin.

Satisfactory control cannot be secured by simply excluding the infected child from school. The parents must be informed by the school nurse concerning the nature of the illness and its importance. She may also suggest techniques as to how the condition may be handled. Usually the private physician of the family is asked to give the treatment. In order to eradicate the condition from the schools, the school nurse may find it necessary to visit the homes of infected children and to aid the family in the actual administration of the therapy. All of these conditions except ringworm are "family epidemic" diseases, affecting adults as well as children, so that elimination of the disease may require extensive family renovation; sometimes an entire classroom must be treated.

Closing of Schools During Epidemics. In the cities, closing of the public schools is not an effective method in the prevention of spread of infectious disease. In rural areas, particularly where children are transported to school by bus, contacts between children can be greatly reduced during epidemics if the schools are closed for a short time. Presence of an epidemic in a community may warrant delay in opening school in order to avoid exposure of an unexposed group. But in most thickly settled communities, daily inspection and close supervision of school children by the nurse, teacher, and school physician constitute a much more effective system of control than that of closing the school.

Periodic Health Examinations

The school desires that every child enjoy, in so far as possible, his greatest physical potentialities and that he have the opportunity for optimum physical growth and development. Thus it is necessary:

1. To detect actual disease or physical defects in the individual child as early as possible, and to secure correction.

2. To be sure that each child in school is physically fit to carry the school routine.

To this end, a system of periodic health examinations has been devised. The primary purpose of these examinations is not to give the child a complete physical examination, such as would be carried out in the office of a pediatrician but to determine a child's fitness for the school program and to "screen out" those who are in need of further medical attention. Usually the examination is given in several parts.

Eye Examinations. Good vision is of paramount importance to the school child. Thus every effort must be made to determine defective vision in the children and to correct these defects immediately.

Usually, simple eye tests are done by the teacher or by the school nurse. Some modification of the Snellen eye chart is used. Those children who are screened out by this test, and who seem to have some defect in eyesight, are referred to the private ophthalmologist for further observation. In some communities, the health department maintains a free ophthalmologic diagnostic clinic, where needy school children may be sent for diagnosis. As a rule, the department of welfare provides necessary glasses for correction of eyesight of the children of indigent families. Many schools require annual testing of eyesight, but this is unnecessary. An eye test by the eye chart method every three years is sufficient to meet most school situations.

Tests of Hearing. The group audiometer test is a satisfactory screening device for detecting early impairment of hearing. This test should be done in the school by a trained employee of the school department or health department. Each child should be examined three or four times during his school life. Children screened out by this test are referred to their physician for diagnosis and treatment. Children who are in danger of losing their hearing as the years go by are assembled in special classes for instruction in lip reading *before* they have lost their hearing.

Dental Examinations. The same principle is followed in dental examinations as in tests of eyesight and hearing. A specially trained person, frequently a dental hygienist, examines the teeth of each child and determines which children have defective teeth.* The findings are reported to the family of the child, with an urgent message to have the defects corrected by the family dentist.

Most departments of health maintain dental clinics for the purpose of giving early corrective dental care, either free or at low cost, to needy school children. Dental caries is by far the most frequent and troublesome defect that is encountered in the school child (see the preceding chapter on dental health).

Each of these special group examinations of the school children should be an educational experience for each child and for each parent as well. The children are taught the purpose of the examination and the importance of early correction of any physical defect that might be encountered. The teacher should understand each situation, know what classroom adjustments must be made for the handicapped child. She also can be of great assistance in urging children and parents to have each child's physical defects corrected.

Medical Examination of School Children. The Massachusetts law of 1906, which was copied by so many states, requires an annual medical examination of each school child. The purpose of this law was an excellent one. It was intended to detect physical defects in the school child and thus to secure early correction.

In most schools, these medical examinations have degenerated into a careless, hurried physical inspection of long lines of children who pass in rapid review.

The general trend is to abandon this method of school inspection for a more leisurely careful medical examination of the child in the presence of the parent. The mother can give the physician an accurate history of the whole situation. The physician discusses the child's attitudes and health habits with the mother and inquires about nutrition and food customs. He examines the condition of the eyes, ears, nose, throat, glands, heart, lungs, and skin. Posture and general nutrition are observed. The physician can also discuss with the parent the various procedures to be followed in securing correction of physical defects that are found. The methods that have been developed in New York City have proven of great value and are being followed in

---

*In communities with a high dental caries rate, this procedure is a waste of time. Every child is affected, and effort should be made to secure for each child a continuous dental corrective program.

many parts of the country. All children entering school for the first time must be examined. This examination can be done by the family physician, but when the parent chooses to have the school physician do the examination, the nurse schedules the child for examination and invites the parent to be present. The school physician can be effective in health education with both parent and child, and point up any necessary follow-up care. Following this *new admission examination,* the child returns to the medical roon *only* if and when a teacher, in subsequent months or years, observes something about the child which she thinks should be checked by the school doctor. Having consulted with the school nurse, the teacher then sends the child to the medical room, where the school doctor decides whether or not to send for the parent and to do a complete health examination. In this way only those children who appear to need medical diagnosis or treatment are examined, and all the others, apparently normal, are not examined.

A school examination of this type need be done only three or four times during the child's school life: perhaps twice in elementary school and once in secondary school. The results obtained from these examinations should be fully utilized. It is more important to expend efforts in a good physical examination, at which time the physician, parents, teacher, and child can map out a well-planned health program, with proper arrangement for securing correction of defects, than to make frequent unprofitable examinations of a large number of boys and girls, with little or no follow-up, and no coordination of planning for correction of defects.

Daily Health Observation. The teacher should note the daily progress of each child and refer to the school nurse or physician any child who does not make normal progress in school because of some illness or physical defect. If a child has a poor academic record, effort should be made to determine if the failure is due to some physical handicap. In the elementary schools, quarterly height and weight records are frequently employed as an index of normal growth. Children who have had recent illness or an accident, or who suffer from chronic disease, such as a cardiac or orthopedic defect, require special consideration.

Treatment. Treatment is not a function of school health service. Correction of physical defects should be urged strongly upon the parents and the child, and efforts should be made by the school authorities so that all community resources are made available to those children who require treatment. But the school should not conduct, or assume responsibility for, dental hygiene clinics, posture clinics, eye clinics, or other forms of therapeutic service.

The school nurse should maintain a room in the school for care of sudden illness or injury that may occur at the school, and she should be prepared to give first aid. The nurse should also, in her home visits and follow-up work, give instruction to parents concerning proper care of the children, in order to promote good health and to prevent further illness. But the school should not take the responsibility for treatment of disease in the school or in the home.

Mental Hygiene in the School

One of the most important health problems that is encountered in the schools is the child who is not adjusted mentally and emotionally to his environment. This situation is met most frequently in adolescents of the junior and senior high schools.

One method of aiding these children is the plan of *child guidance* that can be incorporated in the school department. In New York City, the psychiatrist in charge of child guidance aids in the selection of teachers to serve as counselors. They help plan a future career for each student. Those youths who have difficulty in adjustment can be referred by the counselors to the psychiatric social worker, or to the public health nurse who makes the home visits. The most serious problems of maladjustment are referred for consultation with a psychiatrist. The health department might furnish psychiatric consultation service for selected cases. The more important function of the psychiatrist, however, is to aid the school physician, the public health nurses, the psychiatric social workers, and particularly the high-school teachers who serve as counselors, to an understanding of the emotional difficulties and problems of the adolescent boy or girl (see Chap. 28, on mental health.)

Organization of the School Health Service

The school health service is best organized on a cooperative basis. Part of the responsibility for the work rests upon the department of education, and part on the department of health.

The school administrator is directly responsible for the following school health functions:

1. Environmental sanitation of the school.
2. Health instruction.
3. Physical education.

The health officer and his associates can advise in the health education program and perhaps furnish illustrative materials, but he does not assume responsibility for any of the instruction of the students. The sanitary inspector of the health department can also be of great technical assistance in the school sanitation program. In many areas, he is required by regulation to inspect the school buildings and grounds at regular intervals.

The health department should be responsible for the medical and nursing aspects of the school health service. These include:

1. Control of communicable disease in the community, both within and beyond the domain of the school.

2. The periodic health examination of school children.

3. Securing the correction of physical defects in the school children.

The school authorities give all possible cooperation to these health department activities. Certain procedures, such as the daily health inspections and the screening tests for defective eyesight and hearing, can be carried out by school personnel, working under the guidance of the school physician.

School Medical Officer. The full-time health officer acts as school medical officer in the smaller communities (of 50,000 or less) and in the rural areas under county health administration. In cities of 100,000 or more, a full-time physician is selected, as a rule, by the health department, to administer the school health services. The periodic health examinations and other medical aspects of the school health program are carried out by local physicians, working under the direction of the school medical officer.

The school physicians should have special training in pediatrics and in public health. Usually the local practicing pediatricians are asked to do the work on a part-time basis, and are paid an honorarium for their services. A good plan is to assign all school physicians through the bureau of school health before permitting them to work in the schools. They may be requested to attend a six-week course in school health practices for groups of 20 to 30 physicians. The candidates attend daily sessions of informal lectures and discussions and secure field observation and experience. At the end of each course, a number of the physicians who are considered adequate for the work are assigned to a health center area and to a group of schools which they visit regularly.

School Nurses. The public health nurse is a very important adjunct to a good school health program. The school nursing service should be conducted by the health department as a part of a generalized community nursing program. The public health nurse is not assigned to a school but to an area; and she carries out all phases of a well-rounded public health nursing service in that area. Her duties include the school health activities. During the school session, approximately half her time is devoted to the school health work (see the discussion of the activities of the public health nurse in Chap. 44).

In many communities the department of education employs part-time physicians and full-time nurses, who carry out all school health activities, within the budget allotment and under the direction of the school administrator. This plan has certain administrative advantages to the school system, but is a great disadvantage to the whole health promotion plan for the community.

This type of school health service, organized wholly within the department of education, was adopted many years ago when health departments were ineffective and had low standards of personnel and achievement. The more modern and effective type of organization in a well-rounded community-wide local health service is conducted by highly qualified and well-trained medical health officers and public health nurses. The trend is to assign all health promotion activities of the community, including school health work, to one official administrative unit, namely, the health department.

REFERENCES

PRICE, B.: *School Health Services. A Selective Review of Evaluation Studies.* Children's Bureau Publication No. 362. Washington D.C.

School Health Services. Responsibilities of State Departments of Education and Health. Association of State and Territorial Health Officers. Washington, D.C., 1959.

Qualifications of School Physicians. Report of Committee on Professional Education. American Public Health Association, 1790 Broadway, New York City.

LESSER, A. J.: *Children,* January-February 1958.

25. *CONSERVATION OF VISION*

FRANKLIN M. FOOTE, M.D., DR. P.H.*

Extent and Importance of Visual Handicaps

In 1961 it was estimated that there were 365,000 blind men, women, and children in the United States and that each month the visual acuity of more than 2,000 persons diminishes to 20/200 or worse in the better eye after use of correcting lenses (the legal definition of blindness). At least 400,000 persons have markedly reduced visual acuity (between 20/70 and 20/200), and 1,500,000 Americans have useful vision in only one eye (see Tables 26 and 27).

Prenatal Care

Sight-saving efforts should begin during the prenatal period. Good medical care, including sound advice about nutrition, is just as important to ensure good vision for the unborn child as for his general health. Routine maternal tests for gonorrhea and for syphilis, with adequate treatment when indicated, will help reduce the infant blindness caused by these preventable infections.

German measles and possibly other virus infections in the expectant mother during the first three months of pregnancy can produce congenital cataracts and other defects in the offspring. The expectant mother should be cautioned to avoid exposure to these infections early in pregnancy. If a susceptible expectant mother is exposed during this period, early administration of potent gamma globulin may prevent development of the infection.

Premature babies weighing less than 3.5 lb at birth are likely to develop the blinding eye disease, retrolental fibroplasia, if lifesaving

*Formerly executive director of the National Society for the Prevention of Blindness.

oxygen is administered improperly. In such cases, the retinal blood vessels hemorrhage, and subsequent scar-tissue formation produces gross retinal detachments and disorganization. Research conducted prior to 1954 proved that excessive use of oxygen is the precipitating factor. It is now recognized that oxygen should be given only under the most carefully controlled conditions. The content of the incubator should be tested at least every eight hours to be sure the oxygen concentration is kept under 40 per cent. Each day a test should be made to see if oxygen administration can be discontinued without producing hypoxia.

TABLE 26

Causes of Blindness by Etiologic Factors*

Etiologic Factors	Percentage of Total (all ages)
Infectious diseases	9.7
Trauma	4.9
Poisons (including oxygen in retrolental fibroplasia)	2.7
Neoplasms	1.2
General diseases	15.9
Prenatal causes	13.5
Unknown to science	38.1
Undetermined or not specified	14.0

* Source: 1957 Estimates, National Society for the Prevention of Blindness.

All state laws require the use of prophylactic medication at the time of birth to prevent blindness from *ophthalmia neonatorum.* Since 1909, when Wisconsin adopted the first such state regulation, there has been a decrease in blindness from this cause of over 90 per cent among new admissions to schools for the blind. When suspected gonorrheal eye infections do develop, immediate treatment with penicillin will prevent loss of sight. In some communities, the newer antibiotics are replacing silver nitrate as a prophylactic.

The Child's Eyes

Strabismus. Periodically, the mother should bring her baby or child to the family physician for a general check-up, for examination prior to entering school and prior to going to camp. At each examination the eyes should be checked not only for signs of inflammation but also for any imbalance of the external ocular muscles. Coordination can be tested by circling a bright object about 12 in. in front of the child and then moving the object in toward the nose. After the infant is six months of age, he usually follows such an object reasonably well. If an eye shows any tendency to turn in or to turn out after the twelfth month, prompt referral to an ophthalmologist is indicated.

Formerly it was believed possible to delay referral of a preschool child with strabismus in the hope that he might outgrow it. Selective service records of World War II revealed that thousands of young men had vision of only 20/100 or 20/200 in one eye. In these cases amblyopia from disuse resulted from too late or improper treatment of strabismus in childhood. Ophthalmologists now prefer to see these

TABLE 27

Causes of Blindness by Site and Type

Site and Type		Percentage of Total (all ages)
Whole eye		26
(glaucoma)	(15)	
(other)	(11)	
Cornea		5
Iris and ciliary		4
Lens		24
Choroid and retina		27
Optic nerve, paths, cortex		12
Other and not specified		2

*Source: 1954 Report on 27,079 Persons, Commission for the Blind, New York State Department of Social Welfare.

children as soon as a tendency for the eye to deviate is recognized. Successful surgery can be performed even on infants, and glasses can be worn when necessary by children as young as one year. Early treatment prevents loss of vision in the deviating eye and shortens the time required to patch the good eye. Early treatment also corrects the condition before the child suffers the thoughtless gibes of playmates which may affect profoundly his personality development.

There may be a tendency for an eye to turn up, in, or out, which is sufficient to cause the child trouble even though the eye does not ordinarily deviate. Muscle imbalance of this degree can be recognized if the examining physician will routinely do a "cover test" after checking muscle coordination. In this test, the child is asked to focus on a bright object held about 12 in. directly in front of him. While both eyes are open, one eye is covered and uncovered slowly five or six times, at intervals of one or two seconds, with a 3-by-5-in. card. Any shifting of the covered eye when the card is removed indicates a muscle imbalance which may require treatment. About one child in 25 has a muscle imbalance sufficient to cause headaches, reading difficulty, or even outright strabismus. The general practitioner and the pediatrician can be of great help to the child and his family by looking for imbalance of the extraocular muscles and, if necessary, putting the family in touch with a competent ophthalmologist.

After the child is three years old, he should be tested yearly for distance visual acuity. With the preschool child, the symbol E chart may be used. After the child becomes familiar with the large E, he may be asked to play a game, pointing in the direction in which the legs of the smaller symbols point. Because the eye is still growing and there is a short attention span, the average three-year-old child may have only 20/40 vision. After he becomes six, however, he should be able to read the 20/20 line with each eye. Patience is required in testing the vision of preschool children. It is helpful to have an assistant stand at the chart to uncover the letters while the physician stands with the child to occlude each eye and to observe him for straining or squinting. The time taken for these screening tests is well rewarded by the help that can be given the 10 to 25 per cent of children at different ages who will be found to need glasses in order to see clearly.

Injuries. An important cause of loss of vision among children, particularly boys, is eye injury. Parents of small children should be urged to keep scissors, knitting or crochet needles, pencils, and other sharp objects out of reach.

Hazards to older children's eyes are bows and arrows, darts, slingshots, and BB guns. In 10 states, legislation has been adopted (in 1950) to permit use of an air rifle only under the supervision of an adult. In 29 states, legislation restricts the use of fireworks to public displays. Where these measures have been enforced, there has been a great drop in blindness from trauma.

School Vision Problems. About one fourth of the children of school age require eye care in order to see clearly. Since most of our education comes through the sense of sight, each child should have a competent eye examination before entering school. In practice, some kind of vision testing or screening program is necessary so that children with seriously defective vision may be referred for eye care.

The simplest screening test is the Snellen chart for distance acuity. The teacher who gives the test should have instruction in proper use of this chart. Usually, the teacher may obtain this instruction from the public health nurse who is assigned to the school.

Occasionally, some test for near vision is urged on the grounds that a great deal of school work requires vision at 14 in. Actually, the child's reserve power of accommodation is so great that he can read very fine letters for a minute or two at near sight; yet, after a half hour's study, he may suffer considerable eye fatigue, with resultant constitutional disturbances, because of hyperopia.

More elaborate testing devices, such as the Massachusetts Vision Test and the Telebinocular, are used in some communities, in order to be sure that every child who needs eye care will be detected. An adequate follow-up program for care of those being screened should be established before these elaborate techniques are instituted. Too often the school vision program merely screens the same children year after year and devotes little effort to secure necessary treatment. In most schools the follow-up part of the program needs greater emphasis.

About one child in 500 will be found to have vision of 20/70 or worse in the better eye after correction, and needs some kind of special educational adjustment. In cities, classes for the partially seeing (erroneously called "sight-saving" classes) are established in which are provided correct lighting conditions, large-type books, typewriters, and other aids. Such children go to the special classroom only for close eye work or special help, and participate in most other activities with their more fortunate normally seeing fellows. These children should not be sent to schools for the blind but should attend regular schools where they can be taught how best to use their limited sight.

Adult Eye Problems

Although blinding eye diseases may occur at any age, they are much more common after 40. During the forties also, presbyopia begins to trouble the average person. All too often considerable sight is lost from uveitis, glaucoma, and other serious eye conditions while the individual attributes his lack of clear vision merely to the need for a pair of glasses. It is particularly important that practitioners who examine individuals in this age group make use of the ophthalmoscope, which will often uncover not only signs of eye disease but also evidence of such general conditions as hypertension, diabetes, arteriosclerosis, nephritis, and the leukemias.

In view of the success in treating certain inflammatory eye conditions with cortisone and ACTH, it is particularly important that the general practitioner be alert to refer patients with possible iritis and choroiditis to an ophthalmologist.

Cataracts are responsible for about one fifth of all blindness. In over three fourths of these persons the lens opacities are associated with the aging process. Blindness from cataracts frequently has its onset in the forties and fifties. These patients should be referred promptly to the ophthalmologist so that surgery may be performed at the best time.

Injuries. It is estimated that 1,000 eyes are still lost in industry each year. Most eye hazards can be controlled either at the source or by furnishing eye protection to the worker. In a shop where there are eye hazards, it is essential that everyone in the shop—even a casual visitor or a representative of top management—be required to wear safety glasses at all times. Incorporating needed corrective prescriptions in the safety glasses, providing measures for cleaning them, and other aids to eye protection recommended by the National Society for the Prevention of Blindness can reduce eye loss in a plant to practically zero.

Glaucoma. About 12 per cent of all blindness in the United States is caused by glaucoma, and the incidence of this condition appears to be increasing as public health measures lengthen the span of life.

Chronic simple glaucoma develops so gradually, so insidiously, that the individual often loses considerable peripheral vision before he develops symptoms sufficient to take him to a doctor. There may be occasional headache or eye pain in dim light, in the evening, looking at a television set, at the movies, or at other times when illumination is reduced. There may be headaches or eye pain upon awakening in the morning. Rarely is eye trouble suspected at this stage unless the family doctor is alert to the possibility of glaucoma. Usually, it is not until later that the patient complains of halos or rainbows around light. Sometimes, in the early stages the patient is not quite satisfied with his glasses and will have them changed several times. One patient had nine pairs of glasses within a one-year period before the possibility of glaucoma was finally investigated.

The patient may also have an uncomfortable feeling in his eye, blurred vision, or tearing at times of excitement or worry, since emotional upsets appear to produce an elevation in the ocular tension of glaucoma patients. This dangerously mild course may last for months or even for two or three years before the patient becomes aware of a defect in side vision or before there is loss of central vision. Some patients go to an ophthalmologist with the field of vision in one eye reduced to that which might be seen through a mailing tube or through a gun barrel, yet with a central visual acuity of 20/20.

Acute glaucoma is usually characterized by excruciating pain in and around the eye, blurring or loss of vision, one-sided headache, nausea, vomiting, dilation of the pupil, and cloudiness of the cornea. The patient may complain of halos or rainbow effects around lights. This kind of stormy onset and course usually results in the patient's seeking medical care. Unfortunately, however, the eye signs or symptoms may be overlooked and the clinical picture be so confused that the family physician might make the diagnosis of sinusitis. There have been a number of instances where the eye symptoms were so minor and the constitutional symptoms so pronounced that the family physician has mistakenly made a diagnosis of acute abdominal emergency for which surgery has been performed. This can be avoided if the physician keeps the possibility of glaucoma in mind even though the symptoms bothering the patient most are nausea and vomiting.

Case-finding studies have been carried on in Philadelphia and elsewhere to determine the incidence of early, unrecognized glaucoma among the general population. Based on these studies it is estimated that 1 out of 50 men and women over 40 years of age has this condition. If glaucoma is recognized and treated properly in the early stages, the patient has an excellent chance of preserving useful vision, although he will require observation and treatment for the rest of his life.

There is much that the general practitioner can do, particularly among his patients who are over 40 years of age, that will lead to earlier detection of glaucoma. Six points which have been recommended are:

1. Ask patient about occurrence of occasional blurring or clouding of vision, seeing rainbow effects around a distant light, one-sided headaches, discomfort in or around the eyes after excitement or worry or under reduced illumination. Inquire if he experiences difficulty in reading despite prescribed glasses.

2. Ask if there is a case of glaucoma in the family.

3. Measure acuity of vision. Causes of lowered vision in one or both eyes should be investigated.

4. Note size of pupils and their reaction to light. Unequal or sluggish reaction to light should be investigated.

5. Examine each eye with ophthalmoscope to see if optic disks appear pale or cupped.

6. Check ocular tension and test visual fields if tonometer or perimeter is available. Digital palpation for tension and confrontation test for fields are crude and of value only in advanced cases.

Above all, tact should be exercised so that the patient will not be unduly alarmed. However, if the physician suspects anything at all abnormal, he should arrange for an ophthalmologic consultation. In acute glaucoma the loss of even a few hours' time can be very serious.

If a patient has chronic glaucoma the family physician should remember that belladonna, atropine, and other mydriatics should not be prescribed without a consultation with the ophthalmologist. Cases of glaucoma have been made worse, and apparently even precipitated, by the prolonged use of belladonna or its derivatives; it is recommended that prescriptions for these drugs be marked "not to be refilled." One ophthalmologist recently reported six cases in which belladonna derivatives given for peptic ulcers, colitis, or hyperacidity had been followed by attacks of acute congestive glaucoma. When any of these drugs are to be prescribed, the patient should be questioned about symptoms of eye diseases; if he is under treatment by an eye physician, inquiry should be made as to the nature of the condition.

When the patient with glaucoma requires surgery for hernia, appendicitis, or other condition, his medication for glaucoma ordinarily should be continued throughout his hospital stay.

Public Education. In reviewing briefly some of the causes of blindness, it becomes apparent that it is possible to prevent loss of sight by promoting early diagnosis and by eliminating the cause. To accomplish these objectives in a democracy, general public education is essential. The National Society for the Prevention of Blindness, with its state and local affiliated organizations, for many years has carried on a broad program which includes:

1. Promotion of eye research.
2. Educational activities.

3. Provision of preventive services, including case-finding and follow-up.

State governmental agencies in health, welfare, and education departments, as well as medical society committees, are making great contributions to the national program to prevent blindness.

SECTION II

Accident Prevention

26. ACCIDENT PREVENTION

By very definition of the word, an accident cannot be prevented. "An accident is an event, occurring to an individual without his expectation, and without possibility of prevention *at the moment of its occurrence.*"

Thus, it is clear that all preventive measures must be applied with the intent to alter the series of events which lead inevitably to accidents.

All accidents have certain effects — some negligible, others leading to terrible destruction and death. It is necessary to study these effects in order to understand causes of accidents. Our tendency in the past has been to limit our observations to accidents involving serious injury. In fact, fatalities are the major indices of our statistics of accidents. This is logical, of course, since fatalities are so definite, measurable, and final. We now realize that for study purposes the important individual in the accident is not the man who died but the one who survived, with little or no injury. In instituting preventive measures we must learn not only why a man was killed, but why, under an apparently similar chain of events, another man escaped with little or no injury.

Epidemiology of Accidents

Accidental injuries and accidental deaths have a true epidemiology. These conditions can be studied and evaluated in the same way as are factors that produce illness and death from an infectious agent. The analogy holds further since it is only through our understanding of the epidemiology of accidents that we can institute appropriate preventive measures.

Main Groups of Accidents. In 1959 the total number of accidental deaths in the United States was 91,000.* Nonfatal accidental injuries

*For years the National Safety Council has collected and published extensive epidemiologic data relating to accidents, and has been most effective in promoting measures for prevention of accidental injury and death. The authors are most grateful to the National Safety Council for permission to utilize data from their annual publication "Accident Facts," 1906, 425 North Michigan Avenue, Chicago, Illinois.

numbered 9,200,000, a ratio of about 1 death to 100 injuries. Accidents now rank fourth in leading causes of deaths in the United States.

The major groups of injury are classified in Table 28:

TABLE 28

Major Causes of Accidents — 1959

	Motor Vehicle	Home	Nonhome, Nonmotor Vehicle	Occupational
Injuries	1,400,000	3,900,000	2,050,000	1,950,000
Deaths	37,800	26,000	16,500	13,800

The importance of accidents as a cause of death in the younger and older age groups is shown in Table 29.

TABLE 29

Accidents as a Cause of Death
1959 — United States

Age (years)	Relative Importance	Deaths per 100,000 Population in the Given Age Group
Under 1	6th	103
1-4	1st	31
5-14	1st	19
15-24	1st	56
25-44	2nd	42
45-64	4th	51
65 and over	6th	165

Sex Ratios in Accidents. Fatal accidents are much less common in women than in men, in all age groups except in infancy. Boys are much more prone to serious accidents than girls, and industrial accidents in the adult males are the concomitants of the hazards of their occupations. Furthermore, it is probable that men are more reckless and more accident-prone than women.

Classes of Accidents. The principal types of fatal accidents, including occupational accidents, in 1959 were:

Motor vehicles	36,981
Falls—all ages	18,248
Burns	7,291
Drownings	6,582
Railroad accidents	2,480
Firearms	2,172

For all ages under 65 years, motor vehicle accidents were the most common cause of accidental death. In persons over 65 years, falls exceeded motor vehicle fatalities. Mechanical suffocation was next most important in the age group 1 to 4 years. Drowning was second most important in children from 5 to 14 years. This was true also of young adults from 15 to 45 years. Falls were the second cause of fatal accidents in persons from 45 to 64 years.

Season of Accidents. Accidents vary in seasonal prevalence. Most fatal accidents occur in August, fewest are in April, but motor vehicle accidents are most common in the late fall months and least common in January. Burns cause fatalities most often in January and are least frequent in August; drownings are most prevalent in July and rarest in January.

Geographic Differentials. Considerable variation in the accidental death rate occurs in different parts of the country. The New England and Middle Atlantic states were nearly 20 per cent lower than the average rate of 51.6 deaths per 100,000 population in 1959. The Mountain states averaged 76.1. Motor vehicle death rates show a still greater variation (see Table 30).

The highest death rate from falls occurred in the New England states; burns caused more deaths in the South Central area than in other areas. All these facts are important in analyzing basic causes of accidents and in planning methods of prevention.

Decline in Accidental Deaths. Despite a steady increase in population and a marked increase in industrial activity, and particularly in the number of airplanes and motor vehicles, the death rate per

100,000 population from accidental deaths has declined steadily during the past 20 years. The period of greatest fatality was about 1935 as shown in Table 31.

TABLE 30

United States Motor Vehicle Deaths, 1960

Incidence	State	Deaths per 100,000 Population
Low:	Connecticut	10.3
	Rhode Island	10.4
	Massachusetts	11.3
High:	New Mexico	51.8
	Wyoming	53.0
	Nevada	63.4

Automobile Accidents

Motor vehicles have increased enormously in number in recent years. In addition, their speed capacity has almost doubled. Much has been done to prevent fatalities from motor vehicle accidents, with some success, but the toll of injury and death is still very heavy. These accidents have a distinct and separate epidemiology.

TABLE 31

Decline in Accidental Death Rates in the United States

	Total	Motor Vehicle	Home	Nonhome, Nonmotor Vehicle	Occupational
Average fatalities, 1933-1937	101,388	36,313	33,000	18,500	17,000
Average fatalities, 1949	91,000	31,500	31,000	15,500	15,000
Average fatalities, 1959	91,000	37,800	26,000	16,500	13,800

In 1959, 10,000 automobile accident fatalities occurred in cities and towns (despite the heavy concentration of traffic in the cities), whereas 27,800 occurred in rural areas. The major types of fatal accidents were:

Collision	15,100
Overturning or running off the road	11,600
Pedestrian fatalities	7,750

The chief immediate causes of fatal automobile accidents were, in order of importance: (a) excessive speed; (b) right of way; (c) on wrong side of the road; (d) improper passing.

Alcohol is frequently incriminated as an important factor in fatal automobile accidents. Studies of large series of such accidents have shown that one out of five drivers involved in fatal accidents had been drinking. One out of three fatal motor vehicle accidents involved a drinking driver, and one out of four adult pedestrians killed in a motor vehicle accident had been drinking.

We have already noted that automobile accidents have a seasonal prevalence, being most frequent in the late fall and least frequent in January. In most areas Saturday is the worst day of the week. The daily peak of automobile accidents is reached in the hours of darkness.

Decrease in Automobile Accident Fatalities. The rate of decline in fatalities from automobile accidents can be expressed in various ways. Each gives a different point of view and aids in planning preventive measures.

During the past 35 years, deaths per 100,000,000 vehicle miles have declined from 17 in 1923 to 5.4 in 1960. But the number of deaths per 100,000 population is still high because of the great risk, due to the increased numbers of automobiles, in ratio to increase of population. Through the past decades these death rates for auto fatalities per 100,000 population are as follows:

1920	11
1930	26
1940	26
1950	23
1960	21

A comparison of accidents in public motor vehicle transportation accidents in other forms of transport is given in Table 32.

Broad Conclusions Regarding Accidents

The above epidemiologic data permit the drawing of certain broad conclusions. They show that *accidents are preventable.* The active campaigns for education of the worker in avoidance of accidents while at work have been most fruitful. General adoption of the principles of workmen's compensation by most states has given a strong emphasis on safety campaigns by industry. One reason is that industry pays insurance premiums against industrial hazards in direct ratio to its accident experience, and thus an effective safety plan becomes profitable in every sense. Each industry has organized its safety plan to meet its own particular industrial situation. The theory is that all accidents are avoidable. They occur because of: (a) defects in protective devices; (b) negligence or carelessness of the worker. Each of these factors can be minimized to the point of infinity. The results of these accident preventive programs continue to be most gratifying and become more effective yearly.

A marked decline in fatal accidents in children of school age, which has occurred during the past 35 years, is a direct result of safety campaigns in the public schools. It is an excellent example of the direct gain, in lives saved, of intensive, effective health education.

Unsolved Problems. The greatest deficiency in present accident prevention programs is our inability to prevent injury and death due

TABLE 32

Transport Death Rates, 1959, in the United States

Vehicle	Total Deaths	Deaths per 100,000 Passenger Miles
Automobile	24,300	2.3
Airplane	209	0.69
Bus	106	0.18
Railroad	12	0.05

to the increased propulsion of the human body through space. Speed in transportation has been greatly increased in the past 50 years, but the engineers have not at the same time developed suitable methods of deceleration to prevent the frequent injuries and deaths.

The one exception is railroad transportation. In this field, the development of safety measures has proved that a high degree of safety can be achieved in rapid transportation if proper safeguards are rigidly applied.

Accidents Due to Falls. Accidents and deaths due to falls are the second most common cause of violent death in the United States. The highest death rates occur in the age groups over 65 years, not perhaps because of more frequent falls in elderly people but because falls are so serious to persons in these age groups. The prevention of falls, in fact of all home accidents, is a field that has not yet been exploited. It can be approached from the point of view of the architect who plans the house and by the designer and manufacturer of household equipment and furniture. Active promotion of education in home accident prevention is essential, with special emphasis on the age groups over 65. An excellent measure is the home safety campaign organized as a combined effort of all interested agencies. As prepayment plans for medical care develop, it seems quite probable that the associations administering those funds will be the most active agents in the promotion of education in accident prevention, since such a procedure would pay ample dividends.

Accident-proneness. One important causal factor in accidents that has only recently received attention is accident-proneness. This simply means that a small proportion of the people have most of the accidents. Rawson(1), Dunbar(2), and Alexander(3) have pointed out that some individuals have five times as many accidents as the normal expectancy. They insist that there is an *accident-prone* type of person.

Dunbar has developed the thesis that these accident-prone persons, as a type, are impulsive. They tend to concentrate upon immediate pleasures, they do not plan for the future, but enjoy excitement and adventure.

Rawson has shown that the accident-prone individual tends to be rebellious and resentful. He has a deeply ingrained opposition to the strict regulations of family life. As he reaches adulthood, he has a contempt for law and authority. This author even suggests that many accidents might be "unconsciously intended," in that the victim is motivated by a basic desire for violent and uncontrollable reaction.

Alexander has described the accident-prone individual as an impetuous person who converts immediately into action his momentary impulses without deliberation and planning. He harbors a deep rebellion against the early excessive regulations of his upbringing—a deep resentment against persons in authority. At the same time he has a strict conscience which makes him feel guilty for this rebellion. In the unconsciously provoked accident, he expresses his resentment and revenge, at the same time atoning for his rebellion by his injury.

It is clear that not all persons of this type have frequent accidents. Day and Kunkle(4) have presented the basic factors predisposing to accidents. This analysis balances the influence of the situation against the individual and thus gives the clue for effective preventive procedures.

The Individual:

A. Somatic factors
  1. "Inherent awkwardness" (defective sensorimotor skills without actual structural disease).
  2. Temporary impairment of skill due to fatigue, acute illness, or intoxication.
  3. Chronic impairment of skill due to chronic structural disease, e.g., advanced loss of vision, deafness, lesions in neuromotor system.
B. Psychological factors
  1. Preoccupations (i.e., distractions).
  2. Emotional tension, with accompanying neuromuscular tension.
  3. "Psychiatric equivalents," e.g., unconsciously purposive accident tendencies as expressions of hostility or guilt ("hitting back" or "self-destruction" [Menninger]).

The individual susceptible to these *psychologic* patterns is the *accident-prone* person of primary clinical interest; the individual possessing the *somatic* factors is less likely to be accident-prone because (a) he recognizes and compensates for his deficiencies in skill; and (b) he avoids dangerous situations.

The Situation:

There are accident-prone { situations, e.g., need to meet a deadline in a given activity.
devices, e.g., a sawmill.
occupations, e.g., rodeo performer.

Summary:

When the accident-prone individual meets the accident-prone situation, the accident-potential of this combination is high.

Weinerman(5) has pointed out that the environment plays a very important part in accident-proneness. Defects and inadequacies of industrial equipment, bad housing, long hours of routine work, improper traffic regulations, inadequate playgrounds, poor training for the job, all predispose to accidents. All persons who have accidents are not repressed and frustrated psychotics. Other factors are fatigue, transient emotional stress, press of unfinished work, impaired vision or hearing, underlying disease or physical defects, or the slower reactions of the gradually aging person.

Certain industries such as mining and lumbering have special hazards that produce a high accident rate. In periods of high industrial activity, overcrowding of equipment, unsafe wearing apparel, unskilled workmen, overtime with resultant fatigue, all tend toward an increased accident rate.

Thus Weinerman believes that accidents are not due preponderately to accident-proneness, but are the result of multiple factors, most of which can be modified to bring about favorable results.

Prevention of Home Accidents(4). As we have already noted, the prevention of home accidents is an uncharted field. The essentials of a community-wide program should include the following activities:

1. Education of all the people concerning the causes of home accidents and their avoidance.

2. Epidemiologic studies of home accidents, including the mild as well as severe types.

3. Detection and education of the accident-prone individual.

4. Cooperative planning. This requires the resources of the health department and the school authorities, as well as municipal departments of fire prevention, housing, the police department, and the division of social welfare. All have something to contribute to a community plan for prevention of home accidents.

TABLE 33

Transport Death Rates, 1957 to 1959, in the United States

Vehicle	Deaths per 100 Million Passenger Miles
Turnpike automobile	1.28
Airplane	0.44
Bus	0.19
Railway passenger train	0.13

Gains in Aviation Safety

Great gains have been made in aviation safety in recent years. In the United States the passenger death rate per 100,000,000 passenger miles has declined from 4.70 in 1937 to 1939 to 1.99 in 1947 to 1949 and 0.44 in 1957 to 1959. The rates by type of transport in 1957 to 1959 are given in Table 33.

Careful epidemiologic studies of each airplane accident and stricter regulations regarding airplane structure together with new methods for protection of airplanes at take-off and landing have been most effective in making airplane travel safer.

Crash Injury Research

The epidemiologic studies of the Crash Injury Research at Cornell(6) have developed important information concerning prevention of injury and death in automobile accidents. Tourin(7) states that auto fatalities may be reduced by 25 per cent by use of seat belts and that relatively simple modifications in automobile construction will give a marked degree of added protection to the automobile passenger. Most of the improvements indicated by these studies still remain to be realized.

Summary

Prevention of accidents depends upon cooperative effort of many groups of official and private agencies.

The health department has an important part to play in accident prevention through effective educational measures. These have already proved most effective in diminishing accidents in school children. Industry plays an important role in reducing industrial accidents.

The private physician is important in prevention of disability due to accidents; his educational efforts in prevention of accidental poisoning can be most effective(8).

In Pennsylvania, the State Highway Department, the Governor's Traffic Safety Council, the Health Department and the medical profession work together in preventing automobile accidents(9). In considering the human factor, health standards are set for licensing drivers. There is a physical examination required for initial licensing(10). This is repeated at intervals giving special consideration to eyesight, hearing, and reaction time. Neuropsychiatric tests are applied when indicated. Special consideration is given to the "drinking driver" and to the accident repeater.

Much remains to be done. Many of the measures known to prevent accidents have not yet been widely applied.

REFERENCES

1. RAWSON, A. T.: *Psychosom. Med.*, 1949, **6**:88.
2. DUNBAR, F.: *Psychosomatic Medicine.* Random House, New York, 1947.
3. ALEXANDER, F.: *Pub. Health*, 1949, **64**:357.
4. DAY, E., and KUNKLE, C. C.: personal communication, 1948.

5. WEINERMAN, E. R.: *Am. J. Pub. Health*, 1949, **39**:1527.

6. Reports of Automotive Crash Injury Research of Cornell University. 316 East 61st Street, New York 21, N.Y.

7. TOURIN, B.: *Pub. Health Rep.*, 1958, **73**:381.

8. CANN, H. M., ISKRANT, H. P., and NEYMAN, D. S.: *Am. J. Pub. Health*, 1960, **50**:1914.

9. WILBAR, C. L.: *Am. J. Pub. Health*, 1960, **50**:1349.

10. Medical Guide for Physicians in Determining Fitness to Drive a Motor Vehicle. *J.A.M.A.*, 1959, **169**:1195.

SECTION III

Conservative Medicine

Austin Flint in 1872 clearly delineated the responsibility of the physician and the community in health protection of the adult, and coined the appropriate phase "conservative medicine."* Said Dr. Flint:

Conservative medicine means preservation of the vital forces. It covers everything which prevents the impairment of, or tends to develop and sustain, the powers of life. The practice of conservative medicine is the responsibility of both the practicing physician, and also the health officer who is in charge of community efforts for health promotion.

Chronic disease, affecting an important part, may continue for a greater or less period, and recovery may finally be complete, but during its continuance the powers of life are more or less impaired. It may destroy life by leading to incurable lesions or by its protracted duration.

Under all circumstances, the affection is less likely to be prolonged, serious changes in structure are less likely to take place, and fatal termination is postponed in proportion as the vital powers are preserved.

Conservative medicine therefore dictates measures which tend to sustain the powers of life in chronic disease. It dictates measures to develop appetites, to provide abundant nutritive supplies and all other hygienic measures which invigorate and strengthen the body.

Conservative medicine is particularly applicable to those chronic affections collectively which destroy by gradual inroads upon the powers of life (examples are carcinoma, tuberculosis, diabetes, cirrhosis, and Bright's disease). With a view to prolong life, when recovery is not expected, the great object is to retard, as much as possible, the failure of the vital forces.

Patients with incurable disease are too often abandoned merely to palliative measures, the fatal issue being merely a question of time, and therefore not of much importance. The question, however, may be highly important to the patient and to his friends. To aid in the cure of disease is undoubtedly the first aim of the physician, but when a cure is not to be effected, then comes the prolongation of life, even with health more or less impaired.

*Lemuel Shattuck in 1850 quotes Edward Jarvis as follows: "Our education has made our calling [medicine] exclusively a curative and not a conservative one."

In the management of any incurable affection, conservative medicine dictates the measures which in general terms, will contribute to keep the body in the best possible condition, compatible with the continuance or progress of the disease. In this way, not only the inroads of the disease on the powers of life, but the destructive lesions may often be stayed. An incurable illness is sometimes held completely in abeyance, and the system rendered so tolerant to its continuance, that life may be preserved indefinitely, although a vital organ is affected.*

We have quoted at length from Dr. Flint's essay because we have been much impressed with his vision and understanding of the future role of medicine in the promotion of health of the people. He wrote this essay and developed the concept of conservative medicine almost a century ago, yet we are only beginning to realize the importance of his concept. A great responsibility rests on us: not only to prevent disease but also to conserve the health of those suffering chronic debilitating illnesses and threatened with the destruction of their "vital powers."

Through the years, we have developed a series of procedures in preventive medicine and public health that have met the needs of the community. Most of these have been sound and have had a strong influence in the prevention of illness and the promotion of health. Life has been prolonged, death prevented. Great advances have been made in reduction of the ravages of acute illness, particularly in childhood.

Our very successes, however, have led to new serious public health problems, for which we were not prepared, and for which we had developed no policies or procedures. Chronic illness with its ramifications has become the outstanding unsolved problem in preventive medicine and public health. It is a great challenge.

In Chapter 46 we discuss the various problems encountered by the physician in the field of conservative medicine. The most effective measures to be taken by the doctor and the community for the promotion of public health are also presented.

In essence, the following discussion is on conservative medicine.

---

*Flint, Austin: *Essays on Conservative Medicine.* Henry C. Lea, Philadelphia, 1871.

27. THE PROTECTION AND PROMOTION OF HEALTH IN ADULT LIFE

THE PRODUCTIVE YEARS 20 TO 65

As infectious disease is brought under better control, a larger proportion of the population progresses into the productive period of life. During the early decades, women are subject to the hazards of childbearing. The chief health menace to young men is accidents — related often directly or indirectly to their occupations. During this early period, life habits are established, prejudices are formed, and future health status is determined.

In later years, the adult is likely to be afflicted by one of the chronic illnesses. Once established, these various types of specific illnesses can usually be ameliorated but not cured.

Prevention of Chronic Disease

The life pattern is set in the early decades. It is during this period that most effective measures can be instituted in *prevention* or *postponement* of subsequent illness and perhaps premature death.

Thus the term "preventive medicine" has changed strikingly in its concept since the early years when it connoted simply prevention of illness due to acute infections. Hutchinson(1) has pointed out that "All medical services are preventive services to the extent that they are concerned with altering the natural history of disease." Thus preventive medicine has two major objectives:

1. To prevent the original occurrence of a disease.
2. To prevent progression of a disease.

The success of our efforts may be gauged by the degree to which the measures taken can be shown to alter favorably the natural course of the illness.

369

In order to determine whether progress is made, it is necessary to set up suitable methods of measurement. For each individual case:

1. Make a statement of objectives.
2. Outline a program to fulfill objectives.
3. Set up a control, e.g., would the objectives be accomplished equally well without specific programs?
4. In due time, measure the results obtained.

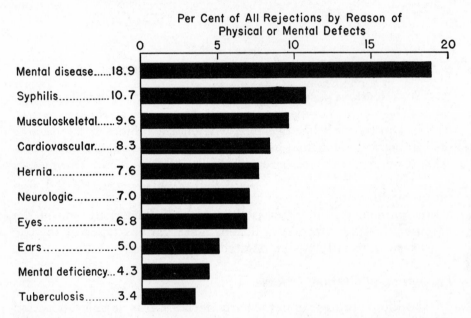

Figure 35. Findings of selective service examinations, World War II. Rejection for physical and mental defects: ten leading causes, as of February 1, 1944.

Early Diagnosis

Often the physician is unable to formulate a satisfactory program in prevention of the progression of a chronic disease, because the patient comes to him late in the course of the illness. This has led to institution of "early diagnosis" programs. One of the most common is the institution of periodic health examinations of presumably healthy adults.

Other methods are: mass methods for detection of a specific disease, e.g., diabetes, tuberculosis, or syphilis. Another technique that has been followed is called "multiphasic screening," in which a battery of diagnostic criteria is assembled and applied to large groups of individuals.

The institution of "early diagnosis" programs is of little specific value unless there is proof that the earlier the detection, the more effective the prevention. In order to benefit from early case finding, a disease must have the following characteristics:

1. Well-established effective therapy.

2. A diagnostic device capable of determining a disease prior to its usual time of detection.

3. One or more critical points at which therapy promptly instituted disrupts the pathologic sequence that would follow if no therapy were applied, e.g., as with rheumatic fever.

4. Such a critical point must occur after accurate diagnosis first becomes possible but before diagnosis is usually made in normal community life.

It is obvious that as the community at large and medical personnel become more alert to early symptoms and signs of disease, the normal community level of case finding may improve to the point that mass screening tests are of no additional value. Conversely, new case-finding tests may make early detection efforts profitable in an area that previously was unrewarding.

One great defect of mass case-finding techniques in the past has been that the cases were found, but no subsequent procedures for health improvement were instituted.

THE PERIODIC HEALTH EXAMINATION

The periodic health examination is now generally regarded as an essential element of sound medical practice. Its purpose is to enable the physician to detect at an early stage any impending chronic illness, and thus be in a position to take necessary measures to prevent further ravages of the disease. It also makes it possible to change environmental factors that might produce or aggravate symptoms. In some instances, cure of the disease can be effected. In most cases it would be feasible to propose measures that will postpone symptoms and prolong life.

A very large series of studies have shown that a carefully planned skilled health examination of a presumably healthy person 40 years of age or over will reveal a significant number of unsuspected conditions that might later result in overt prolonged chronic illness.

Furthermore, as time advances, subsequent examinations at regular
intervals will reveal the development of new conditions that have
evolved since the last examination.

A Periodic Health Examination Program

It is obvious that the plan must be simple, practical, and designed
to secure the highest yield with least expenditures of time and effort
on the part of the physician and patient. Each physician will develop
his own plan, but general experience has shown that the following
procedures are reasonably satisfactory.

Age.

Men: Initial examination — 40 years.
Women: Initial examination — 35 years.

Women are examined earlier because of the hazards of cancer of
the cervix and breast. Some physicians limit their tests to those organs
at first, and begin complete periodic examination of women only at
50 years.

Subsequent Examinations. Men should be given at least two examinations between 40 and 50 years, three during the next decade,
and every other year after 60 years. Many authorities recommend *annual* physical examinations for men over 45 years of age. Some
industrial health services follow this policy for their executives, but
the "yield" is not sufficiently high to warrant this outlay by the
average man.

Scope of the Examination.

1. History. An excellent aid is the Cornell Medical Index,* a
questionnaire prepared in advance by the patient.

2. Physical Examination. This should include tests for vision and
hearing as well as tonometry to detect incipient glaucoma. Procto-
sigmoidoscopy should be done in all males over 50 years, cervical
cytology in all females over 40 years.

3. Laboratory Tests. Six tests are usually employed: hemoglobin,
blood sugar, serology for syphilis, simple urine analysis, sedimentation rate, and X-ray of the chest. Some authorities suggest an electro-
cardiogram in men over 50 years. If of no other value, it furnishes a
base line for future reference.

*Obtained from Cornell Medical College, 1300 York Avenue, New York 21, New
York.

Of abnormalities found, 10 per cent will be furnished by the history, 60 per cent by physical examinations, and 30 per cent by laboratory tests. At least one significant abnormality that could be benefited by medical advice should be encountered in 80 per cent of "normal" persons over 40 years who are examined carefully.

The most frequent abnormalities encountered are:

Condition	Per Cent
Obesity	25-30
Hypertension	14
Rectosigmoidal polyp	7-8
Anemia	7
Gallstones	4-5
Diabetes	2.5

Multiphasic Screening

As the name implies, this is a screening procedure in which large numbers of people are given a battery of diagnostic tests in series, and at one time and place. The procedure is usually organized by the health department. The tests are done by technicians, and the results are reviewed by a physician. If any abnormality is found, the person is so advised and referred to his family physician.

It is an excellent educational method, and promotes the concept of periodic health examinations. The obvious obligation of the health department, however, is to promote the more effective plan of periodic health examinations by practicing physicians as a vital and essential element of private practice.

Prepayment Programs for Periodic Health Examinations

The periodic health examination is becoming an integral part of large organized prepayment plans for medical care, because, in practical terms, early detection and treatment of chronic illness should greatly lower the costs of subsequent medical care. Thus it is to the great advantage of both the patient and the plan to detect chronic illness in its incipiency.

Elson(2) has made an interesting analysis of the results of periodic health examinations with a group of 1,513 executives (1,500 males; 13 females). The average age was 45 years, ranging from 24 to 76 years (the age distribution was not given). Sphygmoidoscope examination was done only in those over 40 years.

Forty per cent of the group was found to have some previously unrecognized abnormal condition. The most common were:

Condition	Number
Hypertension	189
Obesity	179
Prostate	79
Hernia	54

Forty-six per cent of abnormalities had a potential, if unchecked, of producing disability or death. Of diseases discovered in younger age groups, i.e., under 40 years, 65 per cent were insignificant or minor. In the age group over 60 years, 70 per cent of the lesions were significant.

In the following chapters, therefore, we discuss subject matter which relates to *promotion of the health* of the adult, particularly the young adult. We are interested in the prolongation of his life, the prevention of disabling illness and accident, and the provision of *adequate protective* health services in order to reduce, in so far as possible, the toll of sickness and disability in the community.

REFERENCES

1. HUTCHINSON, G. B.: *J. Chronic Diseases*, 1960, **11**:497.
2. ELSON, K. A., *et al.*: *J.A.M.A.*, 1960, **172**:55.

SPECIAL REFERENCES

Bulletin, Hospital Council for Greater New York, August 8, 1947.
DUBLIN, L. I. and LOTKA, A. J.: *Money Value of a Man*. The Ronald Press Company, New York, 1930.
FREEMONT-SMITH, M.: Periodic Examination of Supposedly Well Persons. *New England J. Med.*, 1953, **248**:170.
JACKSON, F. W.: *Canad. J. Pub. Health*, 1941, **32**:491.
LENSON, N.: *New England J. Med.*, 1953, **248**:943.
Periodic Health Examinations, A Manual for Physicians. American

Medical Association, Chicago, 1940.

    PERROTT, G. ST. J.: *Milbank Mem. Fund Quart.*, 1944, **22**:358.

    ___: *Milbank Mem. Fund Quart.*, 1941, **19**:337.

    PREAS, SALLY, and PHILLIPS, RUTH: *Milbank Mem. Fund Quart.*, 1942, **20**:221.

28. PROMOTION OF MENTAL HEALTH

Magnitude of the Problems of Mental Health

Mental health promotion extends into the activities of all health agencies and into the practice of every physician. It requires not only psychiatrists but also the talents of health and welfare officers, physicians, hospital administrators, psychologists, social workers, public health nurses, sociologists, and others who deal directly with people. This includes leaders in the school, the church, and law enforcement agencies.

It has been estimated(1) that one out of every twelve Americans will be hospitalized for mental illness during a lifetime. At the present time one half of the hospital beds of the nation are used for the treatment of mental diseases. Most of this cost falls on the community. Even these startling facts do not indicate the suffering of individuals and families because of the prolonged and disrupting nature of mental illness. Any measure that might possibly prevent mental disease, promote mental health, or aid in treatment and rehabilitation of mentally ill patients is worthy of very serious consideration.

The growing magnitude of the mental health problem is due not to an increase in mental disease but to a realization of existing needs and better understanding of an approach to a solution of these needs. Other factors are the increased proportion of older persons in the community, increased urbanization, and increasing longevity of patients who are mentally ill.

Even the dimensions of the problem are hard to determine. The concept "mental disorder" is not uniformly defined nor are statistics on hospitalization of various categories of the mentally ill adequate.

It seems probable that the greatest needs are: (a) carefully planned and well-supported research in all aspects of mental health, (b) optimum application of the measures already known to be most effective in rehabilitation of the mentally ill.

376

Established traditions in the handling of mental illness are firmly fixed and will be modified slowly. The basic plan of hospitalizing mental patients in large institutions for the purpose of prolonged custodial care without active effort toward therapy and rehabilitation is archaic but well established in most states. This policy is changing in many areas.

TABLE 36

First Admissions and Resident Patients in Public Prolonged-care Hospitals for Mental Disease*

RATES PER 100,000 CIVILIAN POPULATION

Diagnosis	First Admissions		Resident Patients	
	1940	1957	1940	1957
All mental disorders	64.8	70.9	340.6	324.0
Schizophrenic disorders	14.3	16.9	162.8	164.6
Disorders of old age	14.4	17.9	42.6	44.4
Organic disorders Congenital syphilis, epilepsy, mental deficiencies, etc.	10.8	4.2	66.8	50.6
Affective disorders Manic-depressive psychosis, involutional psychosis.	8.5	5.6	35.4	27.2
Alcoholism; drug addiction	6.8	11.0	11.2	11.6
Psychoneurosis	3.4	6.4	9.2	6.8
All others	6.6	9.0	12.6	18.8

*Adapted from *Hospitalized Mental Illness in the U.S.*, Health Information Foundation, 1960, **IX**.

HOSPITALIZED MENTAL ILLNESS IN THE UNITED STATES

During the past twenty years in the United States, a change has occurred in the policy of hospitalizing patients with mental illness. The trend has been to admit more patients and to discharge them more rapidly (see Table 36).

The data from Table 36 show that more than one half the residents of these hospitals suffer from schizophrenic disorders, but this group comprises only a small portion of first admissions. The largest number of first admissions are suffering from the disorders of old age. In fact, in some areas where the proportion of persons over 64 has reached 10 per cent of the population the hospital admissions of elderly persons constitute 40 to 50 per cent of total admissions. This gives us an index of our future problem, since it is estimated that by 1980, the entire population of the United States will have a ratio of 10 per cent of persons over 65 years of age.

Categories of Mental Illness

Since we have no real knowledge of the etiology of most types of mental disease and no clear-cut clinical criteria that aid in differentiation of various types of mental illness, it becomes quite difficult to categorize the diverse mental disturbances encountered by a physician in his medical practice. The following outline is adapted from Lemkau's text, *Mental Hygiene in Public Health*(2):

1. Mental diseases due to brain injury.
   These include infection (e. g., syphilis), trauma, nutritional deprivation, and toxins.
2. Degenerative changes of the brain.
   a. Senile changes.
   b. The effects of cerebral arteriosclerosis.
   c. Certain (rare) neurological diseases.
3. Mental deficiencies of varying grades.
   a. Idiots.
   b. Imbeciles.
   c. Morons.
4. Convulsive disorders.
   Epilepsy and degenerative conditions.
5. Psychoses.
   a. Schizophrenia.
   b. Manic-depressive syndromes.
6. Psychopathic personality.
   This group is not a clear-cut category. Thus comparative prevalence statistics are of no value since the diagnosis is dependent upon the definition of the investigator. A definition sometimes given is: "Difficult persons who repeatedly commit the same type of antisocial acts, who do not learn from past experience, and fail to respond to usual types of appeal." They are said to have a constitutional character deficiency. This is obviously a social, rather than a clinical definition.

Examples are certain criminal types, alcoholics, drug addicts, and sexual psychopaths.

7. Behavior disorders of children and adolescents.
8. Neuroses.
    Psychosomatic disorders.

Preventive Aspects of Mental Disease

Our present knowledge concerning the causes that produce or predispose to feeblemindedness and to psychoses is so limited that there is little utility in speculation upon the value of preventive medicine in these conditions. The administrators of mental hospitals, and particularly the legislators, are most anxious that active community-wide preventive measures be undertaken to reduce the very high cost to the community for the institutional care of persons with psychoses and with mental defectiveness. There are many suitable administrative procedures to assist in cost reduction in the care of mental illness, but these measures cannot have much influence on prevention of mental disease.

However, a limited number of preventive measures can be applied most successfully in specific situations.

Prevention of Mental Disease Due to Brain Injury

Real advances have been made in the prevention of mental disorders due to brain injury. General paresis due to untreated syphilis has almost disappeared from mental disease hospital admissions. Improvements in prenatal care and in the techniques of childbirth have also had a beneficial result. Pellagra and other nutritional deficiencies as a cause of brain injury have diminished, and the industrial toxins that caused so much anxiety in the past are now largely eliminated, e.g., lead encephalopathy.

In this category of mental disease, real progress has been made and we can anticipate further gains.

1. Prevention of General Paresis. Adequate and prompt treatment of early syphilis will greatly reduce general paresis. Beginning about 1930, the U.S. Public Health Service assumed strong leadership in the prevention of syphilis. It has provided aid to all the states in the development of venereal disease control programs. Extensive diagnostic and therapeutic clinic services have been developed, and good epidemiologic work has been undertaken in order to find sources of infection and to bring all cases of syphilis under effective treatment. Already, within 30 years after their initiation, these efforts have resulted in a reduction in admissions to hospitals for cerebral syphilis. The effect undoubtedly will be cumulative. In fact, general paresis will probably be a rare disease in the United States by the year 1975.

2. Heredity. There is definite evidence that the common forms of mental disease have some basis in heredity. The actual disease may not be transmitted directly from parent to child, but the tendency toward mental instability is inherited. It seems not at all improbable for example, that inheritance of schizophrenia and manic-depressive disorders may be comparable, in some degree, to inheritance of epilepsy.

Lennox(3) has shown that epilepsy is not inherited, but that a susceptibility to epilepsy is inheritable.

Electroencephalographic studies have demonstrated a cerebral dysrhythmia which is an index of predisposition to fits. The patterns of these waves have individuality. Lennox studied 312 members of the immediate family of an epileptic: 52 per cent had abnormal tracings. In the general population fewer than 10 per cent have abnormal brain waves. Thus, in a family in which there is a history of epilepsy, the person who has an epileptic predisposition, as indicated by an abnormal EEG, should not marry a person who has a similar dysrhythmia but should select a normal spouse.

Many students of heredity have claimed that certain mental defective conditions are a definitely inherited trait. The conclusion is that the moron should not be allowed to marry and reproduce his kind. But many psychiatrists of high repute have expressed doubt concerning the claim that heredity is an important factor in the production of feeblemindedness.

The Mentally Defective

About 14 children in every 1,000 births in the United States may be classified as mentally defective. The customary classification is:

1. Idiots. They have a mental age of under three years, an IQ of about 25. They comprise 5 per cent of the total.

2. Imbeciles. They have a mental age of more than three years and less than eight years, with an IQ of 25 to 49. Twenty per cent of the mentally defective are imbeciles.

3. Morons. This group makes up 75 per cent of the total. They have an IQ of 49 to 70. They are incapable of receiving instruction in ordinary schools and will require supervision and control throughout life.

It is generally believed that moderate mental deficiency depends upon genetic and, to some degree, environmental factors. The parents may have low intelligence. Many mental defectives do not require institutionalization, and some may be trained to useful and productive lives.

Idiots and imbeciles usually come from normal parents. In most instances the defect is due to perinatal brain injury.

Most mental defectives can be cared for in the community. Approximately 100,000 are institutionalized in the United States. Of these, 20 per cent are idiots, 40 per cent imbeciles, and 40 per cent low-grade morons.

PREVENTIVE ASPECTS OF ALCOHOLISM

Alcoholism is a chronic devastating disease of great import, which is so insidious in its onset that often the patient is not aware that he is seriously sick. In many instances, by the time the patient has reached the hospital or the psychiatrist, the disease has advanced to such a degree that little can be accomplished toward its cure. On the other hand, alcoholism, when properly understood and skillfully treated in its initial stages, is often subject to preventive measures and sometimes to complete cure. No practitioner of medicine can escape the problem of chronic alcoholism. Since the general practitioner is usually the first person who is called upon to treat the disease in its earliest stages, it is most pertinent to present a discussion of alcoholism from the preventive point of view.

Prevalence of Alcoholism

The actual incidence of alcoholism in the United States is not known. Reliable estimates indicate that six or seven out of every 100 adults in the United States seem to find it impossible to be moderate drinkers. One in ten of this group will become a chronic alcoholic. The disease prevails in all walks of life and is not, predominantly, a disease of the poor, the ignorant, and the lower social levels.

Alcoholism is related in some degree to social and economic conditions. There are indications that the disease is more prevalent in the United States than in the Mediterranean countries, or in Belgium, the Netherlands, or England. This might be related in part to higher economic status, which brings about the ability to purchase more alcohol. Racial factors and social customs also have a profound influence upon the incidence of the disease. Some psychiatrists claim that there is a certain type of personality which is predisposed to alcoholism. This might be true, but a person becomes an alcoholic not solely because of his personality but in relation also to the particular life situations and difficulties that he may encounter.

The Nature of Alcoholism

There is no chronic disease less understood, particularly by the relatives of the patients, than chronic alcoholism. No sick person is given less sympathy and aid by his fellow men than the alcoholic addict or the abnormal drinker, largely because the disease is considered a character defect, rather than a pathologic condition.

Alcoholism is not a disease entity but rather a symptom of an underlying condition. Behind all abnormal drinking is some abnormal psychologic process.

A common type of alcoholic is the psychotic person who presents alcoholism as one of his prominent symptoms. This symptom can occur in persons with schizophrenia, with manic-depressive disorder, in epileptics, and in early paretics. The person with manic-depressive psychosis usually drinks excessively only in the downward swing from excitement to depression. Individuals in these categories might be termed pure symptomatic alcoholics because of the obvious relationship of alcoholism to the underlying disease.

Another group of alcoholics drinks because the effect of the alcohol fills a definite personality need.

In some, alcohol furnishes a relief from nervous tension and mental fatigue.

Other alcoholics find that the drug brings relief from an intolerable life situation. They cannot face reality but are able to secure, for a time at least, an escape from an unhappy situation by means of alcoholic bouts.

Perhaps the most common type of alcoholic is the compensating drinker, whose alcoholism is motivated predominately by feelings of inferiority that are on a deep-seated, perhaps quite unconscious, level.

Case 1. C. L. was a chemist who entered the hospital with the complaint of alcoholism and loss of memory.

He worked in one chemical plant for 22 years, rising gradually from assistant chemist to foreman. He expected to be appointed general manager, but instead an outside chemist was selected for the position. On that day he returned home much shaken and weeping. He began to drink immediately thereafter. He dropped his hobbies of carpentry and music, and became irritable, anxious, and insecure. He broke his social contacts but continued his work in the factory. Each evening for the next 14 years, he would go to his basement after supper and drink from a pint to a quart of whisky. He lost his appetite and began to fail physically. During this period he made repeated efforts to stop drinking.

During the past summer he asked his family, before they went on vacation, to throw out all the alcohol in the house, and assured them he would stop drinking. On their return they found he had subsisted almost entirely on alcohol during August, and was becoming disoriented and very forgetful.

The patient was 58 years of age when he entered the hospital. He had been a favorite child, idolized by his mother, who had always given him his own way. His father was a strict disciplinarian, who did not permit the boy to plan a career in opera, as the boy desired, but insisted that he become a chemist. The young man developed a rigid personality, became obstinate, proud, sentimental, autocratic, and emotionally somewhat unstable. He was happily married to a weak, submissive, uncomplaining wife, who has been grief-stricken by his illness.

Apparently the crisis of his life was his failure to realize his personal ambition in becoming general manager of the factory. It left him with a feeling of insecurity and hurt pride, which was compensated by alcohol.

His physical examination revealed a man with marked arteriosclerosis and a peripheral neuritis, which was relieved by treatment with thiamine and niacin. He also had a definite enlargement of the liver.

Through indirect education, the patient began, in retrospect, to analyze his disease in relation to his life situation. He placed emphasis upon his narrow pattern of living, his obstinacy, his desire to succeed, his feeling of hurt pride, insecurity, resentment, and depression, with anxiety, which led directly to recourse to alcohol. Understanding of the situation enabled him to face his life clearly, with satisfactory therapeutic results.

Case 2. A. J. was a young scientist with excellent university connections and real promise of a career in his chosen field. He was independently wealthy, and was happily married with three children. He was somewhat temperamental, "high-strung," and emotionally unstable. During the financial depression his family lost their money, and it became necessary for him to lower his standard of living materially. He had always been a convivial drinker but never became intoxicated. After his financial reverses, he began to drink heavily. He neglected his scientific work, sometimes coming to his laboratory in an intoxicated condition. A crisis was reached when he developed a peripheral neuritis which required hospitalization.

Thiamine and abstinence relieved the peripheral neuritis, but only after some time was it possible for the psychiatrist to aid him in facing the reality: (a) that he was actually ill; (b) that the diagnosis was alcoholism; and, finally,

(c) that his future career was dependent upon self-realization that he alone could initiate the desire to recover from his *illness*. Once the patient understood the situation fully and developed a sincere desire for rehabilitation, his determination, with the aid of sympathetic associates, was maintained, and his alcoholism was cured.

Relapses are common in this type of alcoholism. The patient cannot relax his vigilance for an instant. In order to avoid disaster, he can never take another drink as long as he lives.

The following case represents an entirely different type of alcoholism:

Case 3. J. G. was a 43-year-old white woman who came to the hospital with a complaint of periodic alcoholism.

Twenty years ago, at the time her father died, she began to experience extreme fatigue toward the end of the day. This was overcome by 4 oz of whisky. Four years later, following a period of quarrels with her husband, she increased her intake to a pint or more of liquor daily. This period was marked by her ability to be abstemious for weeks or months at a time.

She began to have sudden episodic anxiety periods, accompanied by severe palpitation and a fear of impending death. Her alcoholism manifested itself by long periods of abstinence, followed by short periods of heavy drinking. Usually the attack was precipitated by some emotional stress, such as a quarrel with her husband.

The patient had a stormy childhood. Her mother had paranoid manifestations of psychosis. The child was sent to a convent at six years, and felt rejected and alone. Her father became a severe alcoholic during his appointment as judge of the state supreme court. Her only brother also became an alcoholic. She was unhappily married at 18 years of age, was sexually frigid, and has had no children.

Extensive psychotherapy proved to be of great value. She was able to determine that her anxiety began in a setting of insecurity, disappointment in her marriage, and her sexual unrest. Her inferiority was traced to sibling rivalry. Her fears of impending death were due to guilt because of an abortion she had had performed, following extramarital indulgence. Psychiatric·care resulted in relief of tension and resentment, with an increase in self-confidence. She has adjusted herself well to her life situation.

Case 4 (the Periodic Drinker). L. S. is a physician of 58 years who holds an important administrative position. He has carried out his duties and responsibilities very well. Since early manhood he has been addicted to periodic bouts of alcoholism. He works steadily and effectively for three to five months. During this period he drinks no alcohol. Gradually he has a feeling of rising tension and a compelling impulse to drink. On these occasions, he leaves his office, and his secretary informs everyone that he is out of town on business. He registers in a hotel in another city, and then, quietly and systematically, he drinks to excess for five or six days. During this time, he eats no food. At the end of this period he emerges from his retreat, thoroughly shaken and in bad physical condition, but with a complete release of nervous tension, and ready for another period of abstinence and excellent administrative work.

There is no satisfactory method of prevention or treatment for this type of alcoholism. The addicts frequently live long and useful lives.

Treatment of Alcoholism

The treatment of alcoholism and the prevention of future attacks depend upon a proper analysis of the underlying cause of the disease.

Drug therapy has been widely used: it consists essentially of the formation of a conditioned reflex, by giving the patient an emetic simultaneously with his alcohol. The taste of alcohol then becomes an unpleasant experience. This form of treatment produces a certain number of cures but is not a satisfactory technique, since it does not remove the basic causes that have produced the condition. Usually the patient returns to the same environment that produced his alcoholism and sooner or later has a relapse.

Alcoholics Anonymous is an organization of former alcoholics that have been cured by a fundamental religious conversion. They work as a group to help each other to maintain the cure. They welcome a drinker into their group if he manifests a desire to be cured, and they help him to build up his self-esteem and to conquer his disease; they aid him in getting a job and in maintaining abstinence. They have effected many cures. The members of this group work very effectively with physicians in helping them with patients who belong to this organization in controlling their urge to drink.

Psychotherapy has advanced enormously in recent years in its effectiveness, and in the understanding of the proper therapy of alcoholism. Psychotherapy determines the underlying cause of the disease and utilizes all procedures which may influence favorably the attitude of the patient toward himself, his illness, and his environment. The great difficulty with psychotherapy is that it is complex, requiring time and money. There are few available hospitals for treatment of these conditions, and most patients do not have sufficient funds to remain in these hospitals long enough to complete their treatment.

COMMUNITY RESPONSIBILITY FOR PREVENTION AND REHABILITATION OF ALCOHOLISM

Most state hospitals for mental illness restrict admission to alcoholics with definite psychoses. Usually the mental disease is the primary cause of illness, and alcoholism is a symptom.

General hospitals, including public hospitals, have in the past refused to accept alcoholics. This condition is changing since tranquilizing drugs and other therapeutic measures make it possible to control the irrational and disturbed patient. The American Medical Association has recommended that general hospitals accept alcoholics where there is a medical need and has prepared a *Manual on Alcoholism*(4) as a guide to general hospitals.

"Halfway houses" have been provided by some communities. These are rehabilitation centers which give an alcoholic opportunity for gradual readjustment to normal community life. These centers are most successful when incorporated into a basic program of community mental health promotion.

Industry has played an important role in prevention and rehabilitation of alcoholism. Many of the large medical services of industrial corporations have made strong efforts to detect early alcoholism in their own personnel. It is estimated that 2 to 3 per cent of the personnel of any large industry can be aided by these programs. The Consultation Clinic on Alcoholism(5) of the Bellevue Medical Center in New York City devotes its entire efforts to this problem. It accepts only those patients referred to it by certain large industrial companies. The clinic has reported highly satisfactory results.

A study by a large industry (6) showed that about 3 per cent of its working force was alcoholic. The alcoholics received 3 times the normal sickness benefits, showed 3 times the normal accident rate, and 2.5 times absenteeism. The company's remedial plan was simple and relatively inexpensive. Nine hundred and fifty alcoholics were uncovered. Each case was treated as an illness; 65 per cent were rehabilitated, 23 per cent improved, and 11 per cent unchanged. Conclusions were that it is important to start treatment in the early stages of the illness, thus preventing serious physical and mental disability.

Community Clinics

Outpatient clinics of many general hospitals have organized special clinics for treatment of alcoholism. Usually the clinic is an integral part of the division of mental health. These clinics can be of great value to private physicians in evaluating the special problems involved with a difficult patient and in outlining subsequent therapy.

In essence, however, the handling of patients with alcoholism, the prevention and treatment of alcoholism, and rehabilitation of the patient are the responsibility of the practicing physician. He should utilize all available community resources, but the responsibility rests with him and depends upon his knowledge, skill, sympathy, and understanding.

General Educational Measures

The entire population should be well informed concerning the great dangers of alcoholism. This information must be presented in a sensible, effective way, devoid of the fanaticism and overstatement that so often accompany the propaganda of the exponents of complete restriction of the manufacture and sale of alcoholic beverages. Alcoholism in each individual must be recognized for what it is — an individual disease which may become a very serious medical problem.

The National Society for Research in the Problems of Alcohol is a serious group of representative scientists and businessmen who are not only studying the social and medical aspects of alcohol consumption and addiction, but are also concerned with the necessity of suitable popular education in relation to the whole nation-wide problem of alcoholic addiction. This organization should, under wise guidance, be of great benefit in the promotion of a real understanding of the various and most complicated economic, social, and medical problems related to the human consumption of alcohol.

Other Drug Addictions

The physician has a great responsibility, in the field of preventive medicine, in relation to prevention of drug addiction. He is the one person permitted by law to prescribe habit-forming drugs for the treatment of illness. He must exercise this function with greatest discretion. The prescription of sedatives and habit-forming drugs can be a very valuable therapeutic measure, but in certain individuals it may, unless safeguarded, lead to serious difficulty and perhaps permanent injury. In such a case the practicing physician is in a position to prevent mental disorder by effective negative measures.

Nutritional Deficiency in Mental Disorder

In areas in the United States where pellagra prevails, psychosis is encountered as a direct complication of vitamin B complex deficiency. Therefore community educational measures in promotion of sound nutrition, as well as mass procedures undertaken by the community to improve vitamin B deficiency states, inevitably aid in prevention of the psychoses resulting from those conditions.

THE SCOPE OF MENTAL HYGIENE

What is the field of mental hygiene, and how can it be of service to the community? Let us approach the field not from the point of view of mental disease but in the interests of the normal people in the nation who at some time or another in their lives have some degree of emotional dysfunction and need assistance and sympathetic understanding. It must be remembered that just as every person is susceptible to acute infectious disease, such as measles or influenza, so also is every individual susceptible to some degree to emotional maladjustment at some time during his life.

Definition of Mental Hygiene

Mental hygiene can be defined as that science and art which aids the individual in securing a satisfactory mental and emotional adjustment to his environment. This definition refers, of course, to all of us — everyone in the community — not only those who manifest actual psychosis. In certain instances, it deals with the individual who actually has mental disease, e.g., home placement of persons who have recovered from mental disease and are ready to leave the hospital — that is a mental hygiene function. This service falls within our definition. But mental hygiene is concerned much more with the potentially normal person, and particularly is it interested in those who constitute the "borderline of psychiatry."

Thus mental hygiene guides the potentially normal individual in understanding himself in relation to others and in meeting his own situation. Perhaps a more appropriate term might be emotional, rather than mental, hygiene since it is not the individual's mental but rather his emotional processes that are most benefited by application of the principles of mental hygiene.

Mental Hygiene in Early Childhood

The practicing physician, the public health nurse, and the well-baby clinic are continually presented with the behavior problems of infants and young children. Seldom are these difficulties serious enough to suggest the necessity of referral to a psychiatrist, yet they are a great trouble and worry to the parent and, if not solved, can result in permanent damage to the life of the child.

The symptoms may at first be apparently insignificant, such as thumb-sucking, bed-wetting, or poor food habits. As the child grows older, the personality difficulty may be evidenced by other more serious functional disturbances, as malnutrition, with anemia, anorexia, and severe constipation. The child may present "behavior" difficulties, with temper tantrums, abnormal fears, or night terror. He may evince cruelty to animals or to small children, destructiveness, stealing, or abnormal jealousy of brothers and sisters.

These manifestations are symptoms of an underlying difficulty: The source of the child's emotional disturbance can almost always be traced to parental attitudes.

The normal child must depend on his parents, or upon some substitute for parents, for the foundation of his emotional balance. He must be able to build within himself:

1. A feeling of competence.
2. A sense of security.
3. A proper adjustment to his environment.

If the parent does not provide the child with these essentials, or if there is a lack of understanding of the needs of the child, or if there is an emotional instability on the part of the parents, then the growing child is under a serious handicap.

Child guidance clinics have found that the great proportion of "problem" children come from broken homes, where one or both of the parents are dead, or where the parents are separated or divorced. It has been noted time and again that if the parents have been unable to adjust themselves to a normal home situation, the children of that home are vulnerable to emotional maladjustment.

The most common faults of parents in dealing with their growing children are overindulgence, oversolicitude, and overprotection. Under these circumstances, the child remains infantile in his emotional development and does not become independent and self-confident. Some parents, on the other hand, are unduly stern and Spartan, with no warmth or affection. This driving, perfectionist attitude, with severe discipline, can crush the spirit of the sensitive child. Lack of attention on the part of parents, their failure to understand the point of view and to sympathize with the child, and inability to realize those things of importance to children can be the cause of serious emotional maladjustment. Quarreling and dissension on the part of parents always bring perplexity, insecurity, and unhappiness to the children.

These simple principles of family management are well recognized by physicians, public health nurses, social workers, and teachers as well as by others dealing with problem children, such as the staffs of child guidance clinics and juvenile courts. But many parents do not realize their own importance in the establishment of the normal emotional development of their children.

Children Unwanted and Unplanned For. We have noted in Chapter 2, on population trends, that in an urbanized civilization each additional child in a family lowers the standard of living of that family. We also noted that many parents did not have sufficient knowledge of contraceptive methods to enable them to work out a successful and satisfactory family plan, with suitable spacing of children in accordance with the family situation. The result is often an unwanted and unplanned-for child. This child may be rejected by the family as a whole or by one or both parents, to the great ultimate detriment of the child.

The family physician is often the key person in the correction of these situations. He is the one consulted first in matters of childhood emotional maladjustment. He deals with these situations in their incipiency. Thus an intelligent and understanding physician, an alert public health nurse, a sympathetic schoolteacher—all can play important roles in the promotion of mental hygiene of the young child.

Juvenile Delinquency. The prevention of juvenile delinquency is a social rather than a medical problem. Nevertheless, the physician practicing in any community has a definite responsibility in this field.

Juvenile delinquency is only an index of an underlying social situation. Increase of juvenile delinquency may represent simply a greater attention on the part of the community to an ever-present situation, or it may indicate an increase in intensity of social and economic factors that tend to disturb the balance of mental and emotional development of the adolescent. It is a social phenomenon, subject to social control; it is not a function of mental hygiene, but the physician with insight and understanding can be of assistance in the prevention of tragedies in the life of the individual child under his purview.

A majority of delinquent children do not belong to a constitutionally psychopathic inferior group. They are normal children who become delinquent because of emotional and environmental stresses with which they are unable to cope. Bad housing, unsanitary living conditions, poverty, and lack of parental supervision are important contributory factors. More than one half of these children come from broken homes; where the parents live together, there is often serious parental maladjustment. A child can feel neglected or discriminated against; he might have difficulties with schoolwork or have some physical handicap that sets him apart from other children. Most delinquents come from particular sections of a city with overcrowding and poor housing. Delinquency occurs to a considerable extent in the families of the well-to-do; it is not limited to the poor. Although it may not be brought to the attention of the police or to the children's court, the situation is frequently presented to the family physician for solution. The underlying factors in delinquency in wealthy families do not differ from those encountered in poor families.

The physician is often asked to examine a child who has been delinquent and to determine the liability of a child toward subsequent delinquency. The initial delinquent should be studied and classified by the physician with care, giving due consideration to the home and parental situation. Is he a mental or physical cripple? Has he a low-grade mentality? Has he a psychosis following encephalitis or other infection? If the child is of the "habitual criminal" type, then measures must be taken to protect society and to protect the patient as well from further difficulty.

The great proportion of these initial delinquents, however, should and do become useful citizens. The primary responsibility for return to normal attitudes rests upon the parents and the home. But the community can supplement the parents' efforts by providing supervised recreational centers and promoting the normal channels of juvenile activity through boys' and girls' clubs. It is important to give the children some community responsibility, such as the Youth Service Corps in England, in which children are made to feel they belong to the community and have a personal responsibility for community welfare.

The school has a definite part in prevention of delinquency, the church also can be of great assistance in this field.

The physician's major job is to determine which of the children are normal and which are feebleminded or constitutionally inferior; then suitable preventive measures for each child can be prescribed in accordance with individual needs.

The important thing to remember is that juvenile delinquency for the most part is a symptom of social, economic, or emotional stress which, if analyzed and diagnosed in its incipiency, lends itself admirably to preventive measures.

Child Guidance Clinics. Although the child guidance community service can be organized in the local department of health, it is more commonly incorporated in the department of education. The usual procedure is as follows:

The teacher selects those children with special emotional or mental difficulties. Perhaps the child has done excellent schoolwork for a period, then begins to lose interest or fails in his school assignments. Perhaps the child is lazy, or a truant, or has been caught stealing. The child is referred to the psychiatric social worker assigned to the school. This field worker then makes a careful study of the situation, including a study of the home. Often the problem is a simple one, readily solved. The more difficult situations are referred to a child psychiatrist. The family may take the child to a private specialist or referral may be made to the psychiatric staff of the child guidance clinic.

Psychiatric Advisory Service. Correction of the more difficult adjustment situations is an important function of the psychiatrist. He can aid only a few of these children since each case requires long hours of study and therapy. Thus the children referred to him must be selected with care.

A much more important function of the psychiatrist in the realm of mental hygiene is the psychiatric advice and training that he gives to schoolteachers, public health nurses, child guidance clinic personnel, social workers, church workers, girls' and boys' club directors, school physicians, juvenile court personnel, private physicians, and all other persons engaged professionally in the care and guidance of children in the mass.

The heavy load of the mental hygiene activities of any community must be carried by those persons who have direct and frequent contact with children. Obviously, as in all other preventive measures, the earlier the techniques are instituted, the simpler they can be and the more easily applied.

Martin(7) has stated that there are no "problem" children but rather "problems of children." All children have problems. His concept is that the "behavior" child is trying to solve his situation by extreme measures. The most common problems of children are:

1. Rejection of the child by one or both parents.
2. Overprotection by parents.
3. Exploitation or excessive demands by parents.
4. Deprivation of parental guidance because of broken homes or the illness of mother or father.
5. Rivalry in the home or school.
6. Male preference on the part of the parent.

7. Erratic discipline by parents.

8. Possessive love, usually on the part of the mother.

The striking feature of this list is that these faults are not the fault of the child but of the parent. The child has to meet a situation with which he is unable to cope, and a "problem" child results.

Mental Hygiene of the Adolescent

The average physician who deals with the adolescent boy or girl in private practice is prone to consider solely the physical health of his patient. School physicians also fall into this same error, forgetting that the behavior of the child, as well as his physical development and mental and emotional reactions, may be dependent upon, or related to, a faulty and insecure social adjustment.

To understand a child, it is necessary to interpret his point of view. What are his attitudes toward: (a) his own body; (b) his classmates of the same sex; (c) his associates of the opposite sex; (d) older people, including his attitude toward work, and his progress in formulating a life plan.

Attitude Toward His Body. Adolescents are always highly dissatisfied with their own bodies. They are too fat or too thin, too tall or too short; their feet are too big, their hair is the wrong color, their skin the wrong texture. This dissatisfaction simply represents a fundamental fact that they are uncertain as to whether they are developing normally and will become successful persons attractive to the opposite sex.

Attitude Toward His Fellows. In early adolescence, the child becomes involved with a group of his fellows—a gang. He is loyal to his group; secret societies are formed from which elders are excluded; he takes on their special language and behavior. This is an attempt on the part of the preadolescent to establish himself as a member of an independent group, and to withdraw from the protection of his family. It is a normal emotional reaction, and should be encouraged and guided rather than checked and misinterpreted by his family.

Parents frequently do not understand the desires of the adolescent to establish himself as an independent person. They are confused because the child tries to develop his independence while wanting to retain the security provided at home. Parents often try to hold and protect their children as long as possible from the outside world and from their outside associates. Quite normally, the parents feel that the other adolescents who associate with their children are "not good enough for them." This leads to conflict between parents and children, with misunderstanding; often with manifestations of bad social behavior or physical incapacity.

The rapidity of growth of an adolescent boy or girl is an extraordinary phenomenon. Mental and emotional development cannot keep pace with physical growth. Out of the discrepancy grow conflicts, since too much is expected of the child. He is expected to perform those physical and mental tasks that an adult can carry out readily, but of which the adolescent is quite incapable. Conflicts arise between the child and his parents—conflicts with associates, with the general environment, sometimes conflicts with community authorities and the laws.

It is the function of the physician to aid the adolescent in understanding himself and in adjusting himself to his own particular situation. For example, the physical examination, carried out in a private office or as part of a school health program, should be an educational experience for the adolescent. Explanation concerning the phenomena of his rapid development is in order, and assurance given that his development has been normal: that he will grow to be a capable man. His home and school situation should be appraised in order to learn whether he has a sound attitude toward his fellows, his elders, and his future career; also whether his family tends to overprotect him or to exploit his talent and ability.

At no period in a child's life is there greater need for sympathetic understanding and help than during adolescence. No greater opportunity will be offered to the family physician to give substantial assistance to a young and potentially splendid individual at a critical period in his physical and emotional development. The wise understanding and personal guidance of a physician in whom the adolescent has confidence can yield an abundant harvest in the field of mental hygiene.

Sexual Guidance.* Sexual guidance should be planned in accordance with the age of the individual. It should therefore include advice to parents so that they are able to handle constructively any sexual interests or activities of their children. Recognizing the frequency of masturbatory activities (especially in minor forms) even in early childhood, parents should be willing to correct them by distraction and the removal of anxiety-producing situations rather than by dis-

*The paragraphs on sexual guidance were kindly prepared for this text by Dr. Oskar Diethelm, professor emeritus of psychiatry at Cornell University Medical College.

ciplinary action. It is a sound principle to answer truthfully every question of the child in such a way that he can understand. It is not wise to offer more than the child can comprehend readily. Books written by physicians and educators can be a helpful guide to child and parents. It is now an accepted fact that every child should be prepared for the occurrence of puberty by his parents, physician, schoolteacher, or other well-qualified person. Comprehensive information can be given to the child at an appropriate time. Additional information should be presented later in adolescence and before marriage.

Sexual hygiene should be based on the fact that physiologic and psychobiologic factors must be integrated, i.e., the physical and the love aspects should be combined. A persistent separation of these aspects leads to sexual maladjustment and dissatisfaction. The resorting to prolonged promiscuity and prostitution should be considered a sign of unsatisfactory mental health. Marriage and the formation of a family unit are therefore the natural goals of sexual desires and activities.

In puberty, sexual information makes possible an orientation to the occurrence of spontaneous erections and seminal discharge, especially with dreams, and to menstruation. The stimulating role of imagination on physiologic functions must be recognized if the person wishes to obtain satisfactory control of sexual unrest. This fact is important for the control of masturbation in adolescence and of promiscuity desires in adult life. The occurrence of a phase of masturbation in practically every male and in a considerable number of female adolescents obliges the physician to include an orientation to this problem in his sexual guidance. He should stress the fact that the occurrence was a passing incident which should not dominate the young person's preoccupations.

In adolescence, a transient inclination to homosexual attachments or even overt homosexual activities are not necessarily alarming. By stressing the essential privacy which should surround any sexual activity, parents can protect adolescents, to some degree, from undesirable involvements. It is obvious that this type of guidance depends more on the instruction of teachers of adolescents than on instruction by physicians of the individual adolescent.

In offering advice on marriage, the physician should emphasize the need to consider the partner's desires and to be willing to space sexual activities. If this rule is kept in mind and if sexual life is not considered of paramount importance, individuals will find spontaneously a sexual life suitable to both partners.

In the fifth decade, many persons go through a period of sexual restlessness which can greatly disturb them. An understanding physician should inform those persons of the general rules of sexual hygiene and offer practical suggestions for indicated adjustments that should solve each person's problem. Menopause is often dreaded because it is believed that it means the termination of sexual life and implies nervous complications. The physician should correct these erroneous beliefs and any others connected with age-old folklore of sex. Education of the population is necessary for better sexual guidance. This education should consider psychologic and physiologic facts. In personal guidance, one must of course consider the individual's ethical concepts and religious convictions.

Career Guidance. A "career guidance" system has been developed in some high schools which seems to offer great merit as a plan for guidance of the adolescent. Several teachers are carefully selected to aid the youths in planning their careers. Each child is urged to lay out a definite plan for his future, then he is guided in accordance with his mental and physical abilities and interests. If a child has difficulty in adapting himself to his life situation, the "career counselor" can be of great help. A psychiatrist might be recommended by the counselor, but here the mental specialist enters the picture as a friend to help in career guidance rather than as an alien trying to determine whether the youth has an abnormal mentality.

Psychiatric consulation is the key to success in this service, but the consultation is given for the most part to the guidance counselors rather than to the children. Only in the more difficult situations is it necessary for the psychiatrist to see the patient. Here again the chief function of the psychiatrist is to give advice and guidance to those responsible for direct care and supervision of the children.

Mental Hygiene at the College Level

College health services usually give complete medical, hospital, and nursing care. The directors of well-organized services have uncovered the essential fact that one of the most important activities of a college health service is mental hygiene. As Fry(8) has pointed out, the college age coincides with the climax of adolescent changes in the physical, emotional, and intellectual spheres. The object of mental hygiene in college is to increase the feeling of security and independence in the individual by aiding in the achievement of mature self-management. The students are sometimes referred to the mental hygiene clinic through the initial physical examination of the freshmen. Many come voluntarily; others are referred by faculty, by friends, by student counselors, or sometimes through the dean's office. Many of the situations encountered are the result of the bad study habits of the student or personal problems of a minor nature, and these can often be handled by the student counselor. Only the more difficult problems are referred to the psychiatrist. The results in this field have been most encouraging and point the way to a broader application of this method of approach.

Mental Hygiene in Adult Life

Neuroses. This category of emotional disturbance is by far the most common type of mental illness. It has been estimated that from 1 to 5 per cent of the population suffers from neuroses to a sufficient degree to reduce the efficiency of daily living. It is three times more prevalent in women than in men and is more common in the lower economic strata of society.

The neuroses are characterized by anxiety and fear, and are magnified by economic and social stress.

The physician encounters this type of emotional disorder in all phases of his medical practice, and his success as a practitioner depends in great part on his ability to handle these situations with sympathy and understanding. It is in this category of mental illness that the physician can receive greatest assistance from psychiatric consultation.

Mental Health in Old Age

The most common types of mental illness in elderly people are senile psychosis and cerebral arteriosclerosis with psychosis.

We do not know the prevalence of this type of illness in the community. As already noted, the new admissions to some of the public, long-term mental hospitals now comprise 40 per cent of the total admissions. There are more males than females, even though females greatly outnumber males in our older age groups. There are also more Negroes than whites, relative to the population, and more patients from the lower economic levels (metropolitan dwellers predominantly). These phenomena are probably due to social factors rather than unbalanced incidence.

For the most part, the aged senile patients are sent to the state hospital for mental illness to receive custodial care until they die.

Rehabilitation of the Patient with Senile Psychosis. It may seem futile even to suggest that an irreversible process such as brain damage due to faulty blood supply can be benefited by rehabilitation procedures. We now have good evidence, however, that maintenance of function by adequate stimulation can be secured so that the atrophy of disuse does not occur. Many authorities now feel that elderly people should not be sent to large state mental hospitals, but should be maintained in their own community; at home, in a foster home, or in a small homelike institution. Nursing care, physiotherapy and occupational therapy should be available.

All the normal aspects of comfortable and dignified living should be available to our senior citizens and can greatly benefit the elderly person who is gradually losing his physical and mental capacities. The emotional crises that occur in some of these patients can be controlled by judicious use of tranquilizing drugs and other adequate therapy.

Perhaps it is true that their senility cannot be prevented nor their life prolonged to any degree, but the elderly do not benefit from commitment to a larger state hospital for final custodial care.

The Role of the Family Physician in Mental Hygiene

The doctor who follows his family groups through two generations is ideally situated to recognize and understand early manifestations of emotional disturbances and perhaps to prevent serious mental breakdown.

All the early manifestations of mental disorders that appear in family life are referred to him; the behavior disorders of the young children and the maladjustments of adolescence are brought to his attention. He is in a key position to understand and aid in the early stages, to correct the minor disturbances, and to refer the more serious cases, when necessary, to a psychiatrist.

The family physician is the repository of confidences dealing with unhappy marriage relationships and with those stresses and tensions of daily life that are a part of a highly competitive social structure. The doctor must insist upon the necessity for attention to a proper balance of work and recreation, and to adequate fulfillment of physical needs.

COMMUNITY RESPONSIBILITY

Trends in Care of the Mentally Ill

In past years, general hospitals did not accept patients with mental illness. A few psychopathic hospitals were organized; some were directly affiliated with general hospitals. The chief purposes of these institutions were (a) diagnosis, (b) prognosis, and (c) initial treatment of mental disease. Long-term care was generally provided by large state hospitals, and the patient often remained in these institutions, under custodial care, for his entire life.

Great advances have been made in care of the mentally ill in recent years. The elements of a community mental health program are as follows:

1. Emphasis should be placed on prevention of emotional disturbances, early recognition of mental disease, adequate diagnosis, and effective treatment.

2. A state-wide comprehensive, well-coordinated plan should be developed through local, state, and federal agencies. This plan calls for continuity in progressive care of the patient.

3. Facilities to meet patient needs should be readily available and accessible to those in need.

4. The facility for care of the emotionally disturbed and the mentally ill should be a part of, or closely affiliated with, the general hospital of the community.

5. Emphasis should be placed on rehabilitation, with return of the patient to his family and community as soon as feasible.

6. Long-term custodial care should be prescribed only when indicated, following intensive treatment.

7. Care of the aged senile, the emotionally disturbed, the mentally retarded, the person with a psychopathic personality, the epileptic, and those in other categories of mental illness should be included in the over-all state and local mental health program.

The General Hospital

The general hospital now plays an important part in the care of the mentally ill. It should accept various types of mentally ill patients, and there should be a qualified psychiatrist on the staff. One great advantage of this plan is that the psychiatrist can serve effectively as consultant to other physicians for those patients in whom emotional stress is an integral part of their physical illness.

In 1949 fewer than 50 general hospitals in the United States admitted persons with mental disease. The number has since risen to more than 1,000; there are also more than 1,500 hospital outpatient departments with facilities for care of emotionally disturbed patients.

The Outpatient Clinic Service

The most important link in care of the mentally ill is the outpatient clinic service. Several large state hospitals have organized "itinerant clinics." A team of staff members makes scheduled visits to communities with no facilities for diagnosis and consultation of patients in need of guidance. These clinics are of special value in follow-up of discharged patients from the mental hospital.

The major functions of the outpatient clinic are early detection of mental disease, consultation with patients who have serious emotional problems, and to a limited degree, therapy. The clinic can be effective in guiding parents in the understanding of emotional problems of childhood. Some clinics have found group therapy to be an effective procedure.

Tranquilizing Drugs

The introduction of a group of tranquilizing drugs has had a most beneficial effect in the handling of emotionally disturbed patients. These drugs do not represent specific therapy for chronic mental disorders. Their chief effect is to control anxiety and tension. They produce calmness and detachment from emotional perturbation. Even incapacitated persons achieve a detached attitude and a feeling of calm and comfort. Once stabilized, the patient can be maintained for a long period.

These drugs have been applied extensively in somatic treatment of mental disorders of both inpatients and outpatients. The use of these drugs has reduced the need of restraint and seclusion in hospitals. The result has been an increase of 25 per cent in discharges from mental hospitals. There is also a diminution in the relapses of those released. Tranquilizing drugs are usually nontoxic and well tolerated, but the patients require constant medical supervision. Side reactions are infrequent and seldom serious, but there are significant exceptions to this rule—under no circumstances should these drugs be self-administered.

The Mental Health Unit

Many communities have established mental health units to aid in the promotion of mental health throughout the area. Many of these units have been established under the sponsorship of the voluntary state and national units of the Association for Mental Hygiene; many others are organized by the health departments. These units serve a different purpose than the outpatient mental disease clinics. The team of this unit consists of a psychiatrist, a psychologist, a psychiatric social worker, and a public health nurse with psychiatric training. The primary function of the unit is to serve as consultant to all the agencies in the area that deal with people. This includes the school authorities, welfare departments, the police and the courts, the church officials, health department personnel, employers of industry, and others.

The major purpose is to aid all these various agencies in dealing with the emotional distrubances encountered in the course of their daily activities.

The mental health unit can accept individuals on a consultative basis, but if it attempts therapy, then it cannot fulfill its more pressing responsibilities. A diagnostic and therapeutic team of this size could not handle more than 200 patients a year, whereas the population they serve is usually from 70,000 to 100,000 people.

Thus major effort must be concentrated in aiding others to an understanding of the emotional problems of the people with whom they must work.

Prevention of Psychosis

Pasamanick(9) seriously doubts our ability at this time to prevent functional psychoses, schizophrenia, manic-depressive psychoses, or psychoneuroses. Furthermore, little can be done at present to prevent the vascular and senile changes of the central nervous system. Pasamanick gives some hope here, however, of delaying the appearance of disabling psychotic signs and symptoms through social stimulation and increased social status. Other effective preventive measures are: (a) prevention of brain injury of the newborn, and (b) aid in social adjustment of deprived children.

Porterfield(10), in discussing prevention of psychoses, states that the ultimate solution probably lies in the realm of biochemistry or psychopharmacology. It is most interesting to note that Sigmund Freud said practically the same thing more than 50 years ago.

Porterfield feels that the most important step in immediate promotion of mental health is to change the concept of hospitalization from long-term, custodial care in overcrowded, understaffed, larger institutions to hospitalization in smaller, well-staffed establishments with facilities for progressive care of patients leading to early discharge. These facilities include a program of: (a) day-care in which a patient goes home at night; (b) night-care, when the person does his work during the day and returns at night; (c) open-door hospitals, where patients are free from close restriction; (d) halfway homes; (e) convalescent homes; and (f) foster homes. The essential element of the patient's progress is gradual advance under supervision back to normal life in the community.

REFERENCES

1. *Hospitalized Mental Illness in the U.S.A.* Health Information Foundation, 1960, **IX**.

2. LEMKAU, P. V.: *Mental Hygiene in Public Health*, 2nd ed. McGraw-Hill Book Co., New York, 1955.

3. LENNOX, W. G.: *Ann. Int. Med.*, 1943, **18**:145.

4. *Manual on Alcoholism. J.A.M.A.*, 1956, **162**:720.

5. PFEFFER, A. Z., *et al.*: *J.A.M.A.*, 1956, **161**:827.

6. *Alcoholism in Industry. Pub. Health Rep.*, 1960, **75**:778.

7. MARTIN, A. R.: *Education*, 1943, **38**:462.

8. FRY., C. C.: *Mental Health in College*. The Commonwealth Fund, New York, 1942.

9. PASAMANICK, B.: *Am. J. Pub. Health*, 1959, **49**:1129.

10. PORTERFIELD, J. D.: *Pub. Health Rep.*, 1959, **74**:303.

SPECIAL REFERENCES

Alcoholics Anonymous. World Services Inc., 305 E. 45th St., New York.

BAHN, A. K., and NORMAN, V. B.: *Pub. Health Rep.*, 1959, **74**:943.

BRIGHTMAN, I. J.: *Pub. Health Rep.*, 1960, **75**:775.

CRUTCHER, H.: *Foster Home Care for Mental Patients*. The Commonwealth Fund, New York, 1944.

HEWITT, R. T.: *Pub. Health Rep.*, 1960, **75**:15.

LOCKE, B. Z., KRAMER, M., and PASAMANICK, B.: *Am. J. Pub. Health*, 1960, **50**:998.

Quarterly Journal of Studies on Alcohol. Williams & Wilkins Co., Baltimore, Md.

The Research Council on Problems of Alcohol, 60 East 42nd St., New York 17, N. Y. (for information about alcoholism and research projects).

Steps in the Development of Integrated Psychiatric Services. Milbank Memorial Fund, New York, 1960.

Tranquilizing Drugs. Mental Hospital and Outpatient Experience. *N. Y. State Health News,* 1957, **34**(5).

29. MALNUTRITION AND ITS PREVENTION

We now appreciate the importance of good food for the health of the individual and of the nation. Formerly it was believed that food was largely a matter of family taste and preference; as long as enough food was available to satisfy the demands of hunger, the situation was considered satisfactory. Natural appetite determined adequate selection of foods.

Under primitive conditions this rule usually holds true. The complexities of an industrial civilization, however, require careful family and community food planning and an exact knowledge of individual needs.

The health officer is interested in the maintenance of community health and vigor. The householder is interested in providing the family with adequate food, well balanced in all its elements, and at a reasonable cost. The health officer knows that if the food supply of the community is not adequate in all necessary elements, then dietary deficiency will inevitably occur. There must be a liberal margin of safety since some persons always get more than their share, and because our system of distribution of food is not perfect in all details.

In recent years, the development of community-wide systems of cold storage and cold-storage transportation has greatly simplified food distribution. Better methods of agriculture and agronomy, increased knowledge in animal husbandry, better types of food animals and grain, vegetables, and fruits, as well as increased family knowledge concerning preparation, conservation, storage, and utilization of foods have completely changed and greatly benefited the nutritional status of the American people. Despite the transition of our economy from an agricultural to a manufacturing basis we have kept abreast of nutritional needs, and it is safe to say that at the present time the people of this nation are better fed than ever before in our history—perhaps better than any other nation or people that ever existed. Better food, and more of it, is available to all people, irrespective of their life station.

404

But the nation still has a long way to go before it can be said to be on an optimal nutritional basis. Large numbers of people in the industrial areas, and also large areas of the country which are predominantly agricultural, actually suffer from lack of certain essential food elements because of peculiar indigenous factors. Chief of these is low economic status, together with ignorance concerning the essential ingredients of a well-balanced diet.

Our growing knowledge of the principles of nutrition, our understanding of the food requirements of the individual, and the basic needs of the community will enable us to correct this situation.

The application of this new knowledge to meet the needs of each individual situation is one of the important advances in preventive medicine and public health that has become the responsibility of physicians, educators, and public health personnel.

Nutrition as the Responsibility of the Physician

Nutrition is an essential element of preventive medicine and is a direct obligation and responsibility of the practicing physician.

In general it may be said that the medical profession has, in the past, given little attention to nutrition. The subject is not presented adequately in many medical schools. One reason is that physicians do not see a significant amount of acute, severe deficiency disease. We no longer have much pellagra. Beriberi is rare. Scurvy is seldom encountered in medical practice. Thus the physician has tended to leave the problems of adequate nutrition to others. He is not interested in nutrition except as it relates to clinically recognizable metabolic disorders or to the therapeutic management of other entities, such as diabetes or coronary disease. Often he does not have the knowledge to enable him to make proper recommendations concerning optimum nutrition.

Extensive dietary studies have shown that, although we do not have many severe cases of metabolic deficiencies in the United States, nevertheless, a substantial proportion of our people are deficient in one or more nutrients. The diet falls short of recognized standards of optimal nutrition. This might not produce overt acute deficiency disease, but it is detrimental to the health of the individual. The physician should be embued with the concept that his patient is entitled to optimum nutrition in order to enjoy optimum health. The doctor should not limit his efforts in nutrition merely to the combating of frank deficiency disorders.

Goodhart(1) has emphasized the importance of the family physician in promotion of nutrition education. The advancement of research and knowledge relating to nutrition constitutes only the beginning of an effective medical and public health program.

People who consider themselves normal frequently make changes in the food they eat, although not generally for health reasons. As an individual advances in economic or social status, his diet tends to change in accord with that section of society with which he wishes to be identified. Other considerations, such as fashions in slimness, educational opportunity, availability of foods, and appearance of food fads, can effect changes in eating habits, but not always in the right direction. These changes are seldom due to a desire to improve one's health.

Community health can be improved through application of our increased knowledge of nutrition most directly by means of: (a) nutritional improvement in available foods; (b) through advances in processing, transportation, and storage practices; and (c) through enrichment and fortification of widely consumed staple foods.

It is the consumer, however, who must make his own food choices. Unless he has some understanding of body requirements and a knowledge of the nutrient value of foods, he is vulnerable to the blandishments of the quacks and food faddists.

Knowledge of nutrition can be presented effectively through instruction in the public school classroom. The child learns the simple principles of adequate nutrition through precept and example. The school cafeteria can be an excellent teaching device in training the adolescent in sound nutritional practices.

Probably the most effective channel of sound education in nutrition is through the efforts of the practicing physicians. It is the responsibility of the physician to keep up to date in this important field of medicine.

NORMAL NUTRITIONAL REQUIREMENTS

It is not possible within the scope of this text to present a full discussion of normal food requirements. The reader is referred for this information to the many splendid books and monographs on this subject. Only an outline of the normal food requirements is given in order to present logically the dangers of deficiency states and the methods of their prevention.

The Committee on Foods and Nutrition of the National Research

Council* has recommended the following daily allowance for the average-sized (70 kg), physically active man, 25 years of age:

Calories	3,000	Vitamin A	5,000 I.U.
		Thiamine	1.6 mg
Protein	70 gm	Ascorbic acid	75 mg
Calcium	0.8 gm	Riboflavin	1.8 mg
Iron	10 mg	Niacin	21 mg

Vitamin D to the extent of·400 IU should be added to this diet if not available in the form of sunshine.

The typical active 25-year-old woman with a weight of 58 kg requires only 2,300 calories and 58 gm of protein; otherwise she needs the same food elements as a man. Caloric requirements can be scaled down with advancing age and degree of inactivity, but the standard basic dietary elements are required throughout life.

Men in active work require more calories and more vitamin B complex. The requirements of an active adolescent boy are greater than those of a grown man. Elderly persons do not require as much food as young children. Particular life periods require supplementation of food. These are, notably, the pregnant mother and especially the lactating mother, the infant, and the adolescent. In these groups the food allowances are higher in proportion to weight than for the very active man.

Translation of these requirements into practical everyday living gives the following dietary for an average individual:

1. Meat or its equivalent, e.g., fish, dairy products, etc. — One generous serving daily
2. Potatoes — One large portion daily
3. Vegetables — Two portions: one green or one yellow, and one other vegetable daily
4. Whole-grain or enriched bread — Two or three slices daily
5. Fruit — Two servings: one citrus, one other, daily
6. Whole-grain cereal — One generous portion daily
7. Butter or margarine — Three average portions (total 30 gm) daily
8. Milk — Adult, 1 pt; children, 1 qt daily
9. Eggs — Three to six weekly

*Recommended Dietary Allowances—revised 1958, National Research Council Reprint and Circular series Number 589.

The balance of energy requirements can be obtained from sugar, whole-grained or enriched cereals, or other inexpensive starchy foods.

Young children and nursing mothers should, of course, have a supplement of vitamin D in the form of fish-liver oil or some concentrate (400 IU daily).

These simple daily requirements can be transformed by intelligent handling into a great variety of diets, depending upon family tastes, racial or national preferences, and available foods.

The body has an extraordinary capacity for storage of necessary food elements, both for its energy requirements and for its maintenance of life. An individual can survive and even procreate and rear a family on a diet that is far below the optimum, represented by the standard requirements listed here. Most of the essential vitamins can be stored in the body for long periods of time. As the supply diminishes, the body utilizes its dwindling reserves very sparingly so that dietary deficiency conditions are almost always chronic and slowly progressive, often with barely preceptible initial symptoms. The final serious physical breakdown can come very slowly, or there might be a sudden and dramatic development of an apparently acute disease, such as the mental aberration in pellagra or the cardiac decompensation of beriberi.

Many persons, sometimes whole communities, pass an entire lifetime under a dietary regime that is markedly deficient in one or several essential food elements. These deficiencies can have a marked effect upon the development of these people. They do survive, however, even though they never have an optimum diet. But fullest potential growth is not reached, illness is frequent, the infant death rate is high, and the life span is short in the groups that habitually maintain themselves on deficient dietaries.

ELEMENTS OF NUTRITION

The problem of nutritional deficiencies requires a knowledge of the variety of food elements that the body must obtain in order to maintain a state of normal nutrition. These essential requirements are summarized briefly here.

Total Calories

We are a most fortunate nation in respect to the availability of foodstuffs. Deficiency in total calories is not a problem of great

TABLE 37

Per Capita Availability of Foods, in Grams per Day

	Countries Included (N)	Milk	Animal Protein	Total Protein
Regions where kwashiorkor is unknown or rare				
North America	2	722	64	94
Oceania	2	642	66	98
Western Europe	15	573	43	85
Regions where kwashiorkor is common				
Latin America	7	222	22	62
Near East	3	93	20	84
Africa	5	93	19	65
Far East	6	30	12	51

importance in the United States. There has been such an abundance of food that it has in many instances been wasted and destroyed. Every person, no matter how poor or improvident, has had "enough to eat." Exceptions to this rule do appear, of course, particularly in the large cities, but they are not of common occurrence. We have never had the great famines that have blighted certain other parts of the world.

Protein

Protein is the most expensive of all essential food elements, and its intake declines in periods of economic stress. Many families cannot afford a daily serving of meat or fish, but capable housewives have learned the value and availability of meat substitutes, so there is little serious danger of nation-wide protein deficiency.

Protein deficiences do occur, however, in the lowest economic and social groups, particularly in periods of unemployment and economic depression. Scrimshaw and Behar(2) have emphasized the fact that protein malnutrition is a major factor in high childhood morbidity and mortality in many underdeveloped areas. The mortality of children 1 to 4 years of age in the United States is 1 per 1,000 population annually, whereas in underdeveloped areas it can reach 50 per 1,000 population. Nearly one half of these deaths is caused by kwashiorkor. This is a clinical entity characterized by pitting edema, hyperkeratosis, and hyperpigmentation. Low total serum protein is a diagnostic characteristic of the disease.

In underdeveloped areas, where protein malnutrition is prevalent, the production of protein-rich foods (particularly those of animal origin) is insufficient to meet the needs of the population. The availability of these foods in different areas is listed in Table 37, which shows that low protein production areas correspond to kwashiorkor prevalence. The per capita availability of protein does not give an accurate index of its distribution among socioeconomic groups. Lack of transportation and preservation facilities results in a decrease in availability of animal foods. Small children suffer most from inequitable protein distribution within the family. Furthermore, intercurrent parasitic infection, severe diarrhea, anorexia, and other factors further deplete the protein absorption of the small child.

The basic treatment of kwashiorkor is the provision of 3 to 5 gm of protein daily per kilogram of body weight. Caloric intake should be high enough to ensure good protein utilization.

Mothers should be taught to utilize locally available sources of protein in the diet of the young children and to appreciate the necessity of adequate protein intake as a preventive measure.

Furthermore, long-term community planning should promote the production of protein-rich foods in order that those essential food elements are readily available and adequate for the entire population.

Calcium

Normal calcium requirements are often lacking in the average American daily diet. This is particularly true in those individuals needing increased amounts of calcium, such as lactating mothers and rapidly growing infants and adolescents. Stiebling and Coons'(3) studies indicated that low income of the family and low calcium intake were likely to run parallel courses. When calcium is not available for normal metabolism, the body must, of course, draw upon its reserves. This results in impairment of growth of bones and teeth. Some authorities believe that defective tooth formation in early childhood, with possible effect on increasing dental caries, and particularly impairment of growth and proper development of the bones, can result from a deficiency in calcium intake in childhood and youth. Excessive intake of calcium has not been shown to be harmful.

Phosphorus

This element is available in sufficient quantities to supply normal body needs. This fact is emphasized in practically all American dietary studies that have assayed this element. Phosphorus is important in normal development of bones and teeth. Daily allowances are approximately 1.5 times those for calcium.

Iron

Almost all American dietaries contain iron in sufficient amounts to supply average bodily requirements. Certain groups, notably infants, adolescents and pregnant mothers, however, are frequently on an iron deficiency basis. Studies carried out in the Department of Preventive Medicine of Cornell Medical College, in conjunction with the U.S. Public Health Service and the Milbank Memorial Fund(4), upon groups of adolescent high-school children, showed that the incidence of substandard hemoglobin values was 1.5 per cent in children attending a wealthy private school; it was 3.3 per cent in the children from a high school where the economic level of the families was low. A parallel investigation of young women from families on the city relief rolls, who were aiding in the study, showed a 69 per cent incidence of substandard hemoglobin values. Women are more likely than men to have an anemia from iron deficiency, because of their special needs for excess iron in menstruation and pregnancy.

Vitamin Deficiency

Our knowledge concerning the role that vitamins play in body metabolism is still in its preliminary stages and is available to us only in fragmentary form. A complete discussion of this most complex subject is not within the province of this text. No subject in medicine in recent years has had a more rapid growth, with greater accretion of information. No field of medicine has been subjected to greater commercial exploitation and haphazard and superficial public health propaganda than that of vitamin requirements and vitamin deficiencies.

Out of a welter of speculation and partial information, certain definite conclusions have been drawn from clear-cut evidence, and certain definite clinical conditions have been delineated, which are produced by a specific vitamin deficiency and which, should proper treatment be given, can be relieved by replacement and supplementation of these elements in the dietary.

Vitamin A. This vitamin is fat soluble and is stored in the tissues, particularly in the liver. Thus, determination of vitamin A in circulating blood is not an accurate index of deficiency or of body needs. The normal body requirements are not known. The National Research

Council has estimated that an average intake of 5,000 IU per day is ample for the average adult. There is good evidence that additional amounts are required for the pregnant mother and the rapidly growing adolescent.

Carotene is the precursor (or provitamin) of vitamin A. The body can manufacture the vitamin from carotene. The chief sources of vitamin A are whole milk and cream, butter, egg yolk, and vegetables — both green and yellow vegetables, but particularly the latter. The heat of ordinary cooking does not destroy vitamin A.

Available data do not demonstrate that vitamin A deficiency is a serious problem in the United States as a whole, though many individuals, because of food habits or idiosyncrasy, undoubtedly do suffer from a lack of this vitamin.

In summary, it can be said that the dietary of special groups, such as infants and pregnant mothers, might require supplementation of vitamin A, but the average American diet, even in the lower-income groups, does not seem to be markedly inadequate in vitamin A.

In animals, there is strong evidence that dividends in health and more effective physiologic function can accrue when quantities of vitamin A are allowed which are well in excess of those required simply to prevent signs of deficiency. The rate of growth and weight increased, reproductive functions improved, and the life span was prolonged.

Vitamin B. This vitamin was once considered to be a single substance. Gradually it has been broken down into its component parts, all of which are not yet completely worked out. Furthermore, the interrelationship of one part to the others is not completely understood.

B₁: Thiamine. Thiamine hydrochloride is a white crystalline compound, soluble in water, and possessing a salty, nutlike taste and a yeast odor. This is a proenzyme which the body requires for carbohydrate metabolism. It acts in combination with phosphoric acid as a coenzyme called carboxylase, which functions to prevent the accumulation of pyruvic acid. Thus, the determination of pyruvic acid in the blood is used as an index of vitamin B_1 deficiency. Since B_1 requirements depend upon carbohydrate metabolism, it is obvious that the greater the muscular activity, the higher the requirement of this vitamin.

Body stores of thiamine are never large and are quickly exhausted by febrile diseases, surgical operations, pregnancy and other stresses.

A minimum of 0.8 mg daily is required to prevent the occurrence of gross evidences of deficiency, such as beriberi. The National Research Council suggests an optimum of 1.5 mg of thiamine daily, for average use.

The symptoms of slight degrees of vitamin B1 deficiency are vague and indefinite. Fatigue, insomnia, constipation, poor appetite, abdominal distress and flatulence, irritability, depression, and weakness are common symptoms. Frank and characteristic manifestations of severe deficiency are polyneuritis, myocarditis, with a final break in cardiac compensation, and all the typical symptoms of beriberi.

Beriberi is widespread in the Orient and in many other parts of the world as well. It is commonly seen where a limited diet, consisting largely of highly milled rice and wheat flour, is consumed. It is not infrequent in Newfoundland and Labrador, where the long winters impose a restricted diet on the people. The milling process of grain removes the pericarp, depriving the food of all vitamin B1. Prevention of beriberi is simple, either through consumption of unmilled rice or whole-wheat flour and other grain cereals, or the addition of B1 supplement to the diet.

Vitamin B1 is found abundantly in the average American dietary. Peas, beans, oatmeal, whole-wheat bread, lean pork, and peanuts are rich in thiamine. It was believed for a long time that B1 deficiency was not an important problem in the United States, and it is true that the typical beriberi of the tropics is seldom seen in this country. Gradually we began to realize, however, that many individuals did not have an adequate thiamine intake, despite its nation-wide abundance. For example, the polyneuritis of chronic alcoholism has been found to be due, not to the toxic effects of alcohol, but to deficiency of thiamine and other essential elements. Alcohol serves as a substitute for the more complex foods and has high caloric value. When it is consumed in quantity, the individual has no appetite for a well-balanced diet; the earliest and most apparent result of this unbalanced diet is a beriberi symptom complex, with polyneuritis, and in the later states, a typical "beriberi heart."

Thiamine is derived from a great variety of foods, each of which contains only a small amount of the vitamin. The aggregate is abundant, so that it is only under most unusual circumstances or under a markedly abnormal dietary regimen that thiamine deficiencies should be encountered. It must be remembered, however, that adequate intake does not always indicate complete utilization.

Thiamine is quite heat stable, but since it is water soluble it can be lost in the cooking process if the fluids in which the foods are cooked are discarded.

When planning family or community dietaries, it is necessary to emphasize the point that whole-wheat bread and whole-grain cereals are excellent and inexpensive sources of B_1.

When individuals are suffering from symptoms of B_1 deficiency, thiamine may be added to the diet in doses of 10 to 30 mg daily. The results of this therapy are almost miraculous, even in those patients who have progressed to a serious stage of illness.

B_2: Riboflavin. Riboflavin is an orange-yellow water-soluble crystalline compound, $C_{17}H_{20}N_4O_6$. It is widely distributed in both vegetable and animal tissues, and thus is contained in a great variety of common foods. It is intimately concerned with the life process in the cell, but its exact function is not understood. Lack of the vitamin in human beings produces cheilosis, with deep fissures at the corners of the mouth and a magenta-colored glossitis.

The National Research Council recommends for optimum nutritional conditions a daily intake of riboflavin, for an average man, of 1.8 mg. This amount is easily secured in the average American diet. Nevertheless, the characteristic clinical symptoms of riboflavin deficiency are seen in widely scattered areas throughout the nation.

Niacin: Nicotinic acid. This is the pellagra-preventive factor. This substance occurs as white, needlelike crystals: $C_6H_5O_2N$. The minimum daily metabolic requirements are about 15 mg for the average adult. The Committee on Food and Nutrition of the National Research Council suggests 17 to 21 mg as optimum.

Tryptophan functions as a precursor of niacin in man. Administration of tryptophan to patients with pellagra results in rapid improvement and healing of all lesions. Sixty milligrams of tryptophan are equivalent to about 1 mg of niacin. Goldsmith(5) has produced symptoms of pellagra in adult human subjects who were maintained on diets which furnished only 4.5 to 5.4 mg of tryptophan daily. Thus a 1,000-mg tryptophan diet would furnish 17 mg of niacin, which is quite adequate for an active adult man.

A mild degree of deficiency in nicotinic acid is accompanied by vague symptoms of distress, such as weakness, loss of appetite, gastrointestinal disturbance and diarrhea, and a sore tongue and mouth; a chronic state of fatigue, irritability, and listlessness. Advanced niacin deficiency results in a clinical condition called pellagra.

Pellagra was widely prevalent throughout the United States 50 years ago, but has almost disappeared. Goldberger and his associates in pioneer experiments(6) showed that pellagra in human beings was not an infection but a dietary deficiency disease. He also proved that yeast was an effective preventive, and he was able to cure experimental pellagra in patients by the simple procedure of adding sufficient amounts of dried brewer's yeast to their diets.

A review of Goldberger's early studies in the light of more modern knowledge concerning vitamins indicates that his patients were suffering from a multiple dietary deficiency. They presented evidences of deficiencies of thiamine (B_1), riboflavin, and niacin as well. In fact, the disease pellagra, as encountered in the rural areas of the South, is undoubtedly a multiple B-complex deficiency disease, and can best be prevented by an adequate well-balanced diet. Excellent pellagra-preventive foods are lean meats and fowl, liver, peanuts, all legumes, kale, green peas, and many other foods. Brewer's yeast in 30-gm doses daily is a splendid therapeutic agent for this disease, and yields extraordinary results even in advanced stages.

Even in areas where pellagra was prevalent, only a small proportion of the people develop typical clinical symptoms. A very large proportion of persons in the households where cases of pellagra are found will be "prepellagrins," in that they are suffering from a moderate, but not a critical, degree of vitamin B deficiency. These individuals, who suffer only vague symptoms of chronic indigestion, weakness, and lassitude, are greatly improved in their general health by modification of dietary habits, with addition of proper amounts of vitamin B complex.

B_6: Pyridoxine, Pyridoxal, and Pyridoxamine. This vitamin has been shown to be essential to animal metabolism. Vitamin B_6 is involved in fundamental biochemical metabolism of the body. Fortunately it occurs in many different foods, such as cereals, milk, meat, and fruits. Except in very unusual circumstances, signs of vitamin B_6 deficiencies have not been recognized in human beings.

Patients have been observed with a rare variety of hypochromic anemia, which responded to administration of vitamin B_6 to their diet, but no clear-cut B_6 deficiencies have been found in humans.

Normal requirements appear to be about 1 to 2 mg daily. It is readily provided by ordinary foods.

Vitamin C. The role of ascorbic acid ($C_6H_8O_6$) in body metabolism is more completely worked out than that of any of the other vitamins.

It maintains intercellular collagen. Mild degrees of deficiency result in increased capillary fragility, with spongy and bleeding gums. In more severe cases a typical picture of scurvy develops.

Scurvy has been recognized as a dietary deficiency for many years, and its prevention and cure have been well understood. Formerly it was the curse of sailors and of explorers. A vivid description of the disease in its severe forms is found in Kane's *Arctic Explorations*(7).

The prevention of scurvy is now so well understood that severe cases of the disease are seldom encountered in adults in the United States. Infants and young children frequently develop scurvy because the parents do not understand the necessity of adding orange juice or other foods containing vitamin C to the baby's diet.

Vitamin C is found in abundance in citrus fruits, tomatoes, raw leafy green vegetables, and potatoes; other vegetables and fruits also have significant amounts. It is water soluble and is easily destroyed by heat and by oxidation. Pasteurization of milk destroys the vitamin. Orange juice that has been stored in the refrigerator even for a day or two loses much of its vitamin C content.

The normal bodily requirements for an average person, as recommended by the National Research Council, are 75 mg daily. Increased amounts are needed during pregnancy, lactation, and adolescence.

Vitamin C deficiency can be determined by a simple assay of ascorbic acid in the blood plasma. A normal level is about 0.5 to 0.6 mg per cent. In the joint Cornell-Milbank-U.S. Public Health Service study(4) of high-school children, it was found that almost all the children in the economically secure private-school group had ascorbic acid plasma levels about 0.6 mg per cent, whereas only one half the school children of lower economic status reached this level. Stiebling's studies(8) also showed that vitamin C intake was directly proportional to income in industrial workers' families. The supply of this vitamin in the population is, therefore, essentially an economic matter. Vitamin C intake is dependent, more than any other food element, upon cheap transportation and cold storage of fresh fruits and vegetables. Kale and spinach lose 50 per cent of their vitamin C if stored at room temperature for a day or two. If these food elements are not readily available at low cost and at all seasons of the year, this vitamin will not be stored in the body, and vitamin C deficiency will result. Ascorbic acid can be added to the diet as a supplement, but the simplest and best method of securing the essential vitamin C is through the use of citrus fruits.

In cases of actual scurvy, excellent and immediate therapeutic results are obtained by the administration of adequate amounts of ascorbic acid.

Vitamin D. This vitamin is essential in the metabolism of calcium and phosphorus. The average person obtains enough vitamin D from simple foods such as dairy products, i.e., milk, cream, butter, and eggs. Vitamin D is manufactured also in the skin by the body through exposure to sunlight, and this yields an excess of the vitamin for all persons during the summer months. In winter, however, when sunlight is at a minimum, rapidly growing children and pregnant and lactating mothers require supplementation of vitamin D.

The best natural source of this vitamin is fish-liver oil (cod or halibut). Normal bodily requirements for infants and children can be met by the administration of 1 tbsp of a good quality of cod-liver oil daily. Synthetic vitamin D, viosterol, can be utilized in 500-unit doses daily, but it is not a perfect substitute for cod-liver oil.

The early stages of vitamin D deficiency can be estimated by roentgenology of the bones, particularly the bones of the wrist and hand.

Vitamin D deficiency does not bear the close relationship to economic status that is encountered in vitamin B complex and vitamin C deficiencies.

No dietary deficiency is so easy to remedy as that of vitamin D. Its control is essentially a function of the practicing physician, supplemented by a general community program of health education. In areas of low economic level, it may be necessary for the community actually to supply cod-liver oil free, or at low cost, to the children of the poor.

Vitamin E (Tocopherol). Experiments with rats have indicated that vitamin E deficiency led to sterility, and vitamin E came to be known as the "antisterility factor." There is little clinical evidence, however, that vitamin E deficiency plays any role in human reproduction. Its utility in prevention of abortion in larger animals or man is controversial. Wheat germ is a rich source of vitamin E. It is also widely distributed in many foods. Since the significance of vitamin E in human nutrition is not known, no standards of human requirements can be set.

Vitamin K. This vitamin maintains the prothrombin level in the blood. A deficiency results in increased capillary fragility, which can produce bleeding from wounds and from postoperative conditions, and sometimes intracranial hemorrhage of the newborn.

The prophylactic use of vitamin K in the prevention of hemorrhage of the newborn is now practiced in many hospitals. Oral administration of vitamin K to the mother before delivery and one dose of 1 to 2 mg administered intramuscularly to the infant immediately after birth have been suggested as practical preventive measures.

Bile salts are essential for absorption of this vitamin from the intestine. Thus, obstruction of the common bile duct leads to great danger from hemorrhage, particularly following gallbladder operation, because of the slow blood-clotting time from lack of absorption of vitamin K. The vitamin is fat soluble. It is found abundantly in green leafy vegetables and is stored in the body. Thus, vitamin K deficiency does not usually result from a lack of the vitamin itself, but is a matter of faulty absorption of the vitamin from the intestine.

Iodine

The body requires a minute amount of iodine in order to maintain the normal function of thyroid secretion. It is effective when administered in any form, and is stored by the body for long periods of time. Fifty milligrams annually are sufficient to meet the needs of the average adult.

Despite these minute requirements, iodine deficiency occurs over large areas of the United States and has been a major public health problem. Iodine is found in the surface water and soils of both the Atlantic and the Pacific coast areas, but in the central plains, particularly about the Great Lakes region, iodine is not found in the soil.

Correction of this situation is largely a public health responsibility. It has been met by:

1. The addition of minute amounts of iodine to municipal water supplies.

2. The use of iodized salt. Potassium iodide is added to all table salt* in the proportion of 1 part in 5,000. Since the average person consumes 5 to 10 lb of salt a year, abundant iodine is secured for each person by these means. Excess beyond the needs of metabolism is excreted.

In areas where goiter is prevalent, prophylactic tablets of sodium iodide are administered to adolescent school children, since it is this age group that suffers most from iodine deficiency.

---

*Usually this is a state regulation in goiter areas.

A total of 2 gm of sodium iodide is administered to each child over a period of a fortnight, on an annual or semiannual basis.

Iodine is found in abundance in sea water and in all sea foods; it is also found in vegetables that have been grown in soil containing iodine.

Recognition of Dietary Deficiencies

The diagnosis and treatment of a well-marked clinical entity, such as pellagra, beriberi, or scurvy, are simple matters. These conditions, however, are the gross manifestations of a long-continued, destructive, and preventable process.

The physician has a much broader responsibility in the field of nutrition than the recognition of advanced dietary disease. He must train himself to observe in his patients all those vague symptoms of ill health that can result from unbalanced diet. He must recognize the fact that dietary deficiency can be produced by many indirect influences, some of which he may have applied to the patient while administering treatment for other conditions. In other words, the physician can actually produce malnutrition in his patients. Furthermore, he must train his clientele in the simple principles of sound nutrition so that each member of the family will enjoy not only an adequate, but an optimum, dietary for his personal and particular needs.

In children, a lack of appetite, listlessness, irritability, with disinterest in play, poor sleep, pale and flabby skin, poor posture, and many other minor symptoms can be indices of malnutrition. Adolescence is a particularly vulnerable period nutritionally, due to greater bodily needs and also to bad eating habits. Loss of weight, poor work in school, weakness, irritability, indigestion, sore mouth, bleeding gums, chronic diarrhea, poor muscle tone, diminished reflexes, redness of the tongue, depression, and many other conditions can occur because of an unbalanced diet, with a diminished intake of one or more essential food elements. It is important to remember that an individual can survive for a very long time and, in fact, carry out a normal amount of activity upon a grossly deficient diet. Both the physician and the community are interested, however, not in mere survival of an individual at a substandard level of efficiency but rather the promotion of optimum health and happiness, with proper provision for maximum growth and development, and the enjoyment of a long life with fullness of energy and buoyancy.

Nutritional Deficiency in the Presence of an Abundant Food Supply*

In certain individuals, a nutritional deficiency occurs despite an apparently adequate dietary intake or the opportunity for a well-rounded food supply. Dr. Jolliffe and his associates(9) in the Cornell clinics in preventive medicine, in a review of case histories of 1,000 patients with nutritional diseases, stated that more than 90 per cent of the conditions that he studied could not be attributed solely to dietary inadequacy, since a variety of other factors contributed to the patients' ill health.

Dr. Jolliffe emphasized some of the important contributing factors in nutritional deficiency:

1. Malabsorption of food. Many individuals do not absorb all the food that they eat. This is particularly true of elderly persons. Atrophy of the intestinal tract can result from an inadequate intake of vitamin-B complex, and this atrophy results in poor absorption of food. In diarrheal diseases, the food is hastened through the intestinal tract, giving insufficient time for complete absorption. Changes in the pH of the intestinal tract, brought about by treatment of disease with alkalis, can result in malabsorption of food. Thus, malabsorption of food can be due to anatomic, to physiologic, or to chemical factors, all contributing to a tissue deficiency.

2. Increased food requirements. Any factor that increases total metabolism will increase the food requirements of the body. With an increase of each degree Fahrenheit in body temperature, the total body metabolism is increased 8 per cent. Thus, a protracted period of high fever draws tremendously upon the food reserves of the body. Since the fever is often associated with anorexia, and sometimes with vomiting and diarrhea, the weight loss can be severe, with a heavy draft upon tissue reserves. Strenuous exercise also increases total metabolism. This is particularly true if the strenuous work is accompanied by heavy loss of sweat. In certain instances, therapy, particularly with thyroid extract, increases total metabolism.

3. Malutilization of food. The conversion of dietary elements into readily available form can be disrupted in liver disease and in diseases associated with liver dysfunction.

Therapy with the various sulfonamides can result in nutritional deficiency. It has been shown, for example, that sulfapyridine interferes with the utilization of niacin unless a sufficient amount of that vitamin is given to counteract this difficulty. Thus, food can be eaten and absorbed but not utilized.

Destruction of Food Elements. An example of the destruction of food elements is in neoarsphenamine therapy, which utilizes some of

---

*From the clinics of the late Dr. Norman Jolliffe, Chief, Nutrition Clinic of the Department of Health of the City of New York, which were presented to students of Cornell Medical College.

of the vitamin C supply of the body as an essential part of the detoxifying process of the drug. Aviators flying at high altitudes must have supplementary vitamin C for the same reason.

Increased Excretion. Increased excretion of food elements occurs in uncontrolled diabetes mellitus and also in diabetes insipidus. Lactation calls on the food reserves to such a degree that thiamine deficiency with typical polyneuritis can develop in the mother who nurses her baby. This condition responds rapidly to thiamine therapy.

Deficient Food Intake. Many patients are given an adequate diet, and yet nutritional deficiency occurs because the individual does not eat his food. Certain illnesses cause anorexia, and in chronic disease, particularly in elderly people, no one gives very much thought as to whether or not the patient consumes all the food set before him. In mental hospitals, pellagra may appear in a patient who has been presented daily with a perfectly adequate diet. The food is put before the patient, but because of his mental confusion he does not eat it.

Nutrition in Illness

The physician has a special responsibility for maintenance of adequate nutrition in illness – acute as well as chronic.

Any person with an illness, (particularly with higher than normal temperature for three or more days) should be given not only a good diet but also supplementary vitamins.

Glucose infusions should include therapy with the water-soluble vitamins, thiamine and niacin.

Individuals with chronic illness, particularly elderly people, must be carefully watched to prevent development of a dietary deficiency state, because of lack of adequate intake of food, greater requirements, lessened absorption and, in some cases, lessened utilization.

Malnutrition can be either acute or chronic. Rapid depletion of the tissues can be relieved quickly by proper therapy, and recovery will be fast. Usually, however, malnutrition is a slow, depletive process, progressing over a long period of years. Permanent tissue damage occurs. Recovery, even with very large doses of vitamin concentrates, will be slow and incomplete. Often there is a combination of the acute and chronic process. When an individual with chronic malnutrition develops an infection, there is a great increase in tissue requirements of essential vitamins. Unless prompt and suitable therapy with vitamin supplements and vitamin-rich foods is supplied, the recovery of the patient will be delayed and further permanent tissue damage will occur.

Subclinical Nutritional Deficiency

Long-continued nutritional deficiency is of greater importance, in the aggregate, than the frank clinical cases of nutritional disease encountered in the community.

Unfortunately we have no simple method of measurement of malnutrition. The following methods have been commonly employed:

1. Individual dietary assays. These are excellent in the individual case if carried out over a sufficient period of time.

2. Statistical studies of the food resources of a country. This method is a satisfactory index of the availability of food, but since food is not equally distributed, malnutrition can occur in the midst of abundant total available food.

3. Family dietary studies. This technique has been used in many of the field studies of malnutrition; from the point of view of the research worker, it is adequate but time consuming.

4. Appraisal of the nutritional status of the individual. This technique is faulty, since we have few clear-cut diagnostic criteria. In the Cornell-Milbank(4) study previously referred to, a great variety of criteria was employed, such as height-weight-age ratio, blood serum-protein ratio, the biophotometer, capillary fragility, roentgenogram of the long bones, and estimates of the chemical constituents of the blood such as phosphorus, calcium, phosphatase, ascorbic acid, and iron. No single test or combination of tests gave exact criteria of the nutritional status of the child.

Certain broad conclusions can be drawn from our knowledge of the American situation. By and large, nutritional deficiency in the United States is not a result of:

1. Lack of essential food elements.
2. Faulty distribution of food.
3. Low purchasing power (seldom an important factor).

The difficulty is that we fail to utilize readily available foods. This results from:

1. Lack of knowledge concerning the basic principles of normal food requirements.
2. Failure to understand the great importance of proper nutrition upon optimum growth and development.
3. Failure to recognize nutritional deficiencies when they occur.
4. Poor judgment in expenditure of food budget.

Correction of this situation is the joint responsibility of the department of health, the practicing physician, and the nutritionist, particularly those nutritionists engaged in research and in health education.

The important function of the physician is to recognize potential or actual malnutrition when it occurs and to correct nutritional defects when they are discovered.

Correction of nutritional defects is carried out on an individual basis by the physician, the family dentist, and the public health nurse, through:

1. Correction of improper food habits in children.
2. Parent instruction concerning the food requirements of children.
3. Special diet instruction for certain types of patients, such as the diabetic or the person with food idiosyncrasy.
4. Solution of problems of infant feeding.
5. Provision for the special requirements of the prenatal and maternal period.

Promotion of Normal Nutrition

The promotion of normal nutrition is a community responsibility. The nutrition division of the health department is responsible for the community educational program in nutrition. This is a slow and difficult task, for it entails the translation of scientific knowledge into popular terms with a sufficient degree of authority and conviction so that this new knowledge can be transformed into action. Various media that have been used are:

1. School-wide nutritional projects.
2. Popular instruction through newspapers, magazines, posters, radio, and television.
3. Group instruction of mothers.
4. Family budgeting instruction.
5. Instruction of community leaders who, in turn, influence their own groups of people.
6. In certain circumstances, direct aid can be given. Seldom is it necessary to supply a complete diet. Supplemental foodstuffs are given in order to provide a well-balanced and complete intake for each member of the family.

REFERENCES

1. GOODHART, R. S.: *1960 Annual Report: Report of Scientific Director.* Natural Vitamin Foundation, 149 East 78th St., New York, N.Y.

2. SCRIMSHAW, N. S., and BEHAR, M.: *Science,* 1961, **133**:2039.

3. STIEBLING, H. K., and COONS, C. M.: *Food and Life.* U.S. Dept. of Agriculture Yearbook, 1939.

4. *Medical Evaluation of Nutritional Status.* Series of reports beginning in 1940 published by the Milbank Memorial Fund, 40 Wall Street, New York, N.Y.

5. GOLDSMITH, G. A.: *J. Am. Dietetic Assoc.,* 1956, **32**:312.

6. GOLDBERGER, J., *et al.:* Bull. 153, U.S. Pub. Health Service, 1929.

7. KANE, E. K.: *Arctic Explorations.* Childs & Peterson, Philadelphia, Pa., 1856.

8. STIEBLING, H. K.: Circular 507, U.S. Dept. Agriculture, 1939.

9. JOLLIFFE, N., TISDALE, F. F., and CANNON, P. R.: *Clinical Nutrition.* Paul B. Hoeber, Inc., New York, 1950.

SPECIAL REFERENCES

Control of Malnutrition in Man. Am. Pub. Health Assoc., New York, 1960.

COOPER, L. F., BARBER, E. M., MITCHELL, H. S., and RYNBERGER, H. J.: *Nutrition in Health and Disease,* 13th ed. J. B. Lippincott Co., Philadelphia, 1958.

Food: The Year Book of Agriculture, 1959. U.S. Dept. Agriculture, Washington, D.C.

J. Am. Dietetic Assoc., 620 North Michigan Ave., Chicago, Ill.

Recommended Dietary Allowances. National Academy of Sciences, National Research Council. Publication 589, 1958, Washington, D.C.

Suggested Guide for Interpreting Dietary and Biochemical Data. Interdepartmental Committee of Nutrition for National Defense. *Pub. Health Rep.,* 1960, **75**:687.

30. OCCUPATIONAL MEDICINE

Occupational medicine or industrial hygiene is that community function which deals with the protection of the health of the wage earner while he is actually at work. It is an important part of the all-inclusive, community-wide plan for health promotion of all age groups and of all elements in the community. In practical terms it is a subdivision of adult hygiene, with a special interest in the age groups of 20 to 65 years.

The element that sets occupational medicine apart from the other health activities is that the responsibility for the success of this work is threefold: the burden rests primarily upon the official health administration of the community but it is shared by the employer and the wage earner.

Since each wage earner spends approximately one third of each day at his work and is engaged for at least two thirds of his total life span in active labor, and since there are many special hazards of life and health directly due to occupation, it is obvious that the community program for protection of the health of the industrial worker is a subject of wide extent and great importance.

Only recently has the community begun to realize that each of its citizens is a potential asset, which might easily become a heavy community liability if proper care is not taken to prevent wastage. Thus, disease, injury, accident, or premature death of the worker from any cause, particularly from preventable causes related to his occupation, is a community disaster. Obviously, conservation of manpower is sound community economy. Thus the community should place particular emphasis upon proper protection of men and women at work. The community also has the responsibility of teaching the worker to protect himself and to aid the employer in providing health safeguards. It must also require industry to provide healthful and satisfactory working conditions for its employees.

HISTORICAL DEVELOPMENT OF INDUSTRIAL HYGIENE

Ramazzini, the great Italian clinician, has been called "the father of industrial hygiene." His text, *De Morbis Artificum Diatriba*, was published in 1700. It dealt extensively with the diseases of occupation. The subject was of continuous interest to all of Europe throughout the nineteenth century but received little attention in the United States because the nation was primarily agricultural at that period.

During the first half of the nineteenth century, there were passed in various states, a few labor laws relating to child labor and also to hours of work for women; in 1869, F. A. Walker published an article on *Occupations of People*. The Lomb Prize Essays were published by the American Public Health Association in 1886. One of them, by J. H. Ireland, was entitled *The Preventable Causes of Disease, Injury, and Death in American Manufacture*. This essay considers very few matters that are of interest to us today and contains very little information. The author gave chief consideration to sanitary construction of factories. Such questions as the hazards of dusts, fumes, and toxic substances now used in industry are barely mentioned.

Caisson disease was well studied and given its name by Andrew H. Smith in 1873 in a prize essay for the Alumni Association of the College of Physicians and Surgeons in New York, but little investigation in the field of industrial disease in America occurred until 1900.

The first decade of the twentieth century was marked by much activity in the United States in the field of industrial hygiene. Dr. Frank Fulton of Providence was the first to plan for medical examination of employees. Within a few years, more than 20 states passed laws bearing directly upon factory sanitation. New York passed a law relating to the prevention of caisson disease. By 1910, six states required notification of industrial diseases—California was the first in this field.

Gilman Thompson, professor of medicine at Cornell University, published the first complete American text, *The Occupational Diseases*, in 1914.*

The U.S. Public Health Service organized a Division of Industrial Hygiene in 1912 and began to stimulate the development of official state industrial health services. Great impetus was given to this movement through the Social Security Act of 1935, which granted subsidies to each state for the purpose of developing state-wide

---

*George M. Kober had published his monograph, *Industrial and Personal Hygiene* (169 pages), in 1908, but it did not deal extensively with occupational diseases.

industrial health services. By 1940, almost every state and several large cities had established special divisions of industrial hygiene as an integral part of the community health service(1).

Industrial Accidents

The death rate from work accidents (death per 100,000 workers per annum) has declined gradually from the peak of 43 in 1939 to 22 in 1958. The frequency of injury and the severity of work injury have also declined markedly. In 1958 the injury frequency rate was 53 per cent lower than the average rate from 1935 to 1939. Nevertheless, there were 1,800,000 disabling injuries of workers during 1958 with 13,300 deaths. Highest rates occur in the construction industry, with transportation and the mining industry following closely. This gradual reduction of the rate of injuries and deaths related to work causes is due in great part to the increasing degree of preventive measures that have been employed.

Occupational Diseases

Occupational disease is defined as any illness that develops in an individual which is peculiar to the occupation in which he is employed, and which is due to causes in excess of the ordinary hazards of employment as such.

The New York Court of Appeals(2) defined occupational disease in similar terms:

An occupational disease is one which results from the nature of the employment, and by nature is meant, not those conditions brought about by failure of the employer to furnish a safe place to work, but conditions to which all employees of a class are subject, and which produce the disease as a natural incident of a peculiar occupation, and attach to that occupation a hazard which distinguishes it from the usual run of occupations, and is in excess of the hazard attending employment in general.

It is almost impossible to evaluate the exact loss of manpower due to occupational disease. Work can actually cause or aggravate illness, or it can bring about a chain of related factors which exerts a profound influence upon the health of the employee.

The type of work and its interest or monotony can indirectly influence the health of the worker. The work itself might not be injurious, but the conditions under which the employee is compelled to work might produce irreparable harm.

For many years the courts have held that the employer is legally responsible for accident injury incurred during occupation, but only recently has the philosophy developed that industry owes the worker complete protection against both injury and illness that might be due directly to the nature of the job. This theory results in the corollary that if injury or illness is produced by occupation, then the worker is entitled to suitable compensation from the employer.

These concepts necessitated a positive plan of action, which has resulted in an extensive industrial hygiene service in all parts of the nation.

Reporting of Occupational Disease. In 1950, the reliable reporting of occupational disease for the nation as a whole was virtually non-existent. Methods of reporting by the various states varied widely, and in some states no effort was made to collect these data.

An experiment on the feasibility of instituting a nation-wide system of uniform collection of reports on occupational disease was initiated by the U.S. Public Health Service in 1950. This was done in conjunction with ten industrial states which had divisions of industrial hygiene and which agreed to use standard forms for reporting, which would be forwarded to the Public Health Service for tabulation and analysis. This plan has been so widely adopted that almost all states now record the incidence of industrial disease in a uniform manner.

The American Industrial Hygiene Program

The major activities of an industrial hygiene program are:

1. Measures that are taken in order to prevent accidents that may be produced by the nature of the job.

2. Measures taken to prevent diseases that are the result of specific toxic substances or other harmful materials employed in industry.

3. Promotion of a hygienic environment for the employee.

4. Medical and nursing service, together with other medical activities that are undertaken by industry to promote the health of employees.

5. Health education measures. These are planned to enable the worker to take measures to protect his own health and that of his family.

6. Research into the causes of industrial hazards and disease, with development of appropriate preventive measures.

7. Promotion of state-wide and nation-wide legislation in which the most modern knowledge of the principles of industrial hygiene is incorporated.

PREVENTION OF INDUSTRIAL ACCIDENTS

The National Safety Council states that in 1958 there were in the United States 1,800,000 injuries resulting from occupational causes, with more than 13,300 deaths due directly to the hazards of occupation. The cost of occupational injury during that year constituted over one third, or 32 per cent, of the total cost of all types of accident in the nation, including motor vehicle accidents. This destruction of manpower, enormous as it may be, is not as serious as it has been in the past. Only a generation ago, there was almost no special provision for accident prevention in industry. Progressively more attention has been given to this matter so that in recent years there has resulted a steady decline in the frequency rate of accidents, i.e., number of disabling injuries per million man-hours worked, as well as in the severity rate, i.e., number of days lost from work per thousand man-hours worked.

Industrial accidents are seldom the result of a single cause. It is estimated that two thirds of all accidents have both mechanical and personal causes. The American Standards Association Code has classified accidents as the result of:

1. Personal causes. Unsafe acts, such as:
    (a) Unnecessary exposure to danger
    (b) Improper starting or stopping machinery
    (c) Operating at unsafe speed
    (d) Lack of skill or knowledge
    (e) Improper attitudes
2. Mechanical causes, such as:
    (a) Improper guards for movable parts
    (b) Hazardous arrangements or procedures
    (c) Unsafe apparel worn by the worker

Dunbar(3) believed the personal element in accidents was paramount. She has even suggested that certain people have the accident habit. She stated that less than 20 per cent of all accidents are due solely to mechanical causes, and describes in some detail the characteristics of the unstable, impulsive individual who is "accident-prone."

The currently accepted theory that most accidents are sustained by a small fixed group of "accident-prone" individuals is criticized by Schulzinger(4). His investigations lead to the conclusion that it seems to be more correct to speak of varying degrees of "accident-proneness" in every individual. If the period of observation is sufficiently long, the "small group of persons who are responsible for most of the accidents" is essentially a shifting group of individuals with new persons constantly falling in and out of the group.

Administratively, and legally as well, management of industry has been held directly responsible for accidents; but, as just stated, in most accidents the employee is at least partially responsible. Thus any plan for prevention of accidents must be based on certain basic policies, as indicated by Bushnell(5):

Management must assume sole responsibility for physical conditions of the plant, the mechanics, and the tools.

Training and job instruction is a direct function of management.

A simple safety organization should be set up which gives due recognition to the employee's interest in his own safety, by providing for employee participation in and joint responsibility for the success of the plan.

Usually one man in the organization is appointed as safety director. A safety committee is appointed from the supervisory personnel, with representation from the workers. The work of the committee is threefold:

1. To investigate accidents as they occur in order to apply the lessons learned therefrom.

2. To follow a continuous plan of application of the principles of safety.

3. To conduct a continuous educational program among the workers so that each employee will assume his share of the responsibility in the prevention of accidents to himself and to his fellow workers.

OCCUPATIONAL DISEASES AND THEIR PREVENTION

Accident prevention is basically a problem for the safety engineer rather than the physician. On the other hand, occupational disease, its diagnosis, treatment, and, to a considerable degree, its prevention, is the province of the doctor; this function is assigned both to the industrial plant physician and the general practitioner of medicine in the community.

Diseases directly related to occupation are the result of a great variety of causes. These etiologic agents have been grouped by McCord(6) as follows:

1. Occupational diseases from infections.
2. Occupational poisoning, usually chemical poisoning.

3. Occupational asphyxiants.
4. Occupational diseases due to mechanical pressure, injury, or irritation.
5. Occupational diseases due to chemical rays and to faulty illumination.
6. Occupational diseases produced by abnormal atmospheric conditions.
7. Diseases caused by thermic conditions incident to the occupation.
8. Fatigue.
9. Noise, vibration, and monotony.

Occupational Diseases from Infections

All infections that occur while a man is at work are not due, necessarily, to the occupation. In certain instances, however, the infection is a direct effect of occupational exposure. An excellent example is anthrax. Often this disease is acquired in handling raw hides from South America or Central America. Woolsorter's disease is also an occupational anthrax infection. Tularemia in butchers, from handling infected rabbits, is another example of this class.

Occupational Diseases from Poisonous Substances Used in Industry

Occupational Dermatosis. More than 50 per cent and some authorities state over 70 per cent of all occupational diseases are due to substances which irritate the skin. The chief materials that produce these lesions are solvents, greases, oils, alkalies, and acids. In some instances, vegetable products, such as the castor-oil bean, or animal products such as furs, and other organic substances are at fault.

The disease does not have special diagnostic characteristics, except that the distribution of the lesions on the skin often gives a clue to the etiology. The diagnosis can be confirmed by a patch test, using the suspected substances for the test. It must be remembered that many individuals who are insensitive to the skin irritants can become sensitive following repeated exposure.

The mode of prevention of occupational dermatosis depends upon the nature of the irritant as well as the industrial process involved. Major measures are:

1. Protection of the skin by gloves, boots, etc.
2. Use of protective ointments.
3. Complete enclosure of processes that are common causes of skin irritation.
4. Liberal provision for showers, lockers, and facilities for cleansing the skin after exposure.

5. Substitution of noninjurious substances in industrial processes.

6. Determination of hypersensitivity of certain individuals and, if necessary, change in the nature of their employment.

Poisonous and Injurious Dusts. Silica is the most serious occupational dust hazard. Other important toxic dusts are lead and mercury. Of lesser importance are arsenic, copper, cobalt, brass, nickel, silver, and cadmium. Textiles and vegetable fiber dusts are of relatively less importance as occupational hazards.

Silicosis. This disease is acquired in occupations such as granite cutting, sandblasting, mining ore and pottery work.

The tiny silica particles in the dust penetrate the natural defenses and reach the air spaces of the lungs. They set up a proliferation of fibrous tissues which results in the formation of characteristic fibrous nodules in the lungs. The disease is dependent upon the intensity and duration of exposure to the microscopic dust. An excess of 5,000,000 particles of silica dust per cubic foot of air is considered dangerous. Exposure must occur intensively over a period of several years to produce true disability from this cause. Ultimately dyspnea and gradually increasing disability occur. In many instances, tuberculosis becomes superimposed upon the silicosis, with fatal outcome.

The diagnosis of this disease is based on the history of exposure and on the evidence of chest roentgenograms.

Prevention of silicosis is chiefly a problem of industrial engineering. The disease has been markedly reduced, following the recognition of its importance, by the development of methods which:

1. Measure dust density in industrial processes.

2. Utilize methods of removing dust from the air, or protect the worker so that he is not subjected to a dangerous degree of exposure to silica dust(6).

Asbestosis. This disease is a pneumoconiosis produced by inhalation of asbestos dust. Like silicosis, it is a slowly progressive condition resulting from long and continuous exposure to a high density of asbestos dust.

The pathology in the lungs is quite distinct from silicosis in that the asbestos particles are deposited in the respiratory bronchioles, around which they produce a fibrotic process. Nodules are not produced, and tuberculosis is not a common complication. The disease is progressive, with dry cough and dyspnea. The diagnosis is made by the history of exposure together with the roentgenogram of the chest, which shows a characteristic "ground glass" appearance, most marked in the lower third of the chest. "Asbestos bodies" in the sputum are found in asbestosis, but are only of supplemental diagnostic aid.

Dust control methods are quite practicable in the prevention of this disease. A workman with asbestosis should be removed from further exposure. In some cases, the disease progresses to a fatal end, but in other instances, it remains stationary if there is no further exposure to the dust.

Plumbism. Lead poisoning is equally as important as silicosis as a serious industrial hazard. Lead has been recognized for centuries as an important cause of "colic" and "palsy."

In industry, the chief danger from lead is the inhalation of lead dust and fumes. The characteristic symptomatology is a syndrome of gastrointestinal disturbance, anemia, and nervous manifestations. There are a loss of appetite and marked constipation, with paroxysmal attacks of severe colic. The blood shows a characteristic polychromatophilia, poikilocytosis and a marked basophilic stippling.

The lead "palsy" usually is first noted as localized paralysis involving the small muscles of the hand or the extensors of the wrist and fingers, producing the characteristic "wrist drop." The localization of the palsy depends upon the degree to which a given group of muscles is used in the occupation. The condition develops slowly, with very slow recovery.

Lead Encephalopathy. This is the cerebral form of plumbism and is the result of an excessive exposure to lead fumes. It produces a rapidly progressive form of convulsions, wild delirium, insanity, and death. When tetraethyl lead was first blended as a fuel, there was a series of fatal accidents among the blenders due to the fact that the substance is so readily absorbed and so highly soluble in fats. The symptoms were those of an acute mania, with death in a few days from exhaustion.

Diagnosis of Lead Poisoning. The diagnosis is dependent upon a history of exposure to lead, together with a characteristic blood picture of basophilic stippling of the red cells (300 stippled cells per million), with a typical history of lead colic and loss of muscular strength. For confirmation of the diagnosis, determinations of excess secretion of lead in the urine and feces are made. Hematoporphyrinuria is also a characteristic sign. In children, roentgenograms of the epiphyses of long bones can be of some aid. The lead line at the gums is an important sign if present, but it is often absent. Not one symptom or sign, but the whole picture must be put together in reaching the diagnosis of lead poisoning and the degree of disability produced by the disease.

The Prevention of Lead Poisoning. Prevention of exposure to lead dust and fumes is a relatively simple matter in large industrial establishments that use lead in manufacturing processes. It is an engineering problem, and requires the development of mechanical processes that give the worker complete protection. It is also necessary to educate the worker concerning the danger of lead fumes and to obtain his cooperation and understanding in the prevention of inhalation.

Absorption of lead by the gastrointestinal tract is a long and slow process, but is a definite source of chronic low-grade plumbism. Mercury, arsenic, chrome, phosphorus, or cadmium poisoning is incurred by the inhalation of dusts or fumes of these substances. There are a large number of occupations in which these substances are used.

Many toxic substances are employed in industry, and these are used in a variety of ways. A list of 128 toxic substances used in various industries, together with the type of occupation which offers exposure to each poison, is given in Chapter 6, "Industrial Health Exposures," in C. O. Sappington's book(1). That author gave over 150 occupations in which lead and its compounds serve as an occupation hazard.

Gases and Fumes. In addition to silica and the heavy metals, there is a large group of substances used in industry which, if inhaled, can result in serious and sometimes fatal disease.

Benzol is an excellent example of this group of poisons. Acute benzol poisoning is not common, but chronic toxemia from prolonged exposure to low concentrations can produce severe injury to the blood and to the blood-forming organs. Blood examination of exposed persons shows a diminution of both red blood and white blood cells. Disability occurs because of the anemia, with subsequent involvement of the central nervous system.

Other solvents, such as carbon tetrachloride, tetrachlorethylene, toluol, xylol, turpentine, nitrobenzol, and many other substances can produce poisoning by inhalation if a sufficient concentration of the substance is allowed to escape into the workers' environment.

Many industrial poisons can produce a severe hepatic necrosis. Trinitrotoluene, lead, bismuth, mercury, antimony, tannic and picric acids, chloroform, and many other substances have been incriminated as factors in acute or delayed liver damage.

Perhaps the most important of all is carbon tetrachloride because of its extensive use in industry and the household.

Carbon tetrachloride (CCl_4) can be inhaled or ingested. Three or four milliliters are frequently given in the treatment of hookworm disease without ill effect. However, if the individual has taken alcohol just previous to ingestion of the drug, a dosage of 1 ml of carbon tetrachloride can cause a severe central necrosis of the liver, with probable fatal outcome. This striking characteristic of sensitization of liver cells by alcohol for subsequent destruction by carbon tetrachloride is an important factor in the high case fatality rate from carbon tetrachloride poisoning.

Occupational Asphyxiants

Injury from occupational asphyxiants belongs in the classification of occupational accidents. Administratively, these conditions are handled as accidents, utilizing the first-aid facilities of the industry for immediate relief. The most important gases in this group are carbon monoxide, hydrogen sulfide, and hydrogen cyanide. It is important to remember that exposure to small but continuous concentrations of any of these poisons can result in occupational disease and disability.

Occupational Diseases Due to Mechanical Pressure, Injury, or Irritation

Many industrial processes, because of long-continued point pressure of friction, or because of vibration, will produce characteristic occupational injuries and chronic arthritis. The rheumatism of elderly men is often the result of long years of hard physical labor, resulting from continuous wear and tear upon the joints.

Diseases Due to Chemical Rays

An excellent example of a disease of this type is a radium workers' disease. This dreadful disease caused havoc in girls who made illuminated dials for watches. They "pointed" their brushes by putting the tip in the mouth, thus leading to a heavy radium absorption, with subsequent terrible destruction of the bones in which the radium was deposited. Welders are particularly exposed to ultraviolet and infrared rays, and workers in roentgenology are also subject to special hazards.

The industrial engineers have devised suitable equipment to prevent exposure to all these hazards, but often the goggles, masks, helmets, and shields are hot and uncomfortable so that it is difficult to get the complete cooperation of the worker in the protection of his health.

Occupational Diseases Produced by Abnormal Atmospheric Conditions

Caisson disease is produced by the effect of the release of increased atmospheric pressure; it is a common condition among divers and tunnel workers. The worker can absorb the compressed air of his environment rapidly, but he must be decompressed very slowly. The reason is that although oxygen of the air is given up rapidly by the tissues, the nitrogen is transferred very slowly. Hours after decompression, the worker can suffer a sudden attack of illness from the expansion in the tissues of a bubble of the retained nitrogen gas. If he is placed in a compression chamber and recompressed immediately, the effects of the local gas pressure will disappear. Thus, all tunnel workers wear a tag stating that if they become unconscious, they must be taken immediately to a given address where there is a compression chamber.

The substitution in diving bells of helium as an inert gas instead of nitrogen has greatly simplified the problem of diver's disease, since helium is rapidly eliminated from the tissues.

The development of high-altitude flying has opened a whole new field of study upon the effect of low-atmospheric pressures upon the health of aviators. The reader is referred to special texts in aviation medicine for complete information on this subject.

Occupational Cancer

These lesions result from long and continued exposure to physical or chemical carcinogenic agents within the working environment.

Most of the occupational cancers occur on the skin. Other organs affected are: the respiratory system, the eye, the urinary system, the blood-forming organs, the bones, and possibly other parts of the body.

Frequently the patient does not know that he has even been exposed to carcinogenic agents, or he has forgotten that he worked in a potentially dangerous environment. The latent period in occupational cancer is long; in the case of radium it can be as long as 20 years.

It is, of course, very difficult to prove that a certain carcinogenic agent produced cancer in a patient when the latent period is a matter of years. Furthermore, individual susceptibility plays a role in occupational cancer, as in all other diseases. A group of persons can be exposed equally to the same hazards and only one might develop the disease.

Thus, a very careful history is required in attempting to appraise the etiology of a presumably occupational cancer. One must know precisely what the patient's occupational exposure was, what chemical or physical agents he was exposed to, and for how long a period. The intensity of the exposure is also important. Furthermore, one must not forget that the cancer can develop years after the exposure to the carcinogen has ceased.

Cancer of the Skin. This is the most common lesion produced by occupational carcinogenic agents. Some of the more important agents are arsenic, sodium nitrate, pitch, tar, soot, asphalt, crude mineral oil, aromatic spindle. oils, anthracene, paraffin, radioactive substances, X-rays, ultraviolet rays, thermic burns, and chronic irritation.

Blood-forming Organs. The major carcinogenic substances in these lesions are benzol and (presumably) benzol derivatives, as well as radioactive substances.

The Respiratory System. The chief offenders are the chrome salts and radioactive substances.

The Urinary Tract (Bladder, Ureter, and Kidneys). Beta naphthalene is an important carcinogenic agent in cancer of these organs. There is evidence also that analine, and derivatives, and alpha naphthalene are of significance.

In addition, radioactive substances have produced tragic episodes of cancer of the bones; asbestos has been suspected as a carcinogenic agent in lung cancer, and the chlorinated hydrocarbons in cancer of the liver. As our epidemiologic knowledge increases and as new substances are added to industrial processes, it seems quite probable that in the near future the list of occupational carcinogenic agents will be considerably supplemented.

The prevention of cancer by elimination of exposure to occupational carcinogenic agents is not as simple as might first appear. The great difficulty is the long latent period between the exposure and the appearance of the lesion, and also the difficulty of proving that a given agent actually was responsible, directly, for the lesion.

Diseases Caused by Thermic Conditions Incident to Occupation

One of the best examples of this classification of occupational disease is "steelworkers' cramps." This condition is due, in great part, to excessive loss of sodium chloride through perspiration, and can be alleviated effectively by addition of sufficient salt to the diet in the form of salt tablets, or by other means.

Occupational Diseases Produced by Fatigue, Noise, and Monotony

Examples of this type of occupational disease are "writer's cramp," nystagmus, and neurosis caused by continuous loud noises. They result from long and continuous exposure to unfavorable working conditions and are acquired, as a rule, over a period of years.

The following brief case histories are illustrative of industrial diseases encountered daily in clinics or in private practice. In each instance the diagnosis was puzzling, and the symptoms were vague and confusing. In each inquiry as to the occupation of the patient gave the clue which led directly to correct diagnosis.

M. J., a 33-year-old white man, was a welder by trade. He came to the clinic with a complaint of abdominal pain of two weeks' duration. His past history was not important.

Present illness: Three weeks previously he had lost his appetite and began to have cramplike abdominal pains. These were mild at first, but became quite severe. His temperature was normal. He had been constipated for some time, and his family noted that he was pale. Two days before admission he became extremely nauseated. He was weak, and noticed a tingling sensation in both hands and wrists.

He had been working for the past three months upon the demolition of the Second Avenue elevated railroad in New York. He used a protective hood, but during rest periods, he had been exposed to the fumes from the torch as it cut through the iron girders.

Physical examination: The patient had all the classic symptoms of lead poisoning. The lead line in the gum margins of the upper incisors was well marked. Weakness of both wrists, amounting almost to wrist drop, was found. Abdominal pain was generalized and was relieved by deep pressure. Examination of the blood showed:

    11.0 gm of hemoglobin
    3.5 million red blood cells
    10,200 white blood cells
    poikilocytosis, with stippling in 3.6 per cent of the red cells
Lead was found in the urine: 1.35 mg in the 24-hour excretion.

This young welder had absorbed lead in toxic amounts by inhalation of fumes from the many layers of old paint on the girders that were demolished by his electric torch.

C. C. was a technician in a chemical company. He entered the clinic complaining of a staggering gait and mental confusion. His family history and past history were not contributory to the present illness.

Present illness: Nine days before admission to the hospital, he became nauseated and vomited severely. His temperature was normal, and no cause was known for his gastrointestinal upset.

Six days later he became drowsy and uncoordinated. He was ataxic, clumsy, restless, and disoriented. Tremor of the hands developed, with blurring of vision, diplopia, and transient scotoma. His wife noted a memory loss, slurring of speech, and delay in answering questions.

Physical examination was negative. The patient ran a higher than normal temperature in the hospital, and became quite disturbed mentally. He had apprehensions, then hallucinations, and on the third day developed a violent activity which required sedation.

Careful inquiry revealed that 12 days before admission to the hospital he was given a job of removing methyl bromide from defective ampules. He wore a mask and gloves, but worked in a small, closed room with poor ventilation, and inhaled sufficient methyl bromide vapor to produce severe intoxication. His recovery was gradual, but complete.

F. C. was a 55-year-old stonecutter who came to the clinic because of weakness, shortness of breath, and chronic cough.

Past history: F. C. lived on a farm until 17 years of age, then learned the trade of stonecutting. He worked in a monument factory cutting granite for some 10 to 12 years. He developed a chronic cough, and went to his family physician, who told him he had better quit the granite-cutting trade or he would develop "stonecutter's consumption."

He returned to the farm where he earned a frugal living. He was unable to gain weight, felt weak, and had a chronic cough which was more troublesome during the winter. Recently he had felt worse, with occasional fever and increased weakness. He also had noted blood-flecked sputum.

Roentgenologic examination of the chest revealed a typical chronic silicosis of the lungs, upon which was superimposed a chronic tuberculosis. The sputum was positive for the tubercle bacillus.

PROMOTION OF A HYGIENIC ENVIRONMENT FOR THE EMPLOYEE

The responsibility for healthful working conditions for the employee falls directly upon industry. Proper heating, lighting, ventilation, comfortable working conditions, adequate lockers and washrooms, suitable safeguards to protect the worker against accident, and other matters that affect the worker's health are all essential parts of industrial construction and maintenance. Prevention of fire hazards, provision for recreational facilities, maintenance of well-balanced nutritious lunches on a cost-basis cafeteria plan, as well as many other measures that can be instituted to promote the comfort and welfare of the worker, have been found to improve the production of the plant and reduce days lost from illness and injury.

Most states have established minimum regulations concerning the installation of devices required to protect the worker against industrial hazards. Practically all states also require certain standards of hygiene and comfort for the worker. Usually the state department of labor employs factory inspectors who are assigned the duty, and in some instances given the power, to enforce all state regulations relating to sanitation of the workrooms. In other instances, the state health department is given the responsibility of enforcing state laws that relate to protection of workers against the hazards of employment. The various engineering details concerning measures that can be employed in protection of workmen are technical matters that can be found in suitable texts by those readers who desire to give this subject further consideration.

In general, the responsibility for safeguards and for prevention of accidents within any large industry is in the hands of a safety department, and usually this function is administered by a specially trained industrial engineer. The first-aid station is in charge of the medical division, with an attendant, usually a nurse, on continuous duty. The two departments of safety and medical care have so much in common that they should work together closely and be organized on an interrelated basis.

MEDICAL AND NURSING SERVICE IN INDUSTRY

The major purposes of a medical service in industry are:

1. To prevent injury and disease that could arise as a direct hazard of the job.

2. To give direct emergency aid in case of injury or illness.

3. To aid in placing each man in the position where he can do the most effective work.

4. To maintain good health in the whole personnel by active health promotion and health educational measures.

The Pre-employment Examination

The primary purpose of the pre-employment physical examination is the determination of any physical handicaps in a work candidate that might unfit him for certain types of work. Some industrial health services prefer to call it a "preplacement" examination, which perhaps is a better term.

An equally important function of this examination is to supply the person with proper information concerning his physical defects. Suggestions also can be made as to the means by which corrections may be obtained.

This examination is not a complete physical examination but a specially planned test for a specific purpose. It is rapid yet comprehensive. Tests for sight, hearing, pulse rate, blood pressure, urine examination, and roentgenogram of the chest are done by the nurse or technician who assists the physician. Serologic tests for syphilis are usually done, although there are very few positions in industry where a positive result would require exclusion from work. This test for syphilis is done primarily as a health-promotion measure.

After the preliminary tests have been made, the physician then makes the actual physical examination, testing particularly the heart, the joints and bones, and muscular and nervous coordination. He also examines for hernia and other physical or mental disabilities. The final recommendation concerning the man's fitness for a given position is then made by the physician to the director of personnel.

Periodic Physical Examinations and Other Services

Selected groups of persons subjected to special industrial hazards should be given frequent physical check-ups. Persons working with toxic substances have a special potential risk, and their health must be carefully safeguarded.

Some industries make it a practice to provide an annual physical examination for workers who have been continuously employed and have passed their fortieth birthday.

The physical examination after absence is usually limited to a brief inspection of the employee who has been absent for seven to ten days or more because of illness. Its purpose is to determine the fitness of the convalescent to resume work.

Clinic Service. A clinical service with a nurse in continuous attendance and a physician present at certain specified hours and always on call is conducted for the purposes of: (a) giving first aid, and (b) consultation service.

Medical care is usually limited to medical advice and the simplest form of initial therapy. The employee is referred to his own physician for medical treatment.

Simple symptomatic therapy can be given, such as a sedative for headache, or a laxative. Sometimes symptomatic treatments for a common cold are administered.

Correction of Defects. A few industries have provided facilities on a low-cost basis for correction of certain defects. Examples are the services of dentists, optometrists, and chiropodists.

Complete Medical Care. Certain industries have provided a complete medical service for employees on a prepayment insurance plan. Usually these are mining or construction companies, where the workers live in remote communities and where medical facilities are not readily available. In some instances, provision is made by industry for medical, hospital, and nursing care of the employee and of his family as well, on a prepayment basis. In most instances, a part of the cost of the service is paid by the industry. The inclusion of the whole family of the industrial worker in a comprehensive prepayment plan for complete medical care is one of the advantageous developments of the period of intensive war emergency construction, 1940 to 1945. These plans which grew out of the requirements of a war emergency have gradually developed into solid comprehensive plans for prepayment for medical care.

Organization of Industrial Health Services

The industrial health service has so many functions that are integrated with personnel relations that the health service is usually administered by the personnel department. Welfare activities of the industry, including sickness benefits, are usually correlated with the medical services.

The medical director of a large company should be on a full-time basis and should have had special training for the work. This training should not be in the field of industrial surgery, as is so often the case, for this position does not require a surgeon but rather a physician with special knowledge of the problems of preventive medicine and public health.

Public Health Committee. A public health committee should be organized in the industry. The committee should be composed of representatives of administration, the shop executives, and the workers themselves. The safety department and welfare division might also be represented. This committee should advise the medical director concerning all matters of policy and should interpret his activities to their various groups.

The Industrial Nurse. The public health nurse has won her place in industry. She assists in the first-aid and clinic services, aids in the preplacement examination, and takes an active part in the health education programs. She relieves the physician of many technical and routine procedures and combines the activities of a hospital clinic nursing service with the duties of a district nurse. Her greatest usefulness is in the home contacts, through visits to sick employees and their families, where she carries out all the activities customarily handled by a district nurse.

Medical and Nursing Service for Small Industries. The industrial medical organization that has been described is best suited to large plants with more than 500 employees. One full-time medical director and his staff can readily care for 2,000 or more employees. But many industrial workers are employed in small industries with no more than 50 employees. Obviously, a complete industrial health service with a full-time medical director is not feasible for these small plants.

The solution is a group plan of cooperative service. The Chamber of Commerce of the United States has worked out an interesting and valuable suggestion through its Public Health Committee, Industrial Section, whereby small industries in any given community can pool their resources and thus secure a satisfactory industrial health service for the benefit of themselves and their employees.

Nursing service can be purchased from the community district nursing organization. Medical service can be secured from local physicians on a part-time basis, with one trained coordinator to administer the service for the whole group(7).

State and Federal Industrial Health Services

The Industrial Health Division of the U.S. Public Health Service has been most effective in stimulating the development of industrial hygiene throughout the nation. The Social Security Act of 1935 made possible grants-in-aid to all the states toward establishment of state-wide industrial health programs. Whereas few states had well-formulated industrial health services in 1935, within the past few years practically every state has established, within the state health department or other state agency, an active official state industrial health service with a full-time medical director.

Workmen's Compensation. New York State initiated workmen's compensation in 1910. Within ten years, almost every state that had any industrial problems adopted some form of workmen's compensation. At first it was related to occupational injury only, but later, compensation for industrial disease was initiated (in Wisconsin in 1919) and has been widely extended in all industrial states.

The workmen's compensation movement has had a profound influence upon the development of industrial hygiene as an applied science. Industry has found that it is much better administration, and far less expensive, to take measures to prevent accident and illness resulting from occupation than to pay high premiums for prolonged illness or injury which might be produced by avoidable situations.

Health Education in Industry

The industrial health service can be of special value to the workers if a well-planned and continuous program in health education is carried out within the industry itself. This plan should be worked out in cooperation with the local health department, together with the various interested voluntary agencies in the community, such as the tuberculosis associations, social hygiene associations, and allied organizations. The Chamber of Commerce of the United States is equipped to provide all local chambers of commerce with excellent and selected health education material that can be utilized effectively by each of the industries in the community.

Research in Industrial Hygiene

Research in industrial hygiene is a twofold responsibility. Primarily it is the function of the U.S. Public Health Service and the health departments of the various states to study the special problems of health protection of the worker. A state division of industrial hygiene should serve as a consultant to all industries within its boundaries, and be ready at all times to make industrial surveys, do necessary laboratory studies, and make suggestions for improvement in plant procedure. Each industry also is under obligation to develop safer methods of production and better administrative methods of health promotion for its employees. For example, no new and untried substance should be introduced into an industrial process—such as a new solvent—until its toxic properties have been determined by the industry that has introduced the material.

In addition, the universities and research insititutions under private auspices could be called upon to solve basic problems in the whole broad field of industrial hygiene.

Legislation in Industrial Hygiene

The incorporation of modern knowledge concerning industrial hygiene into the state and federal laws is of paramount importance. Even such a simple regulation as the requirement for reporting of diseases resulting from industrial processes has greatly increased our knowledge of these conditions.

Administration of laws relating to industrial hygiene, including the routine of factory inspection, is usually assigned to the state division of labor. The functions of the division of industrial hygiene of the state health department are, primarily, consultation and advice, coupled with investigation, both in the laboratory and in the field. Its work might be called the "epidemiology" of industrial disease, since its functions so closely parallel those of the division of epidemiology and control of communicable disease.

REHABILITATION

Comprehensive medical care is made up of four essential parts: (a) preventive medicine, (b) diagnosis, (c) treatment, and (d) rehabilitation. This fourth foundation stone has just begun to receive the attention that it warrants.

No one had doubted its importance, but the necessary organization and planning for effective rehabilitation had not been devised. We did not know how to go about the job. Furthermore, the disabled person usually has a prolonged illness; his resources are exhausted, and the long slow road back is an expensive journey. Thus rehabilitation becomes essentially a community function calling on the combined efforts of voluntary and official agencies, including both welfare and public health. We have just begun to understand and to develop suitable plans to meet individual and community requirements in this field.

Importance of Rehabilitation

Rehabilitation is very important to industry. Many disabilities are produced through accidents or injuries that occur while the worker is on the job. These disabilities are subject to workmen's compensation laws. Permanent occupational disability is a heavy drain on industry that rehabilitation often can relieve.

The general principles of rehabilitation can be applied to each age group. It is true that the details of techniques can vary greatly in their application to various ages and to different conditions and varied social groups. Each person is a special problem (though group teaching can be followed effectively). The method of approach is the same in all; the differences of handling are a matter of degree and intensity, rather than a variation in over-all policy.

The nation was awakened to the great importance of rehabilitation during World War II. Highly trained pilots and other skilled airplane personnel were urgently needed. Many of those men had received combat wounds and were spending months of convalescence in base hospitals. It was discovered that an energetic, aggressive, intelligent rehabilitation program greatly shortened convalescence. Rusk(8), who was largely responsible for this military plan, carried his ideas into civilian life at the end of the war. To him and his associates belongs much of the credit for the rapid development that has been made in the techniques of rehabilitation in recent years.

The basic principles are simple. One must begin as early as possible; in fact, as soon as the acute illness or the results of the injury have been alleviated, the patient should be put on his initial rehabilitation activities. This means that every general hospital, as well as the special hospitals for tuberculosis, mental disease, etc., must have a sustained rehabilitation plan. Great care must be taken to prevent deformities. These can occur quickly, even during the acute stages of illness, but they can be prevented.

The patient must understand what is being planned. Without his full cooperation the program will not be effective. The average patient will not cooperate fully unless he understands what lies before him and what is being planned for him. For this reason group training has great value, since one patient encourages the other.

One must begin with simple things. The patient must first learn to live with himself. He is almost completely disabled. To turn over in bed without aid is supremely important. It is his first lesson. Rusk(9) has analyzed the multiple activities of daily living—the chart consists of over 100 items, such as brushing the teeth, washing the face, combing the hair, getting out of bed, going to the toilet, dressing, walking, feeding without aid, getting up and down stairs. Each test is checked off as the skill is acquired. The triumph of achievement in a paraplegic who has been a helpless invalid for years and who learns to do each and every one of these things is one of the greatest of all human satisfactions.

Ambulation is an essential skill for eventual financial self-support. The patient should learn to get in and out of an automobile or a streetcar. Speech therapy often requires a complete re-education of the handicapped person. Sometimes handwriting must be retaught. Each individual must be carefully studied and appraised. Finally, skills are taught so that within the limits of his capacity he again finds his place in the world and becomes a self-respecting, often completely self-supporting person.

All this requires infinite patience, understanding, skilled personnel, ample facilities, and financial support. Rehabilitation is expensive, but the results secured represent a very profitable community investment. It is the best example we have of the value of coordinating all our efforts; the patient himself, his nurse and his physician, the workman's organization, industry, insurance companies, local state and national official and voluntary health and welfare agencies—all contribute to make the program a success.

REFERENCES

1. SAPPINGTON, C. O.: *Essentials of Industrial Health*. J. B. Lippincott Co., Philadelphia, 1943. (Chapter I has an interesting summary on the development of industrial hygiene.)

2. *Accident Facts*, Report of the National Safety Council, Chicago, Ill., 1959. *Goldberg* v. *Marcy Corp*. 12 N.E. Rep.: p. 211.

3. DUNBAR, FLANDERS: *War Med.*, 1943, **5**:163.

4. SCHULZINGER, M. S.: *Indust. Med. Sur.*, 1954, **23**(4):151-152.

5. BUSHNELL, P. N.: *Organization and Administration of the Company Safety Program*. Portland Cement Association, Chicago, Ill. Meeting, May 19, 1942.

6. McCORD, C. P.: *Industrial Hygiene for Engineers and Managers*. Harper & Brothers, New York, N.Y., 1931.

7. *Organization of an Industrial Health Service*. U.S. Chamber of Commerce, Washington, D.C., 1944.

8. RUSK, H. A.: *Ann. Internat. Med.*, 1947, **26**:386.

9. _____: *Arch. Indust. Hyg. & Occupational Med.*, 1950, **1**:411.

SPECIAL REFERENCES

FAIRHALL, L. T.: *Industrial Toxicology*, 2nd ed. Williams and Wilkins, Baltimore, 1957.

FLEMING, A. J., and D'ALONZO, C. A.: *Modern Occupational Medicine*, 2nd ed. Lea & Febiger, Philadelphia, 1960.

JOHNSTONE, R. T., and Miller, S. E.: *Occupational Diseases and Industrial Medicine*. Saunders, Philadelphia, 1960.

KEHOE, R. A.: *J.A.M.A.*, 1960, **172**:435.

POOLE, F. E.: *J.A.M.A.*, 1947, **133**:91.

Publications of Industrial Hygiene Division, U.S. Public Health Service, Federal Security Agency, Washington, D.C.

Scope, Objectives and Functions of Occupational Health Programs, *J.A.M.A.*, 1957, **164**:1104.

SHEPARD, W. P.: *J. Occupational Med.*, 1960, **2**:255.

WOODWARD, L. C., and RENNIE, T. A. C.: *Jobs and the Man.* Charles C Thomas, Springfield, Ill., 1945.

31. PREVENTIVE ASPECTS OF METABOLIC DISEASES

OBESITY

Overweight, particularly in individuals past middle life, is a burden many persons carry about without reason. In many instances, this heavy burden results in a definite shortening of the normal life span. Extensive data collected by the large insurance companies indicate that overweight persons past middle life are more likely to succumb to premature death from coronary thrombosis, from diabetes, or from infections, such as pneumonia or colicystitis, as well as many other diseases, than are persons in the same age group whose weight is average or below average. Furthermore, the obese individual suffers from unnecessary fatigue, heat intolerance, arthritis, and many other serious discomforts much more commonly than do persons of normal weight. Thus, the prevention of obesity and the maintenance of normal weight are matters of importance in the field of preventive medicine.

Normal Weight

In the United States the Metropolitan Life Insurance Company has compiled a convenient table of desirable weights for men and women over 25 years old, according to height and frame (see Table 38).

The etiology of obesity is, in most instances, not obscure. It has been attributed to:

1. A lower basal metabolic rate in the obese person.
2. A lessened specific dynamic action of food in the fat person.
3. The fact that obese persons absorb and utilize food more readily than do thin people.
4. The lipophilic theory, which assumes a hereditary constitutional trait of the adipose cells in fat individuals which enables the tissues of the obese person to accumulate an excessive amount of fat.

449

TABLE 38

Desirable Weights for Men and Women*

ACCORDING TO HEIGHT AND FRAME: AGES 25 AND OVER:
WEIGHT IN POUNDS (IN INDOOR CLOTHING)

Men

Height (in shoes)		*Small Frame*	*Medium Frame*	*Large Frame*
Feet	*Inches*			
5	2	112-120	118-129	126-141
5	3	115-123	121-133	129-144
5	4	118-126	124-136	132-148
5	5	121-129	127-139	135-152
5	6	124-133	130-143	138-156
5	7	128-137	134-147	142-161
5	8	132-141	138-152	147-166
5	9	136-145	142-156	151-170
5	10	140-150	146-160	155-174
5	11	144-154	150-165	159-179
6	0	148-158	154-170	164-184
6	1	152-162	158-175	168-189
6	2	156-167	162-180	173-194
6	3	160-171	167-185	178-199
6	4	164-175	172-190	182-204

Women

Height (in shoes)		*Small Frame*	*Medium Frame*	*Large Frame*
Feet	*Inches*			
4	10	92- 98	96-107	104-119
4	11	94-101	98-110	106-122
5	0	96-104	101-113	109-125
5	1	99-107	104-116	112-128
5	2	102-110	107-119	115-131
5	3	105-113	110-122	118-134
5	4	108-116	113-126	121-138
5	5	111-119	116-130	125-142
5	6	114-123	120-135	129-146
5	7	118-127	124-139	133-150
5	8	122-131	128-143	137-154
5	9	126-135	132-147	141-158
5	10	130-140	136-151	145-163
5	11	134-144	140-155	149-168
6	0	138-148	144-159	153-173

* Prepared by the Metropolitan Life Insurance Company; derived primarily from data of the Build and Blood Pressure Study, 1959, Society of Actuaries.

5. The related theory which claims that in fat persons there is not only a more rapid storage of fat, but also delay in release of fat from the fat deposits, whenever these tissues are required for energy purposes.

These factors play a small part in the over-all picture. The important factor in production of overweight is simply a daily caloric intake which exceeds the energy requirements of the body — in brief, the fat person eats too much rich food. There are a few exceptions to this rule, particularly the so-called cerebral or neurogenic types of obesity and the cases of Cushing's syndrome, in which the pituitary functions abnormally. Some authorities also believe that there is a definite tendency toward inheritance of obesity. It is true that fat children are often seen in homes where one or both parents are obese, but this condition can be due to family customs of overeating rather than to inheritance of family characteristics.

A positive energy balance can be due to a variety of causes: one of the important factors is familial or cultural dietary habits. People of certain nationalities tend to eat excessive amounts of starchy or fatty foods. The overweight of persons past middle life is almost always the result of the decreased energy output of the individual, as the years advance, with no compensative diminution in diet intake. People over 50 eat as much as they did at 20, although their activities are greatly curtailed. Automation has reduced energy expenditure of the worker by 10 per cent. Furthermore, many individuals overeat as a compensation for an emotional maladjustment. Probably the most common cause of overweight is the fact that individuals overeat because they enjoy food, and do not realize that there is any risk in overindulgence.

Prevention

Prevention of overweight begins with teaching each individual that overweight, particularly with increasing age, is an unnecessary hazard. The person must be convinced that the "normal" gain of weight with increasing age is injurious, in a direct ratio to the degree of increase of weight to increasing age. That is to say, a person of 45 years with a 20 per cent increase in weight over normal has increased his mortality risk 30 per cent, whereas an increase in weight of 40 per cent over normal in the same person increases the comparative mortality risk by 80 per cent. Furthermore, in a person of 55 years of age, there is more than proportionate risk with the same overweight. The other essential educational feature that must be emphasized is that weight reduction can best be secured by maintaining a slow and gradually progressive negative energy balance. In other words, the daily consumption of food should be slightly less than the energy demands of the body. Thus, the body burns the excess fat in place of food.

Many people do not have the determination or the intelligence to continue their regime. Many physicians are unable to present these facts to their patients in a convincing manner. Their patients find it much easier and more pleasurable to avoid the discomfort and self-control of a restricted diet and to pursue the numerous attractive and highly lauded "reducing" devices, such as electric therapy, massage of various types, (both active and passive), applications of heat, exercises of great variety, hot baths, colonic irrigations, hormone creams, and a thousand other "reducing methods" that are limited only by the imagination of the therapist and the gullibility of the obese person. Some persons have resorted to drugs, such as dinitro-phenol, for purposes of weight reduction, with disastrous results. Benzedrine and thyroid extract have also been used to stimulate metabolism, and thus increase the energy requirements. They should never be used for the reduction of obesity except under careful supervision of a physician.

Feinstein(1), in an analysis of methods, results, and factors which influence success in obesity therapy, states that weight reduction involves interaction of three sets of factors:

1. The patient and his attitude.
2. Relationship with the physician.
3. The diet itself.

The dietary program is the least important. The failure is due to the patient's inability to adhere to the program.

A patient's reactions to dietary regimes are manifold. If sufficiently negative, no program is successful.

Standard diets and adjuncts are traditionally prescribed and often followed by failure. New techniques are devised constantly. The highest percentage of success is obtained through the enthusiastic and understanding support of the physician in aiding the patient to maintain his regime.

The Physician's Obligation to Overweight Patients

The patient who comes to the physician for reduction of weight must be convinced that (a) his obesity is due to eating more food than he requires, and (b) the only way that he can return to normal is by the slow, steady, difficult road of a proper diet. The patient should understand the danger of drugs for this condition and the futility of other methods of treatment. He should be told of the hazards of obesity, and perhaps an appeal be made to his vanity or to his pride of his stamina and ability to manifest self-control. It must be explained that results are achieved slowly and are not spectacular. A diet list should be prepared which is as varied and enjoyable as possible, which furnishes bulk and ample vitamin requirements, and which has a caloric value of approximately 1,000 to 1,200 calories daily.

The major contribution of the physician is a genuine interest in and knowledge of the problems of weight reduction, which enables him to give the patient psychological and sympathetic support.

Community Responsibility in Obesity

The health department has a definite responsibility in the prevention of premature death or disability from obesity. Its chief function is educational. It should:

1. Teach the people the essentials of a normal diet.
2. Expose the harmful drugs and other "quack" methods foisted upon the public as obesity cures.
3. Emphasize the fact that overweight is unnecessary and can even be dangerous.
4. Explain the fact that obesity is caused by overeating and that it can be prevented by a properly regulated diet.

The chief responsibility for prevention of obesity rests with the private physician, because success depends upon a personal relationship between patient and physician. The solution of each case can be worked out only on an individual basis.*

DIABETES

There are more than 2,000,000 diabetics in the United States and their number is steadily increasing. Eventually, perhaps within the next generation, about 3 per cent of our total population will become diabetic. Thus it is a major chronic degenerative disease.

Diabetes can occur at any age but it is much more common in

---

*Group psychotherapy, in the form of self-help clubs, has been instituted along the general lines of Alcoholics Anonymous. The clubs have had some success.

the older age groups—80 per cent of the cases are over 45 years; 40 per cent are over 65.

In 1960, 28,000 deaths were ascribed to diabetes, but twice this number died with diabetes, in which atherosclerosis, nephritis, or other diagnosis was given as the primary cause of death.

In the Joslin Diabetic Clinic in Boston, the long survivorship of well-treated diabetics is noteworthy. Of patients first examined in the ages from 45 to 59 years, 75 per cent were surviving after 10 years. Early diagnosis is an important factor in survival. If the disease exists more than a year before initiating treatment, survivorship is markedly diminished.

The disease is more prevalent in women than in men. It is more common in the higher economic levels of the community. Jewish people are particularly susceptible to the disease.

Despite better early recognition of the disease, a better understanding of its natural history, and a very much better method of therapy, the deaths attributed to the disease have increased steadily during the past decades.

This gloomy story, when analyzed, is not as disturbing as it at first appears. The life expectancy of a diabetic has been greatly increased since the introduction of insulin. In 1900, a child with diabetes might live 1.3 years. Now its life expectancy is at least 40 years. The apparent increase in the death rate from diabetes has been due to (a) an aging population, and (b) an unrealistic classification of causes of death(2). As Tolstoi, the great diabetic clinician, has stated: "Elderly people now die *with* not *from* diabetes." In other words, diabetes appears on the death certificate as an actual cause, or at least contributory cause of death when, as a matter of fact, the diabetes might have no more to do with the patient's demise than his gray hair or his "arcus senilis."

Diabetes belongs to the group of "degenerative" diseases in that, essentially, it is a disease which occurs in persons who have passed middle life. It is much more prevalent in obese persons than in thin people. Hereditary factors also play an important role in diabetic incidence. Joslin and his associates(3) have stated that the familial tendency to development of diabetes is a mendelian (recessive) characteristic, i.e., if a diabetic marries a diabetic, then all the children are potential diabetics, and in all probability will develop diabetes if they survive to middle age. Thus, although a diabetic can marry and have children, he should never marry into a family with an immediate family history of diabetes.

Control of Diabetes

At present, we have no methods to prevent the onset of diabetes, in the sense that we can prevent smallpox or diphtheria. Nevertheless, the outlook in diabetes is most hopeful. Much can be done to prevent the ravages of the disease, to prolong life, to prevent the catastrophes of diabetic coma, diabetic gangrene, and diabetic cataracts, and to aid the diabetic in many ways in his efforts to handle a prolonged and difficult life situation.

Diagnosis of Diabetes

Early diagnosis of diabetes is of primary importance in a preventive plan and depends upon several factors:

1. Dissemination of general knowledge to the population of the early symptoms of the onset of diabetes. Particularly, persons over 45 years of age should be taught to see their doctor whenever they suspect that they are not in a normal state of health. An annual routine urine examination is a very simple procedure, and is well worth the trouble it costs.

2. Alertness of the practicing physician to detect diabetes in its early stages. An excellent rule is a routine urine examination on all new patients or all regular patients not seen during the past year.

3. Readily available facilities for accurate determination of blood sugar levels.

If the disease is diagnosed early in its course and brought under proper therapy with continuous medical supervision, the prognosis is excellent for a long and useful life.

Treatment of Diabetes

Each patient must be carefully studied and then treated in accordance with his particular needs. Untreated or poorly treated diabetes results in premature disability, and this frequently leads to disaster.

Joslin has presented extensive data which indicates that diabetics develop arteriosclerosis and particularly advanced coronary disease earlier and more frequently than nondiabetics. The incidence of these changes increases with the duration of the disease, and the degree of severity increases in those who are treated improperly.

Prevention of Disaster in Diabetes

The preventive aspects of diabetes can be divided into two major parts: (a) responsibility of the physician, and (b) community responsibility.

The Responsibility of the Physician. The particular responsibility of the physician is to make the diagnosis of diabetes in his patients as early as possible and to maintain each patient who has diabetes under a continuous regime of adequate therapy. This program must be lifelong and must be varied, as special conditions demand.

Prevention of Gangrene. Diabetic gangrene usually occurs in the feet, almost always following some injury or infection. Thus, every effort should be made to provide for good hygiene of the feet, taking particular care of all bruises and abrasions.

Infections. Diabetics who develop infections require immediate hospitalization and very careful and closely observed therapy. Insulin requirements during a period of infection can be quite at variance with customary needs. Tuberculosis is much more prevalent in diabetic children than in normal children so that special precautions should be taken to prevent exposure of the diabetic to tuberculosis.

Coma. Coma is the major diabetic emergency. All diabetic patients should be taught to be aware of symptoms of impending coma, to call a physician at once, and make all preparations for immediate hospitalization. Minutes count, for treatment should start at once. Hospital facilities should be readily available to all patients in diabetic coma, in order to obtain constant observation of the patient, continuous treatment, and proper laboratory assistance.

The Responsibility of the Community. The community responsibility in a diabetic control program consists of:

1. Provision for adequate and strategically located hospital beds, with laboratory and roentgenologic facilities so that all diabetics are able to obtain an early diagnosis and proper treatment. These necessary facilities must be provided to physicians and to the community because they are essential adjuncts to the proper medical care of diabetes.

2. Visiting nurses should be trained in the therapy of diabetes, and should also be equipped to aid the physician in administration of insulin, and in the techniques of prevention of diabetic gangrene and diabetic coma.

3. The community should furnish insulin, free of charge, to those patients who are unable to purchase the drug.

4. Departments of welfare should make arrangements for immediate free hospitalization of patients with pending diabetic coma, or other diabetic emergency, when so requested by a physician.

5. The health education service of the community should inform the people concerning the importance of the prevention of diabetes and the methods that can be used to control the symptoms of diabetes, and particularly to prevent premature death from this disease.

Mass Diagnosis of Diabetes

Wilkerson(4) in 1947 reported on a mass screening of Oxford, Massachusetts, to determine prevalence of diabetes in the community. Both urine and blood sugar examinations were made on over 3,000 people. Seventy cases of diabetes were found. Thirty of these were newly discovered during the survey. A subsequent selective study(5) was made of 736 blood relatives of known diabetics in Jacksonville, Florida. That study revealed a 5.4 per cent prevalence in the age groups 15 to 75 years.

TABLE 39

General Population Screening Tests for Diabetes*

Age (years)	Persons	New Diabetic Cases (per cent of total)
Under 30	47	0.0
30–39	2778	0.6
40–49	2354	1.4
50–59	1489	2.6
60–69	452	5.3
70+	131	3.8

* Packer *et al.* (5).

Many health departments have devised various methods for screening the general population for diabetes. For example, Packer (5) and his associates have tested 7,294 persons who came to the health department for "health cards." They were presumably normal persons, sent by employment and public welfare agencies. Seventy-five per cent were women; 70 per cent from 30 to 50 years old; and 90 per cent were from 30 to 60 years of age.

The yield of diabetics in blood-testing "normal" persons is given in Table 39.

Sixty-seven new cases were found in persons over 50 years of age (3.2 per cent); 48 cases were found in persons under 50 years (0.9 per cent)

The clinitron technique was followed, using the level of 130 mg per cent.

Bouton and Cortesi(6) have reported the blood-testing by clinitron of 6,308 normal persons. The level used was 160 mg per cent. The yield was 0.9 per 1,000 of newly discovered diabetics; 52 per cent of the persons screened were over 40 years of age; 93 per cent of the new diabetic patients discovered were over 40 years old. Bouton and Cortesi concluded that mass testing should be limited to persons over 40 years of age, and the test should be done within 1.5 hours of an adequate meal. All suspected cases are referred to their physician for confirmatory diagnosis and therapy. Although most patients go to their physician readily, about 15 per cent require sustained follow-up by the public health nurse. Bouton and Cortesi also reported that the cost of finding a new diabetic was about $80.

The great difficulty in this mass procedure is that a single uncontrolled test for the blood and urine sugar of an individual can be quite misleading and often gives a false sense of security or it may give a "fake" positive. It is true that in a large series of examinations of presumably normal people, a small number of undetected diabetics is usually uncovered.

For optimum results, however, the tests should be made not at random but on a selected population. Tests on relatives of known diabetics are most important and the yield is worth while.

Normal persons over 40 years of age give a yield commensurate with the costs involved. The tests alone are of little value unless a program is devised to follow up suspected cases in order that a definitive diagnosis be made and treatment instituted.

Periodic tests of large numbers of people by the health department is not a feasible procedure; nor is the diabetic problem static in any community, for new cases are developing constantly. The solution for case-finding in this disease, as well as in other chronic diseases, is not obvious.

The physician who is trained to incorporate the principles of preventive medicine in routine practice is the one on whom the responsibility falls for early detection of all types of degenerative disease, including diabetes. This requires adoption of a simple system of periodic physical examinations for adults, following the practice that has now been generally adopted for infants and children.

REFERENCES

1. FEINSTEIN, A. R.: *J. Chron. Dis.*, 1960, 11:349.

2. MARKS, H. H.: *M. Clin. North America*, 1947, 31:369.

3. JOSLIN, E. P., *et al.: The Treatment of Diabetes Mellitus.* Lea & Febiger, Philadelphia, 1940.

4. WILKERSON, H. L. C., and KRALL, L. P.: *J.A.M.A.*, 1947, **135**: 209.

5. PACKER, H., *et al.: Pub. Health Rep.*, 1960, **75**:1020.

6. BOUTON, M. A., and CORTESI, J. B.: *Am. J. Pub. Health*, 1960, **50**:524.

32. CONSERVATIVE ASPECTS
OF ARTHRITIS

In this discussion of arthritis, we include those most prevalent diseases that are grouped in the popular terminology of "rheumatism." The most common conditions are:

1. Rheumatoid arthritis (atrophic)
2. Osteoarthritis (hypertrophic).
3. Gout (metabolic arthritis).
4. Infectious arthritis.

Prevalence

The U.S. National Health Survey(1) of Arthritis and Rheumatism secured household interviews on these diseases through 1957 to 1959. It has given us an excellent picture of the prevalence of rheumatism in the general population.

This group of disabling illnesses has a low fatality rate with prolonged disability. This results in a high prevalence which increases year by year because of the aging of our population.

The popular diagnosis of rheumatism is "a disease that produces intermittent or persistent pain in the joints and muscles that has continued over a long period of time"(2). From the patient's point of view the major problems relating to the disease are: (a) loss of time from work; (b) limitation of activity and mobility; (c) bedfast disability; and (d) pain.

Insofar as the limitation of the survey method permitted, the study included only osteoarthritis, rheumatoid arthritis, and lumbago. It did not include in the tabulation rheumatic fever, neuritis, sciatica, or prolapsed disk.

In order to determine the extent of disability produced by rheumatism, certain specific terms were used.

460

1. *Long-term disability.*
   A.   Major. Inability to work in industry or do housework.
   B.   Partial. Limited in amount of activity—household, industry, community.
2. *Chronic mobility limitation.*
   A.   Major. Confined to the house.
   B.   Partial. Need help in moving about outside the house.
3. *Temporary disability.*
   A.   Restricted activity days.
   B.   Bed disability. More than one half of the daylight hours spent in bed because of illness.

TABLE 40

Bed Days of Disability per Person per Year

Age (years)	Days in Bed
All ages over 24	5.6
25 to 44	3.9
45 to 54	4.2
55 to 64	5.2
65 to 74	5.1
75 and over	11.4

The study showed that rheumatism can begin at an early age with a prevalence of 2 per 1,000 in the population at 25 years, increasing gradually to 286 per 1,000 in those over 70 years of age. The mean prevalence was 64 cases per 1,000 population. It has a higher prevalence in women than men in all age groups. This ratio increases with age. The over-all prevalence was: females, 81 per 1,000; males, 46 cases per 1,000.

Bed disability days (with one or more bedfast days per year) increased with age (see Table 40).

The survey estimates that there are almost 11 millions of arthritics in the United States, and that about 10 per cent of them have some degree of bed disability. Over 25 per cent are either completely unable to carry out major activities or are limited in the amount or kind of major or outside activity.

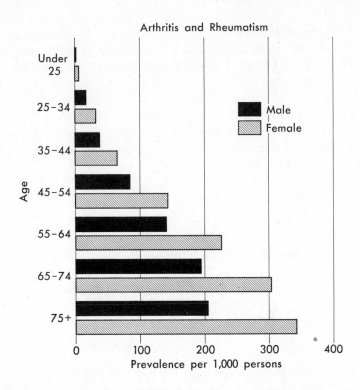

Figure 36. Prevalence of arthritis and rheumatism per 1,000 population by sex and age. (Health Statistics, *Arthritis and Rheumatism*, U.S. National Health Survey. July 1957–June 1959, Series B, No. 20.)

Many physicians have felt that preventive measures in rheumatism are of no avail: we do not know the cause of these diseases; no specific therapy is available; and control is at best palliative and empirical. But the experience of the state-wide rheumatism control programs of Sweden has shown us that this is an unnecessarily pessimistic point of view and that adequate provision for medical and hospital care can check progressive disability of rheumatism and bring about the return of the cripple and the partially disabled person to productive life.

Rheumatoid Arthritis

Rheumatoid arthritis is characterized by swelling, pain, and stiffness of the joints, with slowly progressive involvement that results in ankylosis and spondylosis. The disease begins either insidiously or abruptly as a painful swelling of the joints. It is sluggish and often manifests remission. Perhaps symptoms disappear for several years, but recurrences are the rule—these cyclic bouts eventually result in deformity and disability.

The patients are usually undernourished and underweight. Studies(3) indicate that if a food factor contributes to rheumatoid arthritis, it must be caused by an increase in body requirements rather than deficiency in the diet.

It is a disease of the young adult—often beginning at from 30 to 35 years of age and continuing throughout life.

The disease is much more common in women than in men, and is more prevalent among the poor. It frequently appears at the menopause. States of anxiety or mental stress can precipitate an initial attack or a recurrence of the disease.

Treatment of Rheumatoid Arthritis. Ideally, these patients should be sent to a warm, dry climate, such as Arizona or southern California, at the first appearance of symptoms. There is no better preventive measure. Hydrotherapy and physiotherapy are also of assistance, and orthopedic measures taken to prevent the deformities of ankylosis are often effective. Not knowing how to prevent the disease we try to prevent the recurrences and to ameliorate the ravages and deformities that are produced by the disease.

The patient with rheumatoid arthritis often gives a history of some type of focal, chronic infection, such as sinusitis, chronic tonsillitis, or abscesses at the root of the teeth. Formerly it was believed that the absorption of toxin from these foci was the primary cause of rheumatoid arthritis, but most authorities now feel that these foci of infection play a secondary role in the disease. In some instances, however, a temporary benefit is derived by surgical removal of the foci of infection.

Gold therapy is widely used, on an empirical basis, and if started early in the course of the disease, it often gives relief. The treatment must be given with skilled and experienced hands, as toxic reactions are frequently emcountered. If a relapse occurs at a later period, the second course of gold therapy does not produce as striking results as the first course.

The utilization of cortisone in amelioration of rheumatoid arthritis was considered for a time as an advance in therapy, but many clinicians have found that the benefits derived are not commensurate with the hazards involved in prolonged treatment with this type of drug.

There is a growing appreciation of the fact that an individual with rheumatism can be rehabilitated and trained to reassume a reasonable degree of activity in the community, if the case is carefully handled.

When the disease is once well established, the problems to be solved are:

1. Maintenance of muscular tone.
2. Prevention of ankylosis.
3. Prevention of deformity.

Muscular atropy can be prevented by massage, passive motion, and, later, active motion. The patient should be trained in corrective exercises by an experienced physiotherapist.

Ankylosis can be prevented by proper exercises. In rapidly progressive arthritis, the joints fuse in spite of therapy, but much can be accomplished by patience and perseverance.

Splints and other mechanical devices are used by the orthopedist in the prevention of deformities, particularly in flexions and contractures of the fingers and elbows.

Osteoarthritis

This is a degenerative disease, occurring in persons beyond 50 years of age, particularly in men and women who have spent a lifetime at hard work. It is a disease of "wear and tear." Osteoarthritis occurs generally on the weight-bearing joints. Obesity, with resultant faulty posture, is an important contributing factor in the disease.

Osteoarthritis seldom produces swelling of the joints. In only about one half the cases is there a history of sudden trauma. The lumbar spine is the articulation most frequently involved, and the earliest. Osteoarthritis of the spine is as common in the well-to-do as in the poor, and seems to be more prevalent in certain families.

Some persons inherit good cartilage; others do not. The cartilage wears through with time, and the bone is exposed. In the roentgenograms, lipping and spurs are seen around the margin of the bone — often a considerable degree of osteoarthritis is found in the roentgenograms of the joints of elderly people, without any symptoms of rheumatism.

Osteoarthritis can be greatly alleviated if handled promptly. The first thing to do is correct the obesity, the bad posture, and incorrect walk. A corrective brace often relieves the back pain. Hydrotherapy and physiotherapy often produce relief from symptoms. Avoidance of exposure to cold, and avoidance of hard manual work, heavy lifting, and indulgence in active games are good preventive measures.

Gout

The picture of the country squire, glass of port in hand and great toe swathed in bandages, is a caricature, yet it illustrates some of the salient features of gout. Gout is most frequent in males, is more common in England and France and the temperate zones than elsewhere, and its exacerbations may be related to alcoholic and dietary excess.

The cause of gout is unknown, but its pathogenesis is clearly related to a defect in uric acid metabolism which leads to hyperuricemia and the deposition of urates in the tissues. Gout, the basic metabolic disease, may lead to the sequel of gouty arthritis. Gouty arthritis is first evident as acute attacks of "gout" that may be temporarily incapacitating. Although acute gouty arthritis is not clearly related to deposition of urates, such deposits are characteristic of the chronic deforming arthritis. There is evidence that gout, particularly juvenile gout, has a hereditary basis. Hyperuricemia may appear long before clinical evidences of the disease.

Conservative and Preventive Aspects. Complete prevention of the disease is not feasible because of its genesis in a poorly understood metabolic defect. However, the prompt therapy of beginning or incipient attacks of acute gouty arthritis can abort these recurrences and shorten the period of acute disability. It is possible that prompt treatment may delay progression of the disease. Colchicine is the time-honored drug for such treatment. It is toxic to the gastrointestinal tract so that it cannot be taken for long periods of time.

Rich protein (high-purine) foods are certainly not the cause of gout but increase the metabolic load as purines are broken down to urates. Hence a low-purine diet with limitation of meat to four or five times a week and a high-carbohydrate intake are helpful in reducing hyperuricemia and urate deposition. The provocative effects of alcohol and of the injection of certain drugs (testosterone, penicillin, etc.) are poorly understood, but should be avoided as much as possible. Drugs that promote urinary excretion of urates may be used to good effect (aspirin and certain benzoic acid derivatives). The anti-inflammatory compounds (cortisone, phenylbutazone) used in other types of arthritis may be useful in alleviating the disability of chronic gouty arthritis.

Infectious Arthritis

This disease usually involves a single joint; it is most often a disease of young men but can occur at any age. The most common etiologic factor is the gonococcus. Proper and prompt utilization of the antibiotics has greatly reduced the prevalence and serious import of this type of arthritis.

Better Methods for Control of Rheumatism

The ideal arrangement for care of rheumatism would be for every large hospital to set aside a number of its beds and allocate a part of its facilities for the study and treatment of chronic rheumatism. This would be a better arrangement than the establishment of large state-supported hospitals and government-supported clinics for the care of this group of diseases. Research in chronic rheumatism is expensive; care of the disease is prolonged and requires roentgenologic equipment, laboratory facilities, and physiotherapeutic equipment as well as skilled technicians. The scope of rheumatism control is so great and costly that probably the general plan of the Swedish national hospitals should be followed for the control of chronic rheumatism. This would mean the establishing of national- and state-supported hospitals or state-subsidized hospitals, properly equipped and staffed, and located at suitable centers of population. It seems quite probable as our population ages, and as tuberculosis comes gradually under control, that the government-supported institutions which are now required for treatment of tuberculosis can eventually be transferred to the care of chronic rheumatism and other degenerative diseases.

The trend in development of community facilities for care of chronic illness is "progressive rehabilitation." For this the general hospital constructs a rehabilitation unit for patients in need of rehabilitation facilities rather than acute illness care. The plan includes facilities for extension of rehabilitation into the home (see Chap. 39).

Patients with arthritis benefit greatly from this type of progressive rehabilitation.

Rheumatism is a highly prevalent chronic disease. The proper study and care of the individual case constitute a burden which cannot be borne from the savings of the average worker, or by his family. Since our established policy now is that the care of chronic illness be a governmental responsibility, and since at least 80 per cent of hospital beds for chronic diseases are at present on a government-supported and not a privately supported basis, it seems most logical to take a further step and to include the study and the care of chronic rheumatism in the category of state-supported, or at least heavily subsidized, facilities.

REFERENCES

1. *Arthritis and Rheumatism, Health Statistics, U.S. National Health Survey,* Series B., No. 20, 1957-59. U.S. Dept. of Health, Education, and Welfare, Washington, D.C.

2. JOSLIN, E. P., *et al.: The Treatment of Diabetes Mellitus.* Lea & Febiger, Philadelphia, 1940.

3. BAYLES, T. B., RICHARDSON, H., and HALL, F. C.: *New England J. Med.,* 1943, **229**:319.

33. PREVENTIVE ASPECTS OF CANCER

Cancer is a disease which is predominant in the later decades of life, yet in the United States cancer kills more children between 1 and 15 years of age than any other disease.

For years past, the death rate from cancer has increased steadily, so that in most of the United States it is second only to diseases of the circulatory system as a cause of death. In 1959 cancer was the cause of one out of every six deaths in the United States. The steady increase in cancer has occurred despite our accumulation of knowledge of the disease and despite active efforts that have been put forth for the control of cancer.

Has the increase in the cancer death rate been an apparent or a real increase? Has it been due in part to an "aging" population, since a greater proportion of the people now reach the life periods in which each individual is more susceptible to cancer? Is the increase a result of better diagnosis and better reporting of cancer?

Epidemiology

Epidemiologic studies of cancer prevalence have brought out some interesting facts.

Dorn and Cutler(1) studied ten metropolitan areas for a ten-year period. During that period they found an increase in prevalence of 26 per cent; of incidence, 30 per cent; and of mortality, 19 per cent. When these data were adjusted to changes in age distribution the increase was: prevalence, 10 per cent; incidence, 14 per cent; and mortality, 3 per cent. These data indicate that much of the apparent increase in cancer prevalence is due to changes in the age distribution of our population.

The total incidence of cancer was similar in the two sexes, but there was marked variation in site or origin. One half of the cancers in females originated in the breast and genitals. Cancer of the lung was 4.5 times more frequent in men, and cancer of the larynx was 12 times higher in men. One half of all cancer in men originated in the digestive system. Higher rates for cancer prevailed in the lower economic groups, particularly cancer of the lip, mouth, esophagus, and stomach.

Dorn and Cutler determined that accessibility of organ-of-origin aids greatly in early detection of cancer. Sixty-two per cent of cancers in "accessible" sites were diagnosed while localized. Only 38 per cent of cancers were diagnosed while still localized if the cancer originated in an "inaccessible" site.

For years Connecticut has made a special study of death rates from cancer (see Fig. 37). The crude death rate rose steadily from 1910 to 1950 and then leveled off at 170 per 100,000. Since Connecticut has had a gradual increase in the age groups more susceptible to cancer, this graph indicates a most encouraging decline of deaths from the disease.

Sex differences in cancer death rates suggest important avenues of investigation concerning the etiology of the disease.

Table 41 gives the total deaths by site from cancer in males and females in Connecticut during 1959. There are many more women than men in the older age groups in this state; yet in every category, male deaths greatly outnumber female deaths. These data suggest that there is something related to the activities of males in which females do not, or at least in previous years, have not participated, which eventually results in production of cancer. Investigation of exposures to carcinogenic substances incident to occupation is giving valuable epidemiologic information which relates to this point.

Cancer of the digestive tract is the most prevalent and the most difficult to control. In general, it can be stated that the diagnostic techniques for detecting early cancer of the digestive tract have not been perfected to the point that measures undertaken for control of the disease in these organs can be expected to lower the death rate to any appreciable degree. The best results in control of cancer have been secured in those patients in whom cancer has occurred in the readily accessible organs of the body, where early diagnosis is easily made, and where prompt and radical surgical removal is quite feasible.

Etiology of Cancer

Active and promising research is being conducted in the United States concerning etiologic factors in cancer. John Heller(2), President of the Sloan-Kettering Cancer Center, New York City, noted that certain cancerlike diseases of animals have been shown to be due

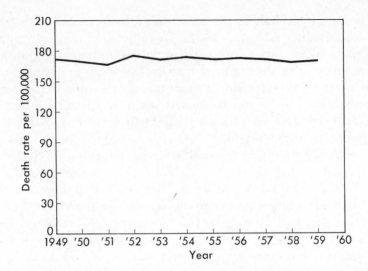

Figure 37. Death rates from cancer for Connecticut. (Data provided by Bureau of Vital Statistics, State Department of Health, Connecticut.)

to specific viruses. Some success has been achieved in developing vaccines against virus agents that have caused cancer in animals. The possibility of producing vaccines to prevent cancer from developing in man offers encouragement.

It might also be possible to develop a virus that will attack and destroy cancer cells without injury to the host. One approach might be the use of a selective drug that would destroy the attacking agent (cancer virus) without injuring the host. Heller concluded that research on viruses might eventually lead to advances in knowledge and skill that will help prevent or arrest the development of many human cancers.*

It has been known for many years that certain agents of the environment predispose to the development of cancer. Most people exposed to these hazards do not develop the disease, but the risk of persons exposed to these agents is much greater than in the general population. Thus these factors can be considered as etiologic agents

---

*The Progress Report XIII of the Sloan-Kettering Institute for Cancer Research, June 1960, presents a comprehensive, detailed, chronological report of cytological research in the cancer field. It concludes: "It becomes increasingly clear that this new flood of interest, knowledge and activity is threatening inexorably to engulf the ancient mystery of cancer."

in cancer and preventive measures taken to reduce the risk of exposure to all persons.

Evang and Pedersen(3) have insisted that continuous efforts must be employed in securing new knowledge concerning environmental factors in cancer. Industrial carcinogens must be determined, and the exposure of the worker minimized. More than 200 industrial carcinogens have already been identified. These include tar, asphalt, creosote, benzol, soot, and shale oil. Inorganic carcinogens, such as various arsenicals, asbestos, and the chromates, are widely used in industry. Physical carcinogens, such as X-rays and ultraviolet rays, are important. Irritants, such as a broken tooth, smoking habits, radiation hazards, and many other environmental factors, can produce cancer in a susceptible individual.

TABLE 41

Cancer Deaths by Site, Males Compared with
Females: Connecticut, 1959

Site of Cancer	Total Deaths	
	Males	Females
Stomach	198	144
Respiratory tract	557	94
Rectum	110	75
Buccal cavity and pharynx	105	13
Bladder	98	28
Esophagus	101	22

Stewart, Webb, and Hewett(4) have shown an apparent relationship of subsequent childhood leukemia with antenatal pelvic radiation of pregnant women.

Influence of Cigarette Smoking

Extensive studies have been carried out on the effect of cigarette smoking in production of cancer of the lung.

Davis(5) has reviewed 267 published papers on this subject, taken from all parts of the world. He has stated that the evidence in favor of cigarette smoking as the major environmental causal factor in epidermoid lung cancer is abundant and consistent. He has pointed out that three fourths of all primary lung cancer in the United States is associated with cigarette smoking.

Dorn(6) has studied the incidence of lung cancer as related to "heavy," "light," and nonsmokers of cigarettes in United States Government Life Insurance policy holders (see Table 42). Most of those observed were men.

TABLE 42

Death Rate per 100,000 per Annum

All Ages to 55		*55 to 59*	*60 to 64*	*65+*
Never smoked	16.0	12.0	14.0	31.0
Light smokers (less than 10 a day)	104.5	48.2	92.5	292.0
Heavy smokers (more than 20 a day)	244.9	174.5	269.4	388.0

It is interesting to note that despite the strong evidence that heavy cigarette smoking is associated with a greater risk of cancer of the lung, and despite the wide dispersal of this information to the public, the national consumption of cigarettes has increased each year in the United States.

Cancer of the Lips, Tongue, and Buccal Cavity

In almost every instance, cancer of the lips and buccal cavity follows some type of chronic inflammation or irritation. Pipe smokers develop cancer of the angle of the mouth which carries the pipe. Jagged teeth can cause an irritation of the tongue, producing leukoplakia, which could eventually result in cancer. It has been claimed that the scar of an old syphilitic glossitis can degenerate into a cancer of the mouth or tongue. These are rare conditions.

The prevention, proper treatment, and, if necessary, the surgical removal of precancerous lesions of the mouth are important methods of prevention of cancer of these organs. It has been estimated that one half of the potential cancers of the mouth can be eliminated and one half of the remainder cured by relatively simple measures if the lesions are treated when first seen. Surgery, electrosurgery, radium and roentgen-ray therapy, either singly or in combination, give excellent results.

Cancer of the Skin

Cancer of the skin results from a great variety of skin irritations. Among the common factors that can initiate skin cancer are:

1. Arsenical keratosis.
2. Irritation of the skin from coal tars, e.g., cancer of the scrotum in chimney sweeps.
3. Scars of old burns.
4. Roentgen-ray and radium burns.
5. Pigmented moles.
6. Exposure to severe weather conditions, such as in sailors and farmers. Ultraviolet rays are regarded by some authorities as of primary importance in production of these tumors. This will be an important finding if substantiated since protection from ultraviolet rays is not a difficult matter.
7. Keratosis senilis.

In all cancers of these types, early recognition and intelligent handling of the precancerous lesion, with prompt treatment of the early cancer, will result in a great saving of life.

Cancer of the Breast and Uterus

Any lump in the breast or any abnormal discharge from the vagina should be a warning sign to a woman to consult her physician promptly. The secret of prevention of death from cancer in these organs is early diagnosis and prompt therapy.

The two most important precancerous lesions of the breast are believed to be chronic mastitis and intraductal papilloma. Pack(7) has stated that approximately 20 per cent of all mammary cancers have their onset in those tissues where chronic cystic mastitis has occurred. He also believes that a considerable proportion of intraductal papillomas become cancerous. Thus, special attention must be given to these two conditions.

Important precancerous lesions of the female genital organs are: keratosis vulvae, leukoplakia vulvae, endocervicitis, cervical lacerations, and endometrial polyps.

Cancer occurs frequently in the injured cervix which has had poor repair, and which presents a picture of chronic infection. Endocervicitis, with the accompanying chronic irritation, also is believed to be an important predisposing factor in cancer of the cervix.

Cancer of the Prostate

The high prevalence of this condition in elderly men has been recognized only recently. It seems probable that as our population ages and more and more men reach the seventh and eighth decades of life, the incidence of this disease will increase. Fortunately, it usually progresses very slowly, and its ravages can be checked by appropriate therapy.

Cancer of the Digestive Tract

Cancer of the more accessible portion of the digestive tract as, for example, cancer of the rectum, offers some hope for amelioration or cure, since the diagnosis can be made early and prompt therapy instituted. Even the less accessible cancers of the large intestine are tardy to metastasize and therefore are susceptible to cure by surgical removal. With the limitations of our present knowledge, cancers of the stomach and intestines do not lend themselves to satisfactory preventive measures. Many researches now under way give promise that diagnostic techniques might be developed to indicate the presence, very early, of hidden cancerous growth in the inaccessible portions of the body.

CANCER RESEARCH AND CONTROL

Cancer research is one of the most important responsibilities that face scientific medicine. The U.S. Public Health Service took the lead in this field and established excellent laboratory facilities in the National Institutes of Health at Bethesda, Maryland. Many universities and private philanthropic organizations have undertaken research in the field of cancer. These studies, though often difficult and discouraging are sure to produce satisfactory results if continued unremittingly.

Community Responsibility for Cancer Control

The essential features of a community-wide program for the control of cancer are simple; they are based on the elementary principles that likelihood of control of the disease rests upon:

1. Prevention of cancer by proper treatment of precancerous lesions.
2. Early and accurate diagnosis of the disease.
3. Prompt and effective treatment.

Diagnostic Services for Cancer. Diagnostic cancer centers should oe established at strategic and readily available locations. In most instances, these clinics require state support. They should be staffed by experts. Patients are generally referred to these clinics by their private physicians. This diagnostic service should be free.

A central laboratory should be provided for the tissue diagnosis of suspected cancerous tissue. This service should be free both to the patients and to the physicians, and organized on the same basis as other state-wide diagnostic laboratory services.

Cancer Detection Centers

The American Cancer Society has promoted the establishment of cancer detection centers throughout the United States. The American College of Surgeons has set minimum standards(8) for these centers and has indicated the purposes and benefits to be derived from them:

1 — Purposes

To provide a complete, thorough physical examination for apparently well persons to:

Detect sooner than would otherwise be discovered early cancer, precancerous lesions, areas of chronic irritation, or abnormal physiological conditions which might lead to cancer.

Discover early manifestations of other diseases.

Inform the public of the early signs and symptoms of cancer.

Lower the incidence of late cancer in the population by detection of early cancer which is so frequently curable.

Document and furnish to appropriate physicians, clinics, hospitals, and other agencies complete, accurate, and uniform records for the purpose of establishing the necessity for this method of approach and education, for follow-up work which is vital to the welfare of persons afflicted with cancer, and for further emphasis on the scientific and economic value of early detection, diagnosis, and treatment.

2 — Benefits

Detection of early cancer or precancerous lesions.

Detection by comprehensive examination of early manifestations of other diseases which frequently are more successfully treated in their early stages.

Encouragement of the habit of regular physical examinations.

Promotion of effective preventive medicine, which provides longer life and prolongs the period of economic productivity.

Direction of people to the correct channel for information, diagnosis and treatment.

Education of the public.

Creation of valuable sources of statistical material for scientific analysis.

Emerson Day(9) has made a summary of results secured in detection of cancer by cancer centers in the United States from 1937 to

1957. He estimated that more than 200 cancer detection centers were in operation in 1957. He collected data from some 21 typical services, which reported 82,216 examinations. Two thirds of the tests were in females. The age distribution was as follows:

Age in Years	Per Cent
Under 40	44
40 to 49	28
50 to 59	19
Over 60	11

Total cancers found in this group were 963, a rate of 117 per 10,000 examined. Many of the cancer centers gave only an initial examination, thus the preponderance of persons examined were women under 50 years of age. In contrast, the University of Minnesota Clinic accepted only women of 45 years or over and men over 50 years, enrolling them in about equal numbers. The Minnesota Clinic insisted on subsequent periodic examinations. The yield of this clinic was 273 cancers per 10,000 persons examined in females, and 272 in males.

Day summarized the sites of previously unrecognized cancer in 18,312 persons. In males, 287 cancers were discovered, a rate of 157 per 10,000 examinations. Cancer of the skin, rectum and colon, and genitourinary tract comprised 70 per cent of the cancers discovered.

In females, 50,466 examinations were made and 677 cancers found, a rate of 132 cancers per 10,000 examined. Nearly 70 per cent of the cancers discovered were of the breast, uterus, and ovary.

Precancerous lesions were found in 10 to 15 per cent of all persons examined. These included skin lesions, polyps of the colon and rectum, leukoplakias, cervicitis, thyroid adenoma, benign breast tumors, etc.

Noncancerous abnormalities were found in 20 to 100 per cent of persons. Major categories were cardiovascular, gynecological, and gastrointestinal. Lung cancer was very seldom found by the cancer detection centers.

Six large centers conducted a screening test that was limited to the Papanicolaou uterine cell test. In more than 250,000 examinations, cancer was found in 1,494 women. The rate in various clinics was consistent: 55 to 67 per 10,000 examined.

In reality, cancer detection is the responsibility of the practicing physician. Every physician should have his own cancer detection service. The chief values of cancer detection centers are that they have clarified the objectives of cancer detection procedures, determined the results that can be anticipated, and developed adequate techniques. The centers are also of great aid to physicians in providing facilities for an initial test, but the responsibility for subsequent periodic health examination of susceptible age groups rests upon the practicing physician. The increasing acceptance by the people of prepayment plans for comprehensive medical care should promote the opportunity for physicians to give adequate periodic health examinations, which include cancer detection.

Hospitalization for Cancer. The community should make provision for adequate hospitalization of all patients who have cancer in order that prompt and adequate therapy can be administered. Provision should be made for free care of the poor, who cannot afford these services.

Adequate provision should be made in general hospitals for cancer therapy, including radium, roentgen ray, and surgery. Special hospitals located in strategic centers of population can be selected for provision of the more technical therapeutic procedures in the treatment of cancer (e.g., radium therapy).

General Education Concerning Cancer. The community should conduct a continuous educational program for the purpose of teaching all the people a few fundamental facts concerning cancer: (a) early recognition of cancer or of precancerous lesions is essential for cancer control; (b) early treatment is the mainstay in prevention of premature death from cancer; (c) the disease is not hopeless and incurable, but prevention requires the alert cooperation of patient, private physician, and the central diagnostic and therapeutic agencies.

The following case histories illustrate good and poor results in cancer control:

A. C. was a 38-year-old, well-educated and intelligent illustrator of children's books. She had been perfectly well. One evening while taking her bath, she noted a small hard painless lump in her left breast. She called her private physician on the telephone at once and told him of her observation. The following morning her physician took her to the surgeon. A radical breast amputation was done the same afternoon. Pathologic examination showed a carcinoma of the breast of about 1½ cm in diameter. It was well localized, with no extension to the axillary glands. She was discharged from the hospital with a good prognosis. There is good reason to believe that this intelligent woman will live a normal life span.

J. M. was a very active and able businessman who gave little thought to his personal trivial ailments. He began to suffer from constipation, which he believed was due to his sedentary life and irregular habits and related to business stress. He took mineral oil and cathartics for relief, but the condition persisted. Three or four months later, he noted a small amount of blood in his stools, and consulted his family physician. No rectal examination was made. The physician made a diagnosis of hemorrhoids and gave a bland diet. He suggested rest and regulation of bowel habits, and gave a palliative ointment.

The patient noted an increase of symptoms, with gradual loss of weight and weakness. He had no pain. After five months, he consulted his physician a second time. A rectal examination revealed a readily accessible annular carcinoma of the rectum which had extended to the adjoining tissues and was inoperable.

H. P., a Negro man of 41 years, came to the clinic in April 1937. He had been badly burned at the age of two years when his clothes caught fire from an open fireplace. The backs of both legs were severely scarred. Four years ago the left popliteal space in the center of the burn scar became ulcerated. The ulcer increased in size, despite ointments and hot applications, and also became painful and very irritated.

Biopsy showed a bilateral epithelioma of the skin in the burn scar. Excision of the tumor and application of skin grafts resulted in cure, with no return in the scar after four years and no metastasis in the groin.

S. T. was an ignorant 47-year-old woman who came to the clinic because she had read an article in the daily newspaper "health column" about cancer. For two months she had noted a hard whitish growth on her tongue. This was due, she felt, to a gold-capped irregular tooth which irritated the area. The irritation disappeared when the tooth was removed, but the sore on her tongue increased.

Biopsy proved the growth to be carcinoma. The growth was removed by cautery, with no recurrence after four years.

These four cases are typical of cancer, and each of them can be duplicated in any clinic. They tell their own stories of suitable methods of prevention and control of cancer.

Effectiveness of Educational Measures concerning Early Detection of Cancer

In recent years, extreme efforts have been expended by health departments, cancer societies, physicians in practice, by newspapers, magazines, and other means to educate the people to the necessity of prompt treatment of cancer. The results of this active propaganda are somewhat discouraging.

Robbins(10) made a study of the lag in diagnosis and treatment, comparing the years 1941 and 1948 with the period 1922 to 1938. Over these years there has been real reduction in the interval between first appearance of symptoms and the establishment of the diagnosis.

Physicians are losing less time between the first consultation and the actual point when diagnosis is established and therapy begins. The interval between symptoms first noted by the patient and the date he first consults his physician still remains discouragingly long. It is clear that the reaction pattern in any given patient is set long before cancer develops.

Robbins concluded as follows:

The patient who is accustomed to face reality or who fears physical pain or disability and who is accustomed to seek medical aid promptly at first symptoms is the one who seeks help quickly when his illness is due to cancer. Conversely, the patient who in the past had to be forced only by extenuating circumstances, by intractable pain, or by the pressure of family or friends to seek medical aid, acts the same way when his illness is due to cancer. Economic status seemed to be of no consequence in the group of patients studied, so far as delay or non-delay was concerned. Better levels of intelligence and education were factors favoring non-delay. Unfortunately, data on those in the age groups 60 and over were the least encouraging, since delay was greater in these patients.

These observations have meaning and are not based on one isolated study. They mean in part that the educational program, which must include propaganda, is the only practical weapon at present to combat inertia and ignorance.

A large segment of the population is never reached or affected by many phases of the educational program. This is not a criticism but simply a statement of fact. One phase of the educational program that will reach a large portion of the population, especially those in the desired age groups (40 years and older), is the type of steady enlightening propaganda that the individual physician can spread. Not the least important measure is the routine annual physical examination. This is too great a task to impose on the cancer detection clinic. Each physician has his own detection clinic in his office and hospital.

Robbins statement is as pertinent today as it was in 1948.

REFERENCES

1. DORN, H. F., and CUTLER, S. J.: *Morbidity from Cancer in the United States*, Public Health Monograph 56, U.S. Dept. Health, Education, and Welfare, Washington, D.C., 1959.

2. HELLER, J. R.: *Pub. Health Rep.*, 1960, **75**(6):501.

3. EVANG, K., and PEDERSEN, E.: *J. Chron. Dis.*, 1960, **11**:149.

4. STEWART, A., WEBB, J., and HEWETT, D.: *Brit. Med. J.*, 1958, 1:1495.

5. DAVIES, D. F.: *J. Chron. Dis.*, 1960, **11**:579.

6. DORN, H. F.: *Pub. Health Rep.*, 1959, **74**:581.

7. PACK, G. T.: Classroom statement to Cornell medical students.

8. *Bull. Am. Coll. Surgeons*, June, 1947.

9. DAY, E.: *A Report on Cancer Detection in the United States — 1937-1957*. Prepared for The International Union against Cancer, Brussels, from Strang Cancer Prevention Clinic, Memorial Hospital, New York.

10. ROBBINS, G. F., *et al.*: *J.A.M.A.*, 1950, **143**:346.

GENERAL REFERENCE

An excellent description of the essentials of a cancer detection examination has been prepared by Dr. Emerson Day,* Professor of Preventive Medicine, Sloan-Kettering Institute. It is highly recommended to all practicing physicians.

*DAY, EMERSON: *The Cancer Detection Examination: C. A. The Cancer Journal for Clinicians*: American Cancer Society, Inc., **11**(3) May-June 1960.

34. PREVENTIVE ASPECTS
OF CARDIOVASCULAR DISEASE

The number of people in the community who die from heart disease each year throughout the United States has increased with startling rapidity during the past hundred years. This striking fact has created great interest in the possible prevention of heart disease; particular attention has been given to a study of means whereby death from heart disease might be prevented or postponed.

The American Heart Association is a national organization for the study and prevention of heart disease with active local chapters in all states and most large cities. The U.S. Public Health Service has established an effective division for study and control of heart disease, and many of the state and local health departments have become actively interested in this field.

This increase in the crude death rate from heart disease has led to conclusions that cannot always be fully substantiated. It is true that heart disease now causes many more deaths than any other single condition and that the actual number of deaths from heart disease is increasing every year. Paradoxically, this fact does not mean that heart disease is on the increase. In fact, there is evidence that heart disease is not increasing but actually is decreasing in importance as a *premature* cause of death. This point is brought out in a comparison of the crude death rate of a community with the standardized death rate (see p. 53).

The following are two main reasons for apparent increase in the cardiac death rate. The first is the great reduction in deaths from tuberculosis and pneumonia, the leading causes of death in 1900, and the almost complete elimination of deaths from acute communicable diseases of childhood. In addition to altering the proportions by virtue of cutting down deaths from these causes, this has meant that many people have survived, to die later from one of the cardiovascular-renal diseases. The result is the progressive aging of the population.

Cardiovascular deaths have been concentrated at the far end of the life span, with more than two thirds of these deaths in 1960 taking place among persons over 65 years of age.

From this simple analysis, it is quite clear that the more intensive our activities for the amelioration of the ravages of degenerative diseases, including heart disease, the higher the death rate from heart disease will go. In other words, the longer a man lives, the greater the likelihood of his finally dying from heart disease.

This fact should not, of course, discourage the official and voluntary health agencies or the private physician from carrying out every possible measure for the prevention of cardiac disease and, more important still, for prevention or amelioration of those factors which affect a cardiac patient adversely.

Furthermore, everything should be done to rehabilitate the cardiac to make his life more fruitful and less of a burden to himself and to his family.

Those who have spent their lives in the field of prevention of communicable diseases and in environmental sanitation, and who have now entered the field of geriatrics, must take a completely new point of view. For successful efforts will increase rather than decrease prevalence of the degenerative diseases. Thus, activities in geriatrics should be directed primarily toward amelioration and rehabilitation rather than toward the actual prevention of disease, which has heretofore been the primary purpose of those in public health.

Furthermore, in attempting to measure the degree of effectiveness of our work we will meet only disappointment, if our scale of measurement is the crude specific death rate. The major effort in geriatrics is to postpone death from degenerative diseases rather than to prevent it; therefore the measure of success can be secured only by the comparative tables of deaths in various age groups or by utilization of the standardized rates. For example, if the death rate from heart disease during the next 20 years declines in the age period from 40 to 65 and increases in the age period from 65 to 90, then our efforts have been fruitful; yet a decline in the total deaths from heart disease cannot be anticipated.

TYPES OF HEART DISEASE

All our data express, in the aggregate, the very high prevalence of heart disease, but they are meaningless unless they are broken down into their component parts. There are many types of heart disease. The most common are:

1. Congenital disease of the heart.
2. Rheumatic fever.
3. Cardiovascular syphilis.
4. Other infections of the heart.
5. Cardiovascular disease: (a) hypertension; (b) coronary disease.
6. Miscellaneous affections of the heart.

Under the last heading are included functional disorders and toxic conditions such as hyperthyroidism.

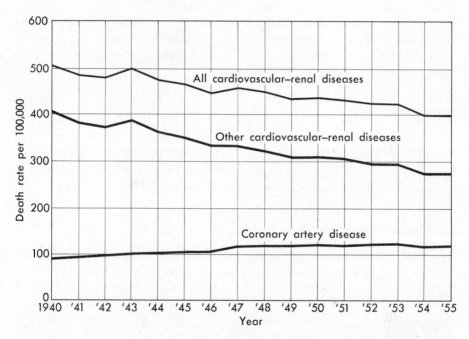

Figure 38. Trend of mortality from coronary artery disease and other cardio-vascular-renal diseases. Age-adjusted death rates. (Deaths classified by Sixth Revision of International List. 1940–1948 Estimated. Age-adjusted on basis of total U.S. population in 1940). Total persons – United States, 1940–1955.

The etiology of each of these conditions is quite different, and the epidemiologic features of each vary one from the other. In some of these conditions, we have little knowledge as to etiology and little concept of methods of prevention. Thus few measures are available for the control of the disease.

In others, preventive measures have a direct application, and control procedures are quite effective.

Congenital Heart Disease

The incidence of congenital heart disease among the newborn is about 3 per 1,000 live births. In the United States this represents some 14,000 cases annually. Sixty per cent die during the first year of life, most of them during the first few days after birth. Five per cent more die before their fifth birthday.

The cause of congenital heart malformation is not known, except for the few cases that are due to an attack of German measles in the mother during the first trimester of pregnancy.

The development of surgical procedures in treatment of congenital heart disease is most promising. Many infants formerly doomed to an early death can now have their heart defects corrected and lead a virtually normal life.

Rheumatic Fever

The heart disease of infants is congenital disease; the heart disease of children is rheumatic fever. This condition is one of the leading causes of death in the age group from 10 to 15 years and is second only to tuberculosis in the next decade, 15 to 25 years.

Cardiovascular Syphilis

When cardiovascular syphilis has developed to the degree that it can be clearly recognized clinically, there is little that can be done by the physician or the health department to prolong life or prevent suffering. The damage has been done. The disease often does not manifest itself until 20 years or more after the initial infection. It is more common in men than in women and appears usually at about 45 years of age. It is more prevalent in Negroes, and appears in this race at an earlier age than in whites.

The prevention and control of cardiovascular syphilis are, in essence, the prevention of, the early diagnosis of, and the proper therapy of syphilis itself. All the various methods employed with increasing effectiveness in the prevention, and particularly in the early diagnosis and prompt and adequate therapy, of syphilis have had a definite effect in reducing the prevalence of syphilitic cardiovascular disease. It seems probable that it is only in the years to come that full benefits of this fine cooperative effort by physicians and the official and voluntary health agencies will be realized.

The basic elements of the syphilis control program are:

1. Case finding of syphilis.
2. Early and adequate treatment of the disease.
3. Preventive methods.

These have been described in some detail in Chapter 14.

H. P. was a 39-year-old unemployed white printer. He came to the hospital one year previous because of progressively increasing orthopnea, dyspnea, and dependent edema.

He had syphilis at 21 years of age, which was inadequately treated because of lack of cooperation on the part of the patient.

Physical examination revealed a markedly enlarged heart in atrial fibrillation, with other signs of decompensation. His Wassermann reaction was 4 plus. The patient responded well to the standard hospital regimen for cardiac decompensation, but was quite uncooperative while in the hospital and was discharged after four weeks.

A roentgenogram of the chest indicated that there was a dilatation of the arch of the aorta, but there were no signs of true aneurysm. It was assumed that syphilis played an important part in the lesion of the heart and aorta, but the patient refused all antisyphilitic treatment, saying that he was "cured."

The social service worker of the cardiac clinic attempted by means of home visits to secure better cooperation from the patient and his family. The report was that "he is unemployed and has been on home relief. He cannot live within his means, and his creditors hound him. He has a nagging wife, who screams at him. He indulges in alcohol and is irritable and disagreeable. His home life is unhappy and financial worries are ever present."

This patient visited the cardiac clinic at irregular intervals, whenever his symptoms became unbearable, and each time responded fairly satisfactorily to simple therapy. He refused hospitalization in a hospital for chronic disease.

This patient illustrates the red side of the ledger in cardiac disease control. It is quite probable that adequate antisyphilitic treatment at 21 years of age would have prevented the present condition. Antisyphilitic treatment at this later date would be of some value, perhaps, but the permanent damage had been done and could not be repaired. He still had a fair degree of cardiac reserve and if he were carried on a proper regime, he might live and work with reasonable comfort and some satisfaction.

But he refused to spare himself. His worry, anxiety, periods of anger, and unhappy home life were compensated for by bouts of alcoholism.

The patient had shown complete lack of cooperation while in the hospital and had been unwilling to listen to, or follow the advice of, the clinic physician and the social worker in arranging for a suitable regime which would make it quite possible for him to live comfortably for a time, at least, within his cardiac limitations.

Other Infections of the Heart

Methods of prevention of infections of the heart resolve themselves into prevention and early therapy of the initial infection, since cardiac complications are practically always a secondary affair. For example, early and adequate administration of antitoxin in diphtheria will prevent myocardial disease.

Treatment of scarlet fever, tonsillitis, pneumonia, and gonorrhea as well as a great variety of septic conditions, with one of the antibiotics will undoubtedly prevent a certain amount of cardiac infection. Subacute bacterial endocarditis usually occurs in individuals with previously damaged hearts, such as congenital defects or rheumatic fever. Those individuals should be carefully watched in case they have any septic foci such as dental abscesses or tonsillitis, for such infections might cause a relapse of their cardiac disease. If they have any surgical operation performed, some authorities believe that they can be saved serious trouble by prophylactic antibiotic therapy.

CARDIOVASCULAR DISEASES

Hypertension

The etiology of hypertension is not known nor are there any satisfactory means now available to prevent or check the advance of the disease.

Early diagnosis may be made, however, and the physician can teach the patient to live within his limitations with reasonable satisfaction and comfort.

In many middle-aged persons, worry, fatigue, stress, anger, distress, and other factors that accompany a hard-pressed hyperactive life will result in an increased blood pressure. The extraordinary results secured in hypertension reduction by a period of simple rest in bed, with freedom from all care and worry, are well recognized.

Normal Blood Pressure

Lasser and Master(1) have made a study of frequency distribution curves of the blood pressures of some 80,000 presumably normal persons from 20 to over 100 years of age. They show that with aging, the mean systolic blood pressure rises until the seventieth year; after that there is no significant change. The mean blood pressure of females is lower than males until the forty-fifth year; after that it is higher than in males. Mean diastolic pressures increase slightly with age, but for all practical purposes remain essentially constant throughout life.

The high standard deviations in this large series of observations of Lasser and Masters indicate that an individual's blood pressure can vary materially from the mean for an age and sex group yet still be within normal limits.

Another frequently made observation is that people, particularly women, in age groups over 55 or 60 years, can have a systolic blood pressure high above the "normal" for her age and yet live a perfectly normal, comfortable life for years.

The conference of the American Heart Association on "Epidemiological Methods in Heart Disease" suggested certain criteria for determination of abnormal blood pressure(2).

Normal blood pressure: systolic below 140; diastolic below 90 in milligrams of mercury.

Hypertension: systolic over 160; diastolic over 95; i.e., either one or both above the specified levels.

Systolic hypertension: systolic over 160; diastolic under 90.

Diastolic hypertension: systolic under 140; diastolic over 95.

This conference stated that "hypertension disease" was a term synonymous with essential hypertension, a clinical entity "in which an unknown pressor mechanism initiates arteriolar vasoconstriction, elevated blood pressure, and vascular sequelae. This clinical entity should not be confused with increased blood pressure due to primary atherosclerosis."

The conference considered various studies under way relating to diet, physical activity, biochemical measurements as well as cultural, societal, familial, psychological, and environmental situations that might be factors in the etiology of atherosclerosis. It was pointed out* that a mere demonstration of statistical association between a given factor and a disease does not establish link causation. A given event shown to be directly associated with a given disease represents only an index of a second factor which might be the true cause. It may be that the clinical entity is due to multiple causes.

It is uncertain whether factors presumed to be related to cardiovascular disease represent primary or secondary etiologies. Are they

*Lew(3) has shown a correlation between mortality from arteriosclerotic heart disease and density of specialists in internal medicine in different areas of the United States. The obvious interpretation is that the higher the quality of diagnostic acumen, the more prevalent the diagnosis.

definite causes or do they provoke clinical attacks in a person harboring a primary cause?

Etiology of Cardiovascular Disease

The etiology of cardiovascular disease is unknown. It is caused by atherosclerosis, but the apparently multiple factors which produce the pathologic change in the arteries are not clearly understood.

Ancel Keys(4) has developed the hypothesis that atherosclerosis is due largely to an overconsumption of animal fat. Cholesterol, a water-insoluble, crystalline alcohol, is essential to metabolism. Normally, the liver synthesizes only sufficient cholesterol to meet body needs for transportation of fat and production of bile. Overconsumption of certain fats, however, will increase blood cholesterol.

Natural food fats fall into three categories: (a) saturated, (b) monosaturated, and (c) polyunsaturated. All have similar caloric values, but saturated fats, such as meat and dairy products, promote cholesterol production in quantities too large for the body to excrete. Monosaturated fats (such as olive oil and margarine) do not increase blood cholesterol levels. Polyunsaturated fats (such as corn, cotton seed and fish oils) actually lower blood cholesterol levels.

No one knows the complex mechanicochemical system that produces deposition of cholesterol on the arterial wall. Keys has stated that there is substantial evidence that high cholesterol blood levels, maintained over a long period, are directly related to arterial disease. Thus, Keys has also concluded that blood cholesterol, which averages 240 mg in the average American of 40 to 60 years, should be reduced. The only satisfactory way to do this is to reduce the dietary fat from 40 per cent to 15 per cent of total caloric intake and to reduce saturated fats from 17 per cent to 4 per cent. This can be accomplished by eating less fat meat, eggs, and dairy products and by eating more chicken, fish, calves' liver, fresh fruits, and vegetables.

Epidemiology

Since the etiology in atherosclerosis is not known, research workers have considered it worth while to use the epidemiologic approach in the study of heart disease in the hope that preventive measures might emerge in spite of our ignorance of exact etiology. The methods used are similar to those employed in the study of infectious diseases, namely, measuring and comparing frequencies and distribution of the disease within defined populations. Various hypotheses have been evolved concerning possible etiologic factors or conditions that cause the disease; these are being tested continually.

Because the preclinical stages of atherosclerosis appear to occur almost universally among the older adult population groups in the United States, an exact comparison of cases and noncases is almost impossible.

Coronary Disease

Attacks of coronary disease are due to atherosclerosis of the coronary artery. It is an important cause of death in the United States. Some authorities believe it is increasing in prevalence.

Lew(3) presented an illuminating discussion on mortality relating to coronary artery disease at the conference of the American Heart Association in 1957.

He stated that 30 per cent of the increase in the crude death rate from coronary disease in recent years is due to aging of the population; 40 per cent of the increase is due to changes in the method of reporting deaths. Thus less than 30 per cent of coronary disease can be attributed to a real increase in prevalence. He noted that there was a higher incidence in young males than in females. The disease seems more prevalent in Negroes than whites. Lew believed that this could be due to better diagnostic facilities for whites. There is a marked geographic variation in the death rates from coronary disease in different parts of the country. Lew again thought that this could be due largely to differences in diagnostic facilities.

Marital status plays a role in prevalence of the disease. Coronary disease is more frequent in widows and single persons than in the married. The disease is also more prevalent in the lower socioeconomic groups than in those with higher income and status.

Many studies have shown a direct ratio between obesity and heart disease prevalence. Several epidemiologists have established a correlation between heavy cigarette smoking and coronary disease.

Master(5) has made a 30-year progress report on coronary thrombosis. He stated that aging of the population is largely responsible for the apparent increase in coronary disease in the United States. Other factors include more accurate diagnosis and changes in medical terminology. His belief has been that coronary disease has multiple causes, such as disturbance of lipoid metabolism, stress, heredity, smoking habits, and physical exercise.

Master has emphasized the relatively good prognosis in coronary disease. In patients under medical guidance, fewer than 5 per cent of initial attacks are fatal. At the end of 5 years, 50 per cent are surviving; 30 per cent after 10 years, and 10 per cent after 15 years. Thus many persons live 15 to 20 years after the initial attack of the disease.

Miscellaneous Affections of the Heart

Certain toxic conditions that affect the heart can be diagnosed early and treated promptly with excellent results. For example, a person with thyrotoxicosis and severe heart involvement can be greatly improved by early diagnosis and adequate therapy.

The influence of vitamin B1 deficiency in the production of heart disease has been discussed in the chapter on nutrition. Only in recent years have we appreciated the extent of the disease and the serious injury that can be produced upon the myocardium by prolonged thiamine deficiency; only now are we beginning to understand the preventive and therapeutic aspects of the condition.

General Measures in the Control of Heart Disease

The community can assume its share of the burden in the control of heart disease by providing proper facilities for the diagnosis and care of these patients. The problem will increase inevitably because of our aging population. Many of those who suffer with heart disease are elderly: many are poor. Part of the cost of their care must be met from public funds.

The community can provide the following facilities for the proper handling of this situation:

1. Provision for readily available facilities for early and accurate diagnosis of heart disease.

2. Provision for domiciliary care. The utilization of the public health nurse in home care of cardiac disease should be advanced.

3. Development of simple nursing homes is indicated for those persons who need limited care and do not require extensive hospitalization.

4. Provision must be made for convalescent care of cardiac patients. It now seems probable that, as tuberculosis recedes, the sanatoriums formerly required for the care of tuberculous patients can be used for the care of the increasing number of patients with cardiac disease.

5. Finally, adequate provision of hospital beds is required to complete the facilities for the care of heart disease.

The Social Security Act, which has provided for unemployment insurance, sickness benefits, and retirement annuities, with old-age benefits, should prove to be a most effective measure in providing for suitable care of persons with chronic disease, particularly those with chronic disease of the heart.

REFERENCES

1. LASSER, R. P., and MASTER, A. M.: *Geriatrics*, 1959, **14**:345.
2. Conference of the American Heart Association: *Epidemiology of Cardiovascular Diseases Methodology*. Princeton, New Jersey, April, 1959. *Supplement to Am. J. Pub. Health*, 1960, **50**:(10).
3. LEW, E. A.: *Some Implications of Mortality Statistics Relating to Coronary Artery Disease. Report of Conference on Atherosclerosis and Coronary Disease*, New York Heart Association, Jan. 15, 1957.
4. KEYS, A., and FIDANZA, F.: *Circulation*, 1960, **22**:1091.
5. MASTER, A. M.: *G. P.*, 1958, **XVII**:123.

35. MEDICAL CARE AND
REHABILITATION OF THE AGED

The well-planned "White House Conference on Aging," January, 1960, gave us a broader and more complete understanding of the special needs of persons over 65 years of age in the United States(1).

The problem is complex, involving many factors: social, economic, hereditary, psychological, and political. This chapter is limited to medical care of the aged. Community responsibilities for provision of adequate facilities to meet medical care needs are considered here with special reference to the role of the physician in care of the aged.

We are an aging population in the United States. In 1900 only 4.1 per cent of the population was over 65 years of age. By 1960 there were 17 millions of persons over 65 years, and it is estimated that by 1980, there will be 25 millions. This will represent almost 10 per cent of the total population. The ratio now varies from 2 per cent to 12.9 per cent in the various states. Several states in the northeastern and middle western sections of the nation now have more than 10 per cent of their populations in the old-age bracket. The older people dwell more often in the villages and rural areas. They have a relatively low income — one third of the men over 65 years have an income of less than $1,000 annually. There are more older women than men, and this ratio increases with age. In 1960 the life expectancy of a white man at 65 years was 12.8 years; a woman had nearly 16 years life expectancy. Life expectancy for a newborn baby has increased 19 years since 1950, but less than 1.2 years for a man at 65 years.

Gains in Life Expectancy After 60 Years of Age

We should not be too optimistic about possible gains in life expectancy in persons over 60 years of age.

From 1930 to 1960, males over 60 gained only 1 year. A reasonable

TABLE 43*
Calculated Life Expectancy Increases

	White Males (years)			White Females (years)		
	60	65	70	60	65	70
Life expectancy 1958	15.7	12.7	10.1	19.2	15.4	12.0
Gain through 10 per cent reduction						
Cardiovascular disease	0.7	0.6	0.6	0.7	0.7	0.6
Malignant neoplasia	0.2	0.1	0.1	0.2	0.1	0.1
Accidents	—	—	—	0.1	—	0.1
All other causes	0.1	0.1	0.1	0.1	0.1	0.1
Total gain (Life expectancy in 20 years with 10 per cent reduction each year)	1.0	0.8	0.5	1.1	0.9	0.9

*Metropolitan Life Insurance Co., *Statistical Bull.*, Nov. 1960.

goal during the next 20 years would be a 10 per cent reduction in the death rate of persons over 65 years.

The Metropolitan Life Insurance Company has calculated the increase in life expectancy that would occur if we could achieve the goal of 10 per cent reduction in the death rate of the elderly in the next 20 years (see Table 43).

Even a 50 per cent reduction in all causes of death over 60 years will not increase life expectancy more than 5 years during the next 20 years.

Characteristics of Aged Persons

Aging is a physiologic process. It is not a disease. Some persons age more rapidly than others. For practical reasons, the chronological age of 65 years can be considered the baseline in discussing problems of the aging. From the point of view of medical care, the major factor in aging is susceptibility to chronic illness and gradually increasing disability.

TABLE 44*

Mortality from Leading Causes

AVERAGE ANNUAL DEATH RATE PER 100,000 POPULATION

	1930	1958	Per Cent Change
White Males			
All causes	5,559	5,067	− 8.8
Cardiovascular and renal disease	3,164	3,180	+ 0.5
Malignant neoplasia	714	912	+27.8
Accidents	243	123	−49.0
Pneumonia and influenza	391	130	−66.0
Tuberculosis	123	43	−65.0
White Females			
All causes	4,651	3,007	− 35.0
Cardiovascular and renal disease	2,610	1,898	−27.0
Malignant neoplasia	700	605	−13.0
Accidents	149	65	−50.0
Pneumonia and influenza	374	63	−83.0
Tuberculosis	89	9	−89.0

*Metropolitan Life Insurance Co., *Statistical Bull.*, Sept., 1960.

The leading causes of deaths in persons over 65 years in the United States are: heart disease, cancer, stroke, influenza and pneumonia, arteriosclerosis, accidents, and diabetes. Three fourths of all deaths are due to the first three causes (see Table 44).

Accidental deaths in persons over 75 years are three times higher than in age groups under 65 years. Accidental deaths are much more common in females than males and are usually due to falls.

From 1957 to 1959, a household survey(2) was make of impairments and disability in the aged (see Table 45).

TABLE 45

Impairments per 1,000 Population in People over 65 Years

Impairment	Age 65 to 74	Age 74 and Over
All categories	376	617
1. Blindness and visual impairment	78	157
2. Hearing	129	256
3. Paralysis	16	34
4. Lower extremity impairment, not paralysis	37	39
5. Upper extremity impairment	24	26

A tabulation(3) was also made of disability in elder people due to chronic illness (see Table 46).

TABLE 46

Disability Due to Chronic Illness in People over 65 Years*

	Age 65 to 74 (per cent)	Age 75 and Over (per cent)
No chronic condition found	24	17
Disabilities due to one or more chronic conditions:		
No limitation	38	28
Partial limitation	27.8	31.1
Major limitation	9.4	23.7

* From U.S. Public Health Service Report(3).

The six common illnesses encountered in people over 65 years were:

1. Arthritis.
2. Heart disease.
3. High blood pressure.
4. Impaired vision.
5. Impaired hearing.
6. Diabetes.

Persons over 65 years have a much higher initial admission rate to mental disease hospitals than the general population (6 per 1,000 population). Three fourths of the nursing home patients are over 75 years of age; two thirds of them are women.

Old people require more medical care than the younger age groups. Physicians' visits total seven per year. More hospitalization is required. In an average community, 1,778 hospital bed days per 1,000 population over 65 years are required, as compared with 660 bed days for those under 65 years.

Most medical care of elderly people can be given on an ambulatory basis in the doctor's office and the clinic, but 5 per cent of them are institutionalized at any given time.

The average length of stay of the aged in a general hospital is 15 days, as compared with patients 25 to 44 years of age who stay only 7 days.

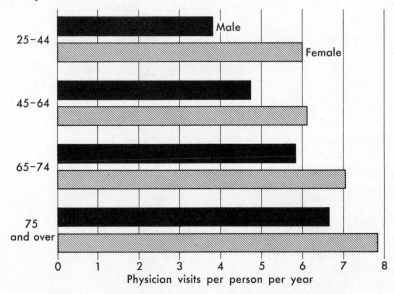

Figure 39. Older persons visit doctors more frequently than do younger people. (Health Insurance Plan of Greater New York, 1960.)

In summary, all these data indicate that elderly people are much more susceptible than the younger age groups to prolonged, disabling illnesses, which increase in prevalence and severity as age advances.

The elderly require medical care facilities different from those needed for the younger age groups, and they are less able to provide for their care from their own resources.

Community Facilities for Medical Care of the Aged

1. Primary Prevention. Since knowledge of the basic etiology of the various types of chronic disease that affect the aged is so meager, there are few preventive measures of value. Accidents are an important factor in disability and death of the aged. The major category is "falls." If educational measures and other procedures that have been successful in reducing the accident rate in the younger age group are promoted, it is quite possible a reduction of the accident rate in elderly people might be effected. Preventive measures employed during the productive years, such as reduction of occupational hazards might prevent subsequent disability.

2. Early Detection of Chronic Disease. This procedure can be most effective when applied to the younger age groups — long before the 65-year mark. For the most part, the chronic disease of the elderly person is already clinically manifest before the seventh decade.

3. Medical Care. Chronic illness is usually progressive, resulting eventually in disability. From the patient's point of view, the major objective is to limit and ameliorate his disability to the degree that he can live a reasonably comfortable normal life.

The elderly patient should be treated not simply to prolong his life but also provide him an opportunity for a more abundant life. The greatest single advance in treatment of the elderly person with chronic illness is the recognition of the degree to which severely disabled persons can be rehabilitated. Harold A. Rusk has been the great leader in this field. He has demonstrated the techniques of rehabilitation of the elderly: the type and amount of treatment as well as the understanding and patience required to return a disabled, bedridden patient to a reasonable degree of self-care.

Even the senile patient, formerly assigned to a large state mental hospital for terminal custodial care, can be maintained at home (or in a foster home) with a striking degree of improvement and can live a relatively normal life.

One of the needs in our community medical care program is the full development of plans to afford the aging person with chronic illness the best opportunity for a decent, dignified, and worthwhile old age.

Facilities for Adequate Care of Chronic Illness

In the United States we have not, as yet, provided proper facilities for care of the chronically ill. The old people do not belong in a general short-stay hospital. Hospital care is needed for acute episodes of chronic illness, but as soon as possible the patient should be transferred to a convalescent unit* or rehabilitation center. Here the patient begins his progressive care.

Organized Home Care

The objective of organized home care is to promote the patient to home care as rapidly as possible. A team is organized by the hospital, consisting of a physician, social worker, visiting nurse, and physiotherapist. A rehabilitation program is set up for the patient at the chronic disease unit or rehabilitation center of the hospital. As soon as is expedient, the patient returns home but his name remains on the hospital roll. He is visited at home at appropriate intervals by various members of the team. His private physician becomes an integral part of progressive rehabilitation and medical care. In some cases, long-term care is required, with continuous nursing supervision. This might not be feasible in the home.

Nursing Homes

The primary function of the nursing home is to give expert long-term nursing care to the patient with a major disability. Ninety per cent are more than 70 years of age; most of them are women. At the present time, almost all nursing homes in the United States are proprietary homes. Many are poorly staffed and inefficient. A strong effort is being made throughout the land to develop state-wide standards for adequate nursing home care, with provision for adequate staff and effective procedure. A system of official periodic inspection of the nursing home is important. We have every reason to hope that the nursing home can play an increasingly effective role in care of the chronically ill.

*This concept is so new that we have not yet invented a suitable term to designate this facility.

Public Health Nurse

The community public health visiting nurse is a splendid asset to the physician, the patient, and the community in home-care of the chronically ill. Her educational and therapeutic visit to the disabled patient in the home is an invaluable part of medical care of the aged. In most communities, this type of work occupies more than 60 per cent of her time.

The Mentally Ill Aged Patient

It has been a custom to assign elderly senile patients for custodial care in large state institutions for the insane. It is now generally agreed that they do not belong in those institutions. The trend is to provide facilities for them in their own communities, in homes for the aged and in foster homes, with close supervision by the mental health center of the local community.

Home-Maker Service(4)

A community facility, called "home-maker services" for supplementary care for the chronically disabled has been developed by voluntary agencies in some communities with great success. Another voluntary agency service called "meals on wheels" is a definite community asset to the house-bound.

Summary

Adequate medical service for the aged is essentially a comprehensive progressive program for the amelioration of the ravages of chronic illness, with emphasis on rehabilitation of the disabled patient so that he can take his place in the community with a reasonable degree of satisfaction and contentment.

The plan requires participation of all the health agencies in the community and development of new facilities to supply rehabilitation needs. The most important person in the development and execution of the program is the practicing physician in the community.

REFERENCES

1. *Report on the White House Conference on Aging.* January 9-12, 1961. U.S. Public Health Service, Washington, D.C.

2. *U.S. Survey, 1957-59,* Publication 584-B9, U.S. Public Health Health Service, Washington, D.C.

3. *U.S. Public Health Service Rep.,* Publication 584-B11.

4. HIGGINS, E.: *Home-maker Service for the Chronically Disabled.* New York Tuberculosis and Health Conference, April 26, 1960.

SPECIAL REFERENCES

Programs for Older People. Federal Council on Aging, Report of the President, 1960. U.S. Dept. of Health, Education, and Welfare, Washington, D.C.

Publications of the National Council on Aging, Inc., 349 East 46th St., New York 17, N.Y.

SECTION IV

Public Health Administration

36. ADMINISTRATION OF
LOCAL HEALTH SERVICES

We have considered in previous pages the various community activities that can be instituted for protection and promotion of the public health. We now consider the methods by which these activities can be administered by the community most expeditiously and effectively. An attempt is also made to allocate the various responsibilities for the given tasks.*

Public health administration has been defined by Dr. C.-E. A. Winslow as the "art and science of preventing disease, prolonging life, and promoting physical and mental efficiency, *through organized community effort.*" This definition emphasizes the important fact that a coordinated community effort is required to secure an effective service.

The official health agencies are directly responsible for the establishment of leadership in community health service, but other official agencies should also play an important role in the health promotion program. Notable in this field are the departments of education, of public welfare, and of parks and playgrounds. The department of public works, which has charge of municipal housekeeping, such as cleaning of streets and removal of garbage and waste, is also a useful adjunct to health protection.

Voluntary community agencies have an essential part to play in health administration too. The local health organizations, such as the mental hygiene committee, the tuberculosis association, the visiting nurse service, and the Red Cross, all work in close cooperation with

*The reader will note much repetition in this chapter of matters that have been discussed earlier. This is done for purposes of coherence. In the previous chapters, we have described various public health activities in some detail. In this chapter, we show how these activities can be correlated in a single over-all administrative plan. The reader who is particularly interested in the details of public health administration is referred to a special text on this subject: Wilson G. Smillie: *Public Health Administration in the United States,* 3rd ed. The Macmillian Company, New York, 1947.

503

the official health agencies. Community organizations interested in promotion of community welfare, such as religious institutions, men's service clubs, the chamber of commerce, fraternal organizations, and the like, all aid in the comprehensive program of health protection of the community. Each has its part to play in the administration of the public health.

It is a basic principle that the direct responsibility for health protection rests upon the official health department of the local self-governing unit—be it village, township, county, or municipality.

The state has an important function to perform in public health administration, and a state health department is organized for this purpose. The federal government also has important nation-wide health responsibilities supplementary to those of the local and the state health departments.

Local health departments function on the social theory that the community is responsible for protection of its members against the special hazards of community life. The usual administrative division of activities is as follows:

1. Communicable Disease Control

Some of the hazards of community life are more obvious than others. Contagious or communicable disease is an obvious menace to all mankind, and thus the control of contagion has been assumed by government for centuries. On this continent, the isolation of those sick with contagious disease, quarantine of the family, and sometimes of the whole community, has been followed as a measure of community protection since the earliest Colonial days. Smallpox and yellow fever were the great menaces to the colonist, and the yellow* quarantine flag was a familiar and dreaded symbol of danger.

Those quarantine activities led to all the other measures that aid in prevention of the spread of communicable disease described in Book One, Section II.

2. Vital Statistics†

The local health department has responsibility for the accurate and prompt collection of vital data, particularly birth and death certifi-

---

*Sometimes the quarantine flag was white; other times it was red.
†See Chapter 3 for a discussion of the collection and interpretation of vital data.

cates. As a rule, the essential information from these certificates is transcribed into the records of the health department office, and the original certificates are forwarded to the state health department. It is the function of the vital statistics division of the state health department to compile, analyze, and interpret the vital data for the whole state. Certain information of nation-wide import is forwarded by the state to the Office of Vital Statistics in Washington, D.C., which analyzes and interprets these data from the national point of view.

3. Environmental Sanitation

The first local boards of health were organized specifically for the purpose of preventing exposure of the community to the decaying debris and wastes of communal life. (It is an interesting fact that a great public-spirited citizen, Paul Revere, was chairman of one of the first local boards of health, organized in Boston in 1798.) Citizens believed, at that time, that disease, particularly "fevers," was due to bad odors which arose from tanneries, pigsties, and stables, from decaying fish and rotting vegetables and other food wastes, from the odors of privies, stagnant ponds, and wells. In fact, all the early local sanitary regulations relate to quarantine and to disposal of garbage and wastes. This led to the more comprehensive idea that it was a community responsibility to provide a safe and healthful environment in which to live. Picken(1) has presented a modern concept of the scope of public health administration in this environmental field that encompasses many and varied functions. He stated that the health department should be concerned with:

1. The condition of houses in which people live.
2. The arrangement of these houses in relation to one another and to the adjacent buildings.
3. The community water supply.
4. The disposal of human excrement.
5. The disposal of offensive and deleterious accumulations.
6. The supervision of trades that could become offensive or dangerous.
7. The prevention of pollution of water courses.
8. The prevention of pollution of the air.
9. The sanitary state of factories.
10. The sale of unsound or adulterated food.

11. The hygienic conduct of places where people congregate to eat and drink.

All these matters relate to sanitation of the environment and have become a part of the official health services.

4. Health Education

Health education is a joint responsibility of the department of education and the department of health. It can also be promoted effectively by the various voluntary health agencies of the community. It must be continuous, keep abreast of modern knowledge, and be so planned and executed as to meet the needs of each particular group that should receive the information. Promotional methods in dissemination of information found so highly effective in merchandising should be utilized in promotion of health education. The information must be sound and true, but it must be presented so effectively and convincingly that it becomes a part of the lives of the people.

5. Promotion of Individual Health

The men who founded American democracy did not realize. that promotion of individual health was a community responsibility, and no provision whatsoever was made for this activity in local, state, or national government administration. Only within recent years have we gained the concept that a healthy individual is a community asset. Contrariwise, a sick individual or a man who dies prematurely represents a community liability. The person who is ill requires community-supported facilities for medical, nursing, and possibly prolonged hospital care. Furthermore, there may be the danger of disabling illness occurring among persons in the employable age groups. Thus people who should be self-supporting might, because of preventable illness, require long-continued community support. Loss of earning and impairment of capacity for productive work represent not only individual loss but community loss as well. Thus it behooves the community to protect its most important asset against damage. In recent years, this concept has led to the development of extensive community-wide public health measures. Many have been quite effective; others are still in the initial, developmental stages.

Maternal and Child Health. The incorporation of this activity as a community health service is one of the great achievements of a modern health program. Perhaps no single activity of the health department has been more fruitful (see Book Two, Section I).

School Hygiene. Community responsibility for the promotion of sound health of the school child has been discussed in Chapter 24. It is a joint function of the department of health and the department of education.

Adult Hygiene. We are only beginning to realize the opportunities for development of health promotion of the adult population as a community function.

1. Control of tuberculosis and venereal disease is of special benefit to the young adult and should be considered adult hygiene.

2. Industrial hygiene is a subdivision of adult hygiene. It is that community activity specially concerned with the health of the man or woman while at work. Particular emphasis is placed upon protection against the special hazards that are an integral part of the particular employment.

3. Cancer control, control of diabetics, amelioration and prevention of heart disease, arthritis, and other conditions incident to the aging process (the degenerative disease) are all a part of adult hygiene.

Undeveloped Public Health Activities

Certain community functions relating to health promotion are, in theory at least, a direct responsibility of the health department or other official health agencies. Many of these theories have not yet been put into practice because of administrative difficulties or because they have not yet been accepted by a majority of the people as a direct public responsibility.

Better Distribution of Medical Care. It is generally agreed that the community should provide medical, nursing, and hospital care for the poor and unfortunate of the community. This is a public welfare function, but the medical aspects of public welfare are frequently assigned to the public health department.

Many farsighted leaders have insisted that medical care is an essential health service and that the proper distribution of medical care, together with provision of adequate facilities for curative medicine at a cost that the individual and family can afford, is a community responsibility and should be regulated and administered by the official community health service. Students of community life also believe that social and economic status has a profound influence upon family and community health and that social work must be combined with public health programs to secure the best results in health promotion.

Nutrition. Recent advances in our knowledge of nutrition show conclusively that the health of a community can be greatly improved when the essential food factors are provided for every family in the community at reasonable cost. Provision of adequate foodstuffs and proper utilization of food are a combined community function in which the health department plays an auxiliary but important role.

Newer Concepts in Public Health. As our understanding of community responsibility changes and as scientific knowledge and social concepts develop, it seems axiomatic that more improvements will be made in the methods of administration of the community health services. Thus, any discussion of a static administrative unit for a community health service is quite unsatisfactory, since our concepts of the functions of government in matters of this sort are continually being modified.

We can only present a plan of health organization for each type of community, in accordance with our present ideas of community responsibility. It must be appreciated that within a short time ideas are modified, and the organization that is presented might be quite inadequate to meet the changing requirements. In the following pages a satisfactory working organization, under our present concepts of public health administration, is given for each type of governmental organization, including local government (both rural and municipal), state government, and federal health administration.

REFERENCES

1. PICKEN, R. M. F.: *Public Health Administration,* printed by Local Government Finance, University of Wales. England, May, 1939.

37. RURAL HEALTH ADMINISTRATION

The National Office of Vital Statistics uses the criterion that a city of 10,000 population or more becomes a municipality; all smaller towns and the adjacent scattered farms are rural areas. For purposes of public health administration, however, a suitable rural unit of population is from 25,000 to 50,000 or more people. This unit is made up of the central marketing community and the surrounding farms. The county is usually the unit of government. Sometimes several counties are combined to secure sufficient population for a suitable administrative health unit. In New England rural areas, the smaller township is the governing unit and does not lend itself satisfactorily to a county health department organization.

Growth of County Health Departments

The county health unit plan originated in Yakima County, Washington, in 1911 as suggested by Dr. L. L. Lumsden of the U.S. Public Health Service. The Rockefeller Sanitary Commission became interested in rural sanitation in the southern states at about the same time and began a system of grants-in-aid to states in order to develop better local health services on a county-wide basis. The U.S. Public Health Service carried out a similar plan concurrently. Various types of administrative experiments were attempted during the following ten years. The great Mississippi Valley flood of 1922 demonstrated that full-time county health services, where they had been established in the valley, were most effective in an emergency; this gave an impetus to the county health unit movement. In 1918 there were only 30 counties with full-time public health personnel in the United States. The Social Security Act of 1935 enabled rural areas to secure substantial federal financial assistance for well-organized health services and gave great momentum to this work. In 1960, almost the entire rural area of the United States had profited by the services of well-organized local health departments that were staffed by trained and competent full-time personnel.

Principles of Organization of a County Health Department*

1. **Integration.** The health unit should be incorporated as an integral part of local self-government. It should be supported by local taxation and become as essential to the people of the county as the department of education, the county road commission, or the department of law enforcement.

2. **Budget.** A substantial part of the budget should be met from local tax funds. Voluntary health agencies can be of great assistance in promotion of new types of services and can aid in supplying additional personnel, supplies, or actual grants-in-aid.

3. **State Aid.** State aid is an important adjunct to local health work. The state health department should assist in planning the local program, give advice in difficult problems, and give guidance in the selection of qualified personnel. In many instances, the state gives a substantial subsidy to the county for maintenance of health activities. Under the Social Security Act of 1935, the U.S. Public Health Service allotted funds to states for direct aid of rural health departments, to be expended in accordance with special needs.

4. **Full-time Service.** The key personnel of the health department should work on a full-time basis. Auxiliary personnel, such as clinic physicians, dentists, and veterinarians for meat-inspection work can be utilized and reimbursed on a per-diem or per-service basis, but the health officer, nurses, and sanitary inspectors should have no outside financial interests.

5. **Training of Personnel.** Each member of the staff should have the proper qualifications and training for his position. The state department of health should establish minimum qualifications for the essential positions in the local health department. Suitable standards of training and experience for various types of personnel of rural and municipal health organizations have been promulgated by the American Public Health Association. These have been a-dopted, officially or unofficially, by many states and municipalities.

6. **Unified Program.** All the health-protection activities of the county should be centralized under the direction of the official county health unit. All the voluntary agencies in the community that take part in public health promotion should correlate their work with that of the county health officer.

*The details of rural health administration will not be presented in this text. The reader is referred for this information to Smillie, W. G.: *Public Health Administration in the United States,* 3d ed. The Macmillan Company, New York, 1947.

7. Generalized Plan of Work. The health department should develop a well-rounded health service and not overemphasize one activity to the detriment of another.

Plan of Organization of a County Health Department

A county board of health should be organized, consisting of from three to five prominent and public-spirited citizens. Not all of them should be physicians. They should have overlapping terms of office and serve without pay. The position is honorary and advisory and without administrative responsibility.

This board makes the general policies, approves the health department budget presented to the governing body of the county, selects the health officer, and approves the sanitary code. It can also be empowered to hold semijudicial hearings on health matters.

Four types of trained full-time personnel are required for a well-rounded health department service:

1. Health Officer. The health officer should be a physician with special preparation for this work. He should understand the psychology of rural people and be familiar with the problems of rural life, but most important is the special training that is required to do his work well.

2. Public Health Nurses. One public health nurse per 5,000 population represents an adequate personnel for rural health work. Many health departments are able to employ only 1 nurse per 10,000 people.

3. Sanitary Inspectors. The sanitary inspector has direct charge of all matters relative to environmental sanitation. If that officer is well trained and competent, usually one or two sanitary inspectors are sufficient for the average county unit.

4. Clerical Services. The trained clerk who understands the community health needs is one of the most important parts of the county health unit.

Laboratory services are usually incorporated in a state-wide system, without a separate county health unit laboratory.

5. Other Personnel. A nutritionist or a social worker can be added to the full-time staff. In some areas, county home demonstrators, working under the state department of agriculture, carry out the nutritional education in the county. They work in close collaboration with the county health units.

As health promotion has become an increasing responsibility of local health services, additional personnel has been added. A well-qualified health educator is a great asset to a rural health service. Some health offices have added a physiotherapist, who aids in the rehabilitation activities of the health unit.

6. Part-time Personnel. Physicians are needed to staff the public health clinics, to aid in the examination of school children, and to help in many other ways. Dental services might be required, and veterinarians for meat inspection. The local practitioners can be selected by the board of health to aid in this clinical work; they should be compensated for their services.

Activities of the County Health Department

The health officer administers the whole program. The medical aspects of the work are his direct province. His chief activity is health education, but he can also act as the clinician in one or all of the clinic services. He also serves as consultant to the physicians in diagnosis of communicable disease.

Clinic Services. These are organized in cooperation with the county medical society. In most instances, the most successful services are: (a) tuberculosis clinics; (b) immunization clinics against smallpox, diphtheria, and poliomyelitis; (c) venereal disease clinics, cancer detection clinics, mental health clinics; and (d) in some communities, dental clinics for children.

The school health program is a joint responsibility of the department of education and the health department. It is participated in by all members of the health unit, including part-time physicians who aid in physical examinations of the school children.

Public health nursing is organized on a generalized basis. Each nurse is assigned to a geographic area, and she carries out all phases of public health nursing in that zone. Her major activities include maternal and child health work, school health promotion, communicable disease control, nutrition, and health education.

In many areas, public health nurses are utilized in rehabilitation services, notably in the fields of detection and care of crippled children, in mental hygiene, and rehabilitation of chronic illness. They are particularly valuable in health promotion of the aged.

The sanitary officer has a great variety of activities. He is a health educator primarily; he has supervision of environmental sanitation, including safety of public water supplies and sewage disposal plants. He makes the dairy inspections, the restaurant and food inspections, and oversees the sanitation of schools and other public buildings together with many other duties. He enforces the sanitary code.

The office work of the clerk or secretary requires a knowledge of methods of statistical analysis. The clerk keeps a record of achievement. She records and transmits vital data, arranges the clinic schedules, maintains laboratory supplies for the diagnostic kits of the physicians, and manages the office while all the other personnel are in the field.

Housing the County Health Department

A separate, well-constructed, dignified health center building should be planned to fulfill all the functions of a health service, in accordance with present needs and probable developments. When building any service structure, it is necessary to plan at least 25 years ahead, anticipating trends and future requirements. This is difficult in health work, since there is divergence of opinion as to the future scope of rural health administration.

Plan 1. The local health unit becomes a center of all clinic activities of the county. This requires extensive development of clinic facilities, with a large health center building which has ample provisions for clinic care, including roentgenology, laboratory, and other diagnostic aids.

Plan 2. In the second system, the health center acts simply as an administrative unit for community health activities. The community hospital in this case not only cares for its bed patients but also houses all clinic activities as well as the diagnostic laboratories and roentgenologic equipment. This plan avoids duplication of roentgenologic and laboratory equipment. Some plans propose domiciliary care by the hospital unit, which includes the nursing care of the sick in their homes, under the supervision of the community hospital.

Combination of Plans 1 and 2. Under the combined plan (sometimes called the health center plan), all administration of health services in the county becomes centralized in one unit. The health center administrator becomes the county health officer. He also administers the community hospital and all the clinic activities of the health service and the hospital. He administers the diagnostic and treatment facilities of the health center for its ambulatory patients. All these activities are carried out under the roof of the community hospital, which thus becomes a true health and hospital center for the area. Any community plan of prepayment for medical and nursing care should, of course, be administered through the health and hospital center.

This plan envisages group medicine, or rather grouping of all facilities, with the practicing physicians carrying out their activities on an independent basis, with free choice of physicians by patients. The preventive clinic services are carried out by the practicing physicians on a part-time basis, for which they receive proper remuneration.

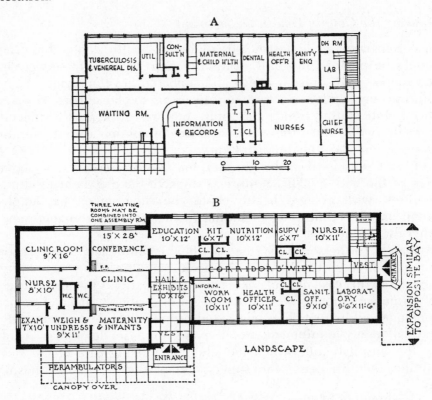

Figure 40. Floor plans for rural health center. (A. Public Health Centers, Building Types Study No. 67, *Architectural Record*, F. W. Dodge Corporation, 1942. B. "Organization of a Rural Health Unit," *Hospitals*, November, 1942.)

Many different types of health service plans should be developed in the rural areas of various parts of the United States, dependent upon local conditions, such as distribution of population, type of agriculture, and per capita wealth. It is quite obvious that no single plan is suitable for all the varied conditions encountered in the rural areas of the United States.

Various concepts of community health service functions are illustrated by the diagrams of health buildings, which illustrate different types of organization and activity (see the floor plans in Fig. 40 A and B).

District Health Organization

In some states, the small township is the unit of self-government. In other areas, the counties are small or are sparsely populated. These situations might necessitate a modification of the county health unit plan to a district plan. The general policies and activities of a district health unit are identical with those of the county health unit, with the same basic personnel, but the organization of the services is modified to meet local conditions. Usually a sufficient number of local government units — counties or townships — are grouped into a health district which will provide a suitable administrative health unit of from 30,000 to 50,000, or even more, people. District health units require more direction and greater subsidy from the state health department than county units. In some instances, the health officer and supervising nurse are supplied directly by the state health department. In a few states, the major part of the budget and personnel of the district health service is under the direct supervision of the state health officer.

Joint County-city Plan of Health Organization

In some areas, the central city of the area has a population of 10,000 or even 20,000. It might be greater than that of the surrounding rural area. In such instances, the municipality should not have a separate health department but should form a joint municipal-rural health department to provide for the needs of the city as well as the needs of the surrounding county.

The Budget of a County Health Department

No specific rules can be drawn for formulating the budget of a community health unit. The salaries of the professional personnel — health officer, nurses, and sanitary officers — must be commensurate with their training and ability, and must be adjusted from time to time to the cost of living of the given community.

The voluntary health agencies of the community usually do not contribute directly to the official community health unit budget. Their function is to give supplementary aid when needed. Primarily they are interested in development of new and untried fields.

It is most advantageous if one half the total budget is obtained from local sources of funds. State and federal social security aid can be of great supplemental assistance, but the local community should appreciate the advantages of health services sufficiently to pay for them.

Further details of organization and administration of rural health services, with indications for allocation of budget items, can be found in textbooks on public health administration.

SPECIAL REFERENCES

EMERSON, HAVEN: *Local Health Units for the Nation.* The Commonwealth Fund, New York, 1945.

HANLON, JOHN J.: *Principles of Public Health Administration.* C. V. Mosby Co., St. Louis, 1950.

"Proceedings of the National Conference on Local Health Units," University of Michigan School of Public Health, September 9-13, 1946. Published by American Public Health Association.

ROEMER, M. I., and WILSON, E. A.: *Organized Health Services in a Rural Community.* U.S. Public Health Service, Federal Security Agency, January, 1951.

See also publications of the National Advisory Committee on Local Health Units, National Health Council, 1790 Broadway, New York 19, N.Y.

38. MUNICIPAL HEALTH ADMINISTRATION

Each municipality has a charter granted by the state, which gives it certain powers to make laws (in so far as they do not conflict with state laws) and to institute self-government. Usually the executive of the city is elected, as mayor, or selected, as in the city-manager system. The governing body is a group of elected and representative citizens which makes the city ordinances, formulates the budget, and determines general policies.

Protection of the public health is one of the functions of this government. The major activities of health promotion in the community are allocated to the health department.

Organization of a Municipal Health Department

Board of Health. Usually a board of three to five citizens is selected by the executive, in concurrence with the city council, to carry out the municipal health functions. The position of board member should be an honorary one, without salary, and should be for a term of three to five years, with overlapping terms of office. In some cities, a board of health has advisory powers only, but in most instances the board has the power to select the health officer, to make policies, and to formulate the sanitary code. In some cities, there is no board of health. The health officer is appointed by the chief executive of the city and is responsible directly to him. In such instances, the city council is responsible for formulation of health ordinances.

Health Officer. The health officer should be a physician who has had special training for his position. The larger the city, the greater the administrative responsibility, and thus the greater the amount of training and experience that is required.* The term of office for the

---

*Minimum standard requirements for health officers for different classes of cities have been formulated by the Conference of Mayors and also by the American Public Health Association. These may be secured by writing to the Committee on Professional Education, American Public Health Association, 1790 Broadway, New York 19, N.Y.

health officer should be for a definite number of years. Five years is suggested as a suitable period.

Other Personnel. The basic personnel of a municipal health department is the same as that of a county health unit, but since hazards of municipal life are greater than in rural areas, the health work is more intensive, and the proportionate cost is greater. The work of

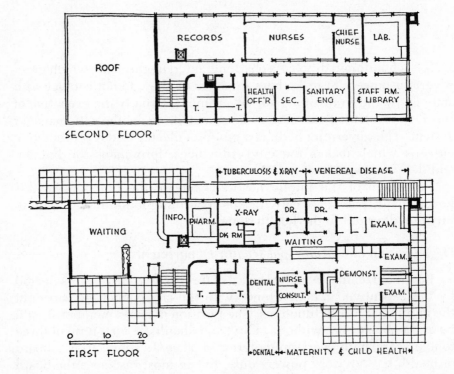

Figure 41. Health center plan for a small municipality. (*Architectural Record*, Reprint 67, 1942. F. W. Dodge Corporation.)

the department is usually organized on a functional basis. The simple chart of the organization of a health service for a municipality of 100,000 people given in Figure 42 illustrates these points.

Each of these divisions should have a full-time person in charge. The health officer himself, in a community of this size, might carry the work of the division of communicable disease control, or he could be responsible directly for division 3. In this case, he would employ a full-time epidemiologist for division 2. Health education is a function of all the divisions, but is often centered in division 3. Nutrition is essentially an educational activity and could be allocated to division 3 or 6. Laboratory services might be incorporated in division 4, since a great deal of the work relates to routine examinations of water, milk, and food. In other instances, the laboratory is in the division of communicable disease control.

Promotion of adult health, particularly as related to rehabilitation of the aging, must also be given consideration. This could be incorporated in a division of medical care which would be closely related to public health nursing, and include personnel for medical social work, physiotherapy, etc.

Personnel of a Municipal Health Department

The major portion of the budget is expended for salaries of personnel. More than one half the personnel is made up of public health

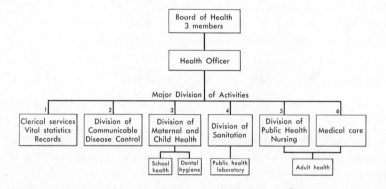

Figure 42. Organization chart of a municipal health department.

nurses. A public health nursing quota that is frequently recommended is 1 nurse per 5,000 population. In a city of 100,000, the usual public health nursing staff is 1 director, with a staff of 12 to 15 nurses. An assistant educational director, who has had special training in the fields of nutrition, health education, or child psychology, is a very useful adjunct to the division.

A suitable system of selection of personnel should be utilized, such as is provided by civil service regulations. These rules, however, should not be so rigid as to preclude selection of the best possible available personnel. Often key personnel, such as a trained health officer or director of nurses, is not available locally so that residence requirements of civil service should be waived when necessary.

Advisory Committee of a Municipal Health Department

The health officer should select an advisory committee made up of representative citizens. He should include representatives of those organizations in the city interested in the public health and welfare. The local Red Cross, the tuberculosis association, the chamber of commerce, church organizations, service clubs, representatives of labor organizations, and others, should be selected to advise the health officer in his work. This committee should be informed of any new developments and should prove to be a potent factor in interpreting the aims and achievements of the health department to the people. The committee should meet at regular intervals and be assigned tasks periodically in the promotion of health education.

Medical Advisory Committee. The health officer may select the medical advisory committee or, better still, the medical society of the municipality may be requested to select a public health committee which will serve as adviser to the health officer in relation to the medical aspects of his program. A leading dentist should also be asked to serve on this committee.

Health Organization in Large Municipalities

In cities of more than 500,000 population, the health administration becomes quite complex, since it is not possible to give direct service to all the people from one central office. Furthermore, the volume of work for a single division becomes so large that the responsibility for the activities must be subdivided.

Certain functions lend themselves to centralization, e.g., the sanitation of water supplies, of sewage disposal, and of milk inspection, and the industrial health services. Collection and interpretation of vital statistics and public health laboratory work are also administered centrally.

Direct services to the people, such as public health nursing, well-baby clinic service, prenatal clinics, tuberculosis clinics, venereal disease control, dental hygiene, school hygiene, health education, and promotion of adult health, should be decentralized.

This type of decentralized health unit organization was initiated in Boston through the energy and imagination of Dr. Charles Wilinsky, director of the Division of Child Health of the Boston City Health Department. It was made possible through the generosity of Charles White, who gave to the city the funds necessary for the erection of the health center buildings.

Other cities have carried these plans still further and modified them to meet local needs. The city is divided into suitable districts, and an appropriate health center building is located in the geographic center of the district. A full-time district health officer is placed in charge of the health activities of the area. The central department of health has the customary functional divisions of health administration: epidemiology, perhaps with separate divisions of tuberculosis and venereal disease control, maternal and child health; health education; public health nursing; and community sanitation. The central divisional directors of functional services determine the broad policies in their various fields and make all necessary plans for the successful achievement of objectives, but the direct administration of the various fields of activity within the health district is the responsibility of the district health officer. Each health center building should be the headquarters for the district nurses and sanitary inspectors. Each of these persons is assigned a definite area in the district which is his special province. The center also has facilities for a tuberculosis clinic service, a dental clinic, a well-baby station, small conference rooms, and a large room for public meetings. Space for voluntary local health and allied agencies as well as for the advisory citizens' committee should be provided. Small substations for prenatal care and infant hygiene clinics could be established out in the periphery if the area of the district is great. (Pregnant mothers, or mothers with infants, cannot utilize a central clinic if it is more than three miles from their homes.)

The health center plan for rendition of direct health services to the people is an excellent one, but its full possibilities are only beginning to be realized. It seems most probable that the health center idea will become a potent force in the life of the community.

Public Health Combined with Public Welfare

Several local communities have attempted to combine the governmental functions of public health with public assistance, in a single division under one director. This type of organization seems quite logical, but is full of pitfalls. The function of public health is, in the long run, far more important and of greater fundamental value to the community than public assistance. The provision of food, shelter, and clothing to the poor is an immediate, obvious, and pressing need; the delinquent boy is in immediate trouble; the homeless orphaned child cannot be neglected. Thus, the tendency is for the over-all public health program to be relegated to the background, because of the overwhelming and immediate necessities of public welfare. Furthermore, public assistance is costly, and the greater portion of the joint budget is assigned to this function. Thus it assumes greater relative importance than public health, whereas in reality public health is paramount.

Usually the director of the joint activity is selected because of his training in social service rather than because of special training and talent in the public health field. In this case, undue emphasis is placed upon public welfare, to the neglect of the public health. Many communities have found it practicable to assign the medical activities of the division of public assistance to the department of public health. In this case, the county (or municipal) hospital is administered by the department of public health, and all the domiciliary medical and nursing care of the sick poor is assigned to the health department.

As communities are assigned greater responsibility for promotion of health and rehabilitation, it seems probable that the medical director of the health services will be asked to administer *all the medical care functions* that are assumed by the community. These matters are discussed in some detail in Chapter 46.

39. STATE HEALTH ADMINISTRATION

The state is the sovereign power in our governmental system. The federal government possesses only those powers that are granted it by the states. Furthermore, local governments, such as municipalities, have limited powers, each of which is specifically granted by the state. Thus, each state has its own laws, and no two states follow exactly the same pattern. For this reason, no one uniform system of state health organization can be presented. However, there are certain broad principles of health administration that are followed by most of the states.

Almost every state has a separate department of public health, with a full-time medical health officer in charge. He is appointed by the governor with the consent of the legislative body or is appointed by the state board of health.

STATE BOARD OF HEALTH

The state board of health is made up of five or more representative citizens who have overlapping terms of office. They are appointed by the governor and receive no salary. The position is one of high honor. The board determines general policies, formulates the state sanitary code, approves the budget, and selects the state health officer.

State Health Officer

The state health officer should be a physician who has superior qualifications. He should possess administrative talent and special public health training and experience. He must have the confidence of the people, the medical profession, and his colleagues in state administration. His chief function is the administration of the work of the state health department.

Activities of a State Health Department

The activities of the state health department are threefold:

1. To advise, and in some degree to supervise, local health departments.

2. To provide direct services in local communities.

3. To cooperate with other states and with the federal government in interstate health affairs.

1. Advice to Local Health Departments. The major function of the state health department is to build and improve local health services. This is done in many ways: by aid in selection of qualified personnel, by aid in planning programs, and by direct subsidy. When difficult situations arise, such as uncontrolled epidemics, the state can send skilled epidemiologists to aid in the solution. Each of the directors of the functional divisions of the state health department, such as the director of health education, nursing, public health laboratories, or state engineering, aids the local health departments in a great variety of ways in the planning and the execution of their programs. If a local health department does not function effectively, the state has the right to step in and give direct supervision of services, and in an emergency can take complete charge of the local situation.

The state health department adjusts intercommunity health problems, such as pollution of the water supply of one community by another. The state also has complete sanitary responsibility for control of facilities to which the whole public has access, such as community water supplies, the sanitation of state parks and recreation grounds, and the sanitary quality of roadside wells.

The state health department determines sanitary standards which are applicable throughout the state. Local communities can promote local sanitary regulations which supplement the state standards but cannot have regulations which nullify the state-wide sanitary law.

The state sanitary code is formulated by the state department of health, and each of the 50 states has its own separate code. There is no national sanitary code, since each state is a sovereign power. This is a matter of constant confusion to health administrators from foreign countries who visit the United States to study our public health procedures.

2. Direct Services of a State Health Department.

Vital Statistics. The state health department has direct responsibility for collection, recording, and interpretation of vital statistics.

The original certificates are filed in fireproof vaults and become a part of the state archives.

Public Health Laboratory. The state should develop a public health laboratory system which supplies a high-grade diagnostic laboratory service for communicable disease to all the people, free of charge. In some states, a diagnostic service for the degenerative diseases also is developed. The manufacture of biologic products is an important activity of some of the larger state laboratories. In addition, the laboratory carries out the necessary bacteriologic and chemical tests required by the state bureau of sanitary engineering for proper control of community water supplies, sewage disposal plants, shellfish culture, milk, meats, and other foods. The industrial division's laboratory work is also centralized in the state laboratory. If the state has a large area, then branch laboratories are established to meet the needs of remote communities, or local laboratories are subsidized and supervised by the state laboratory. The functions of a public health diagnostic laboratory service have been outlined elsewhere in this text.

Hospitalization. Local communities often find it impossible to hospitalize, in an effective way, their needy patients with tuberculosis, cancer, arthritis, or the crippled children, the blind, and other afflicted persons. These functions can often be developed best on a state-wide basis. The state provides the facilities, which are paid for by each local community, usually on a per-patient cost basis.

Sanitary Engineering Service. The state provides an expert sanitary engineering corps which has direct control of the sanitation of all public works, such as water supplies and sewage disposal plants, public bathing beaches, and roadside wells to which the public has access. Supervision of the hygiene of industrial plants is also frequently allotted to the state health department.

Health Education. An over-all health educational service is provided to the people directly by the state health department, in addition to the advisory education services that the state gives to the local health department.

Epidemiology. The details of communicable disease control are carried out by the local health departments. The state furnishes a qualified staff of epidemiologists to aid the local health departments and also to give direct service in tracing outbreaks and in working out sources of infection and satisfactory methods of control.

Adult Health Promotion and Rehabilitation. As our population has shifted to the older age groups, increasing attention has been given to the prevention and early detection of chronic disease and the rehabilitation of persons suffering from prolonged illness. This has led to the establishment within the state health department of a special division of adult health promotion and rehabilitation. Subdivisions include activities in (a) cancer control, (b) heart disease, (c) promotion of mental health, (d) accident prevention, and (e) other important causes of disability and death.

Each of these state activities that are in the category of *direct services* is a cooperative service, since the state and local health departments work together in the development of effective service.

3. **Interstate Health Affairs.** In addition to the activities discussed, the state health department cooperates with adjoining states and with the federal health organizations in promotion of all health programs that require joint action of these various governmental agencies.

Organization of a State Health Department

The work of the health department is assigned to bureaus. Each bureau has a director who is specially trained for his job. The commonly established bureaus, or divisions, are:

1. Administration.
2. Vital statistics.
3. Public health laboratory.
4. Sanitation or sanitary engineering.
5. Epidemiology or communicable disease control.
6. Maternal and child health.
7. Public health nursing.
8. Health education.
9. Industrial health.
10. Adult health.

In the smaller states, various bureau activities can be combined under one director. For example, industrial health can be combined with sanitary engineering; public health nursing with child hygiene. Health education can be administered directly by the health officer. The supervision of local health services is almost always the direct responsibility of the health officer, and may be in the bureau of administration. This function can be delegated to the deputy health commissioner, for it is the biggest task of the department. The chief function of most of the bureaus is to serve as advisers and consultants to local health services. For example, the divisions of public health nursing, maternal and child health, tuberculosis, mental health, dental hygiene, and health education need only small staffs of consultants. Those bureaus giving direct services, such as the public health laboratory and the vital statistics bureaus, can have a larger number of highly trained technical personnel on the central staff.

The Budget of a State Health Department

The budget of the state health department varies markedly in accordance with the population and area of the state. It also varies in accordance with the functions assigned to it. If, for example, the state health department has direct responsibility for hospitalization of the cases of tuberculosis, cancer, arthritis, or other chronic disease, a large hospital budget is required. If the state assumes considerable financial responsibility for the establishment and maintenance of good local health service, then the budget can be relatively large. For these reasons, it is almost impossible to compare the health bureau expenditures of one state with another, or to make suitable estimates of per capita expenditure by the state for promotion of the public health.

SPECIAL REFERENCES

STERN, B. J.: *Medical Services by Government.* The Commonwealth Fund, New York, 1946.

"Symposium on State Health Administration," Reports of Annual Meeting, American Public Health Association, 1946.

Health Departments of the States and Provinces of the United States and Canada, U.S. Public Health Service Bull. No. 184, as revised 1943 and subsequently.

40. NATIONAL HEALTH SERVICES

Apparently the founders of the American Republic did not believe that the federal government had any responsibility for the protection of the health of its citizens. In 1786, governmental functions in health protection were limited to: (a) maritime quarantine; (b) control of communicable disease; and as a corollary of the latter, environmental sanitation, such as disposal of wastes, and control of odors. At that time, all health protection matters were considered a responsibility of local government. There were no state health departments, and each of the ports instituted its own ship quarantine measures.

The federal government, under the Constitution, was given very limited powers in matters relating in any possible way to the public health. The clauses of the Constitution that have some bearing on health functions are:

1. Regulation of commerce with foreign nations and between states.
2. Power of the President to make treaties with foreign powers.
3. Direct jurisdiction of the federal government over territories, national parks, and other federal domains.
4. A short general clause that gives the power to the federal government to *promote the general welfare.*

Thus, the great proportion of the activities of the U.S. Public Health Service and the Children's Bureau, together with the welfare work of the Department of Health, Education, and Welfare rests on the interpretation of the authority that is vested in those few words, *promote the general welfare.*

HISTORY OF THE U.S. PUBLIC HEALTH SERVICE

The U.S. Public Health Service originated as a prepayment plan for medical care of American merchant seamen.

In 1798 a Marine Hospital Service was formed, under the U.S. Treasury, to give medical care to American seamen. Each sailor was required to pay 20 cents a month for this service. The money was deducted from his wages by the Department of Customs, which was in the Treasury Department. For the following 140 years, the major activities of the national government in the public health field were administered by the U.S. Treasury.

The Marine Hospital Service was poorly organized, and functioned haltingly and rather ineffectively for a long period. In 1870, Dr. John Woodworth, a Civil War Army officer, was selected as Surgeon General. He organized the service on semimilitary lines and formulated many of the policies that are followed by the U.S. Public Health Service to the present day. He put the service on a sound and effective basis, with full-time commissioned personnel. When Dr. Woodworth was appointed, the nation had just been through a series of epidemics of cholera and yellow fever that had entered the country at the various ports. Since the Marine Hospital Service was likely to encounter an epidemic at its onset and because of knowledge of illness in seamen, it was given certain maritime quarantine powers in 1878, which were carried out in cooperation with local health departments of the port cities. These related especially to yellow fever and cholera.

The National Board of Health was founded in 1878, and within a short time it was assigned the maritime quarantine powers that had been allocated to the Marine Hospital Service.

The founders of the National Board of Health were farsighted and public-spirited men, but they made many mistakes. They missed a great opportunity to place health on a national level. Their failure was tragic, but was probably unavoidable, for the nation was not yet ready to accept nation-wide unification of health procedures(1).

The Marine Hospital Service resumed the maritime quarantine services after the National Board of Health expired in 1882, and was given increased powers in 1893.

In 1902 the U.S. Public Health and Marine Hospital Service was formed, and the National Hygienic Laboratory established. Finally in 1912 the U.S. Public Health Service was authorized by Congress. It was given increased functions:

1. Investigation and research.
2. Improvement in methods of public health administration.
3. Distribution of federal aid to state and local health departments.
4. Interstate control of sanitation and water pollution.

Physical and mental examination of all aliens entering the United States was instituted in 1917, and medical officers of the service were sent to foreign countries to make these examinations of the emigrants. The National Leprosarium at Carville, Louisiana, was established the same year.

Mental hygiene was added as a function in 1929, and the medical care of federal prisoners and narcotic addicts was also assigned to the Public Health Service.

The Social Security Act of 1935 gave a tremendous impetus to the U.S. Public Health Service. Title VI, which was administered by the service, included substantial grants-in-aid ($8,000,000 was the initial annual appropriation) to all the states for the purpose of strengthening state and local health departments.

The National Cancer Act was passed in 1937, and the National Venereal Disease Control Act in 1938.

In 1939 the U.S. Public Health Service was removed from the Treasury Department and placed in the Federal Security Agency, but no other changes in its organization occurred at that time.

The Public Health Law of 1944(2) represents an epoch in the U.S. Public Health Service, since it entailed a reorganization and consolidation of the service, with a revision of national laws relating to the public health.

Federal Security Agency

The Federal Security Agency was founded in 1944 and organized with four main operating divisions:

1. Social Security Administration.
2. Education.
3. Public Health.
4. Special Services.

Social Security Administration controlled three major activities: (a) old-age insurance, (b) unemployment assistance, and (c) the Children's Bureau.

The Division of Food and Drugs, formerly operated by the Department of Agriculture, was transferred to Special Services. The Vocational Rehabilitation Division was also allocated to Special Services.

Department of Health, Education, and Welfare

The Reorganization Act of 1953 replaced the Federal Security Agency. The director of this new department has cabinet status. It was organized as follows:

1. Public Health Service.

2. Office of Education.
3. Social Security Administration.
    Office of Commissioner.
    Bureau of Federal Credit Unions.
    Bureau of Old Age and Survivors' Insurance.
    Bureau of Public Assistance.
    Children's Bureau.
4. Office of Vocational Rehabilitation.
5. Food and Drug Administration.
6. St. Elizabeth's Hospital for the Mentally Ill.

The great proportion of federal government health promotion activities is centered in the Children's Bureau and the U.S. Public Health Service.

The Children's Bureau. This bureau carries out three major activities: (a) maternal and child health promotion; (b) care of crippled children; (c) promotion of child welfare. Grants-in-aid to states are provided by the Children's Bureau for the development of state and local services in these three important fields.

The important functions of the Children's Bureau are:

1. To investigate and report upon all matters pertaining to child health and welfare.
2. To administer federal grants-in-aid to states under Title V of the Social Security Act.
3. To administer funds appropriated by the federal government for emergency maternity and infant care for families of enlisted men in the armed forces.*
4. To cooperate with the other American republics (and with the World Health Organization) in the world-wide promotion of maternal and child health

The Children's Bureau is organized with a central office in Washington, D.C., and has eight regional offices.

The crippled children's aid program is particularly important. A national registry of crippled children is maintained. Consultation service and grants-in-aid are provided to the various states to secure:

1. Suitable methods for locating crippled children and providing services for them.
2. Establishment of standards for physicians, surgeons, and hospitals that participate in the crippled children's program.
3. Provision for rehabilitation and social aftercare of the crippled child.

*A special World War II assignment.

ORGANIZATION OF THE U.S. PUBLIC HEALTH SERVICE

The Surgeon General is the administrative officer of the service. He is advised by a National Health Advisory Council, consisting of 14 members. Ten members at large are appointed by the Surgeon General for a period of five years. The Director of the National Institute of Health, and three experts, one each from the Army, the Navy, and the Bureau of Animal Industry, are ex-officio members of the council.

In addition, there is a National Advisory Cancer Council, consisting of six members appointed by the Surgeon General; an Advisory Board for Control of Biological Products; a Federal Advisory Board of Hospitalization; and such other advisory boards as may be authorized. Membership on one of these advisory boards is a position of great honor and responsibility. They are not salaried positions and are not subject to civil service laws.

The Regular Corps of commissioned officers consists of physicians, dentists, sanitary engineers, and public health nurses, as well as specialists in such fields as entomology, chemistry, and zoology. The great proportion of the personnel is made up of medical officers. All commissioned officers are appointed by the President with the consent of the Senate. A Reserve Corps is provided for, in order to have a suitable body of trained men available in time of national emergency. In general, all appointments, grades, ranks, pay, allowances, and retirement of the commissioned officers of the Regular Corps of the U.S. Public Health Service, and of the Reserve Corps as well, correspond closely to those of the U.S. Army. However, the titles of the commissioned officers are different from similar grades in the Army.

The major functions of the Public Health Service are allocated to four departments:

1. Office of the Surgeon General.
2. National Institutes of Health.
3. Bureau of Medical Services.
4. Bureau of State Services.

Office of the Surgeon General

The Office of the Surgeon General includes a variety of activities which can be broadly classified as the administrative functions of the Service.

National Institutes of Health

The Institutes are located in Bethesda, Maryland, and are organized as follows:

National Institutes:
   Allergy and Infectious Diseases.
   Arthritis and Metabolic Diseases.
   Cancer.
   Dental Research.
   Heart.
   Mental Health.
   Neurological Diseases and Blindness.
Clinical Center
Divisions:
   Biologics Standards.
   General Medical Sciences.
   Research Grants.
   Research Services.

The National Institutes of Health are essentially research institutions. They have developed tremendously in the years since 1902. At that time the major purpose of the National Hygienic Laboratory, as it was then called, was the standardization and control of biologic products that were intended for interstate shipment. The ramifications of the National Institutes of Health now encompass research in all the major phases of medical science. In addition, the Surgeon General is empowered to make the research facilities of the Institutes available to scientists and public health authorities. He also maintains research fellowships in the service, and makes grants-in-aid to universities, hospitals, laboratories, and other institutions for research in projects recommended by the National Advisory Councils.

Bureau of Medical Services

This bureau has charge of all the marine hospitals and their outpatient clinics. This very extensive activity is an outgrowth of the former division of medical and hospital care of American seamen. In general, all other medical activities of the U.S. Public Health Service in which direct service is rendered are assigned to this bureau. Foreign quarantine, including maritime quarantine, airplane quarantine, and medical inspection of immigrants, is organized in the Bureau of Medical Services.

Maritime quarantine is still an important function of the Public Health Service. All ships from foreign ports must be cleared when they enter an American port and must be able to give assurance to the officer of the Public Health Service that there is no contagious disease aboard. The most important diseases subject to quarantine are: plague, cholera, yellow fever, leprosy, smallpox, typhus fever, and anthrax. The development of international airplane travel has greatly complicated the duties of the service in prevention of entrance of contagion from foreign countries through means of the airplane.

Other medical activities include care of federal prisoners, as well as provision of medical and public health services to many other federal bureaus. Examples of this function are: the medical care of the Coast Guard, the U.S. Employees Compensation Commission, and the Office of Indian Affairs. The administration of the National Leprosarium at Carville, Louisiana, is the responsibility of this bureau.

Bureau of State Services

This bureau is concerned with all those matters relating to federal aid in promotion of health through the health departments of the various states. This includes grants-in-aid.

The Bureau of State Services has two major components: (a) Division of Community Health, and (b) Division of Environmental Health.

The National Center of Health Statistics is a separate division.

Hospital and Medical Facilities Division. The Hospital Survey and Construction Act of 1946(3) authorized grants to states for surveying existing hospital facilities and for planning and subsidizing additional facilities. This division has been of great value in stimulating construction of suitable hospitals in rural areas and in improving the standards for hospital care for all the people.

It is less than 50 years since the U.S. Public Health Service, as such, was founded in 1902. At that time, it was a minor governmental bureau that was responsible for maritime quarantine and the medical care of American seamen. The growth of the service, its increase in prestige, and the magnitude of its accomplishments are phenomenal. It has more than kept pace with the developments in medical science and public health. It has shown a strong leadership and has been directly responsible for many of the advances achieved in epidemiology, sanitary engineering, public health administration, and the basic medical sciences. The end is not in sight. There is every reason to believe that the U.S. Public Health Service will continue to grow in influence and enhance its potentialities in all the fields of medical science and health administration.

In conclusion, it is important to re-emphasize the fact that the federal government is not the sovereign power in the United States. It has only those powers that are granted to it by the various states. Each state is sovereign. Thus the federal government has direct jurisdiction only in limited areas such as territories, the District of Columbia, the Panama Canal Zone, and the national parks. Thus the major public health activities carried out by the federal government do not take the form of direct services but must be consultative and advisory, giving assistance when necessary and arbitrating between states in public health matters when occasion arises. When authorized to do so by Congress, the federal health officials may make grants-in-aid to states, in order to aid in improvement of local and state health services, but the actual administration of the work is the direct responsibility of the state and local authorities.

REFERENCES

1. SMILLIE, W. G.: *Am. J. Pub. Health*, 1943, 33:925.

2. Public Health Law No. 410: To Consolidate and Revise the Laws Relating to the United States Public Health Service, July 1, 1944.

3. Public Law 725–79th Congress (S. 191). An act to amend the Public Health Service Act to authorize grants to the states for surveying their hospitals and public health centers and for planning construction of additional facilities, and to authorize grants to assist in such construction. August 13, 1946.

SPECIAL REFERENCES

BRADBURY, D. E., and ELIOT, M. A.: *Four Decades of Action for Children: A Short History of the Children's Bureau.* U.S. Dept. Health, Education, and Welfare, Washington, D. C., 1957.

Public Law 487–79th Congress (H.R. 4512). An act to amend the Public Health Service Act to provide for research relating to psychiatric disorders and to aid in the development of more effective methods of prevention, diagnosis, and treatment of such disorders, and for other purposes. July 3, 1946.

41. THE WORLD HEALTH ORGANIZATION

The World Health Organization (WHO) is an integral part of the United Nations, with headquarters in Geneva, Switzerland.

It consists of a policy-making body, the World Health Assembly, which meets once a year. Each of the member states is entitled to three delegates to the Assembly. The Assembly selects an Executive Board, which has 24 members, and which meets twice a year in Geneva.

The activities of the WHO are directed by the Secretariat, which is headed by a Director General, who is elected every three years.

In addition to the headquarters in Geneva, there are six regional offices in Africa, Southeast Asia, Europe, Eastern Mediterranian area, Western Pacific area, and the Americas. (The Pan-American Sanitary Bureau, which functioned effectively for many years in promoting public health throughout the Americas, is now the American Division of WHO.)

The Director General of the Secretariat has a strong and capable permanent staff. In addition, he often selects highly skilled scientists in special fields to aid him, on a temporary basis, in the solution of a special problem in some particular area of the world. Thus he is able to call on the most highly skilled public health personnel, physicians, and scientists from any country to aid WHO in prevention of disease and promotion of health in any part of the world.

The functions of WHO are very broad and its activities are widespread. They include:

1. Regulations to prevent international spread of disease.
2. International statistical and epidemiologic services.
3. International promotion of maternal and child health.
4. Coordination of international health activities.
5. Advice and aid to individual governments, on request, in study of specific disease problems as well as aid in strengthening their health services.
6. Research in a great variety of fields, including studies of administrative and social measures that might affect medical care and the public health.

7. The Fellowship Program is one of WHO's most effective activities. These fellowships are granted on request from interested governments. Over 10,000 had been awarded by 1960; 59 per cent for health services; 28 per cent for communicable diseases; and 13 per cent for medical education.

Broad fields of preventive medicine given high priority by the WHO are: (a) malaria control, (b) control of tuberculosis, (c) malnutrition, (d) maternal and child health, and (e) environmental sanitation. International research in health has become an increasingly important function of WHO. At the Twelfth World Health assembly in 1959, Dr. L. T. Coggeshall, an American delegate, stated: "The World Health Organization has both a responsibility and opportunity to play a vital role in health research which could be played by no other agency." This is gradually becoming a major function of WHO.

The reader who has a special interest in the achievements of the World Health Organization is referred to the *WHO Chronicle,* which is published monthly. The breadth of interest, the dedication of effort, the imagination, enthusiasm, and intelligence expended by the staff of WHO in promotion of health throughout the world, and particularly in those areas in greatest need of help, are truly heartening.

It should be stressed that WHO utilizes the existing national public health administrations in the implementation of its goals, wherever possible. Because of its relatively small staff and budget — and for obvious political reasons — its primary functions are essentially advisory, educational, and investigative.

SPECIAL REFERENCES

Publications of the World Health Organization, Palais des Nations, Geneva, Switzerland.
Particularly:
   (a) *WHO Chronicle,* published monthly (in English)
   (b) *Technical Report Series.*
      Examples: 1. #137, 1957, Measurements of Levels of Health (Report of a Study Group)
             2. #194, Local Health Service (By An Expert Committee on Public Health Administration)
   (c) *World Health,* a popular magazine published bimonthly in English, Spanish, French, and Portuguese, by the WHO Division of Public Information.

42. VOLUNTARY HEALTH ACTIVITIES

The voluntary public health agency is a unique American institution that has developed out of the national character as a direct result of the pioneer spirit of helping a neighbor in the event of trouble and illness in the home. It is an admirable trait when properly developed and well directed.

In pioneer days, voluntary community health activities were concerned primarily with the care of the sick. Dorothea Dix, who was a crusader for better care of mental disease during the early part of the nineteenth century, was one of the first American voluntary health workers. The National Sanitary Commissions that functioned during the Civil War were forerunners of the Red Cross, and the soup kitchens of the depression period of 1872 to 1878 led directly to the establishment of milk stations for babies in the various large cities.

National Voluntary Health Agencies

The first nation-wide voluntary public health organization was the National Tuberculosis Association, which was founded in Philadelphia in 1892 and put on a national basis in 1894. Other national health organizations followed, such as the American Social Hygiene Association, the American Society for the Control of Cancer, the National Society for the Prevention of Blindness, the National Foundation for Infantile Paralysis, the National Committee for Mental Hygiene, the American Heart Association, and many others.

All these organizations have certain points in common:

1. Each has a specific public health purpose.
2. All are organized on a national basis, with a central governing body.
3. Each has local chapters or units. Services can be organized on a state basis also; some have local chapters only.
4. The budget is dependent upon current contributions. They have small endowments.

The central governing body is responsible for general policies of the organization. Leadership has been excellent through the years. The policy of each of the national health organizations has generally been to cooperate with local official health agencies in carrying out the special programs of community health service.

The chief functions of the local chapters of the national voluntary health agency have been:

1. To render advisory and consultation services.
2. To provide direct services for a temporary period, in conjunction with the official health department. Usually the direct service is a demonstration of the value of an improved technique.
3. To aid the local health department in specific community-wide instruction.
4. Research is sometimes carried on by a local chapter. In general, research in the special field of interest is a function of the national body rather than the local chapter. Investigations are frequently conducted by an official health organization or a university research department, under a subsidy that is supplied by the voluntary organization.

The great difficulty that has been encountered in the field of voluntary health work is that the organizations do not recognize when their work is done. They have no "terminal facilities." For example, a local tuberculosis association may have sponsored and perhaps supported entirely a tuberculosis diagnostic clinic in the community. The clinic serves a fine purpose, but it is a demonstration only, for a tuberculosis clinic is the function of the official health agency. The demonstration of the value of the clinic by the voluntary agency should therefore be a short one, and the work should be turned over to the health department as soon as possible. Too often the local voluntary agency is reluctant to give up a direct community service because it fears that the work will not be "done as well" by the official agency.

Local Voluntary Health Agencies

Many voluntary health activities have developed on a purely local basis. Most notable are the visiting nurse associations.

Visiting Nurse Associations. The visiting nurse association was established more than half a century ago as a philanthropic effort to bring skilled bedside nursing care to the sick poor. It was successful from the very onset. The nurses soon discovered, however, that their efforts were of little avail unless preventive measures were combined with actual nursing care of the sick. Thus the visiting nurse became a forerunner of public health nursing activities. Official public health nurses were first used in school health work and in maternity and infant hygiene. This activity has grown so rapidly that at present the major part of the personnel and nearly half the budget of a municipal health department are assigned to public health nurses.

The assumption of the responsibility for public health nursing by the official health agencies did not supplant the visiting nurse, but it did modify her program.

The visiting nurse association has developed as an organization giving expert nursing care to the sick on an hourly basis. These services are provided free to the poor; at cost to those who can afford to pay for them. Practicing physicians have discovered the value of these services in the care of their private patients. It now seems clear that the future of the visiting nurse association is secure as a self-supporting community activity, which serves all economic groups rather than limiting its activities to nursing care of the sick poor. It is probable that necessary hourly nursing care will be included with hospitalization and other medical services in the prepayment plans for complete medical care. In addition, industries that require a nursing service, but with too few employees to warrant paying a full-time nurse, have found it profitable to contract with the visiting nurse association for the required nursing services for their industrial employees.

Currently, the deficit in the budget of a visiting nurse association resulting from the free nursing services given to the poor is met by philanthropy.

The average man on the street finds a dual nursing system very confusing. He cannot distinguish between an official public health nurse and a private "visiting" nurse. Oftentimes there is overlapping of activity. A good nurse who gives bedside care to the sick gives instruction in preventive medicine as well.

It has been suggested frequently that a unified system of nursing service should be provided by the community from taxation funds. Such a plan, however, requires one nurse per 2,500 population. This results in an unbalanced health department budget. The costs of the nursing service would be so heavy that all other necessary health activities might be submerged.

The programs of the private visiting nurse association should be closely integrated with that of the official community nurses to avoid duplication of services. The health officer should be on the board of directors of the voluntary nursing association; if a health center building is established, the voluntary nursing organization should be provided with headquarters there.

Other Voluntary Organizations. Other community organizations, such as men's service clubs, churches, and fraternal organizations, are often interested in community welfare and desire to aid in health protection in specific ways, particularly in child health promotion. The chamber of commerce might be interested in industrial hygiene. In some instances an organization provides for the care of crippled children; another pays for dental care or for the glasses of needy children. This work is helpful and most effective when coordinated with the activities of the official health and welfare organizations.

The Public Health Council. The public health council is a very successful device for coordinating all the official and voluntary health activities of the community.

The council is made up of representatives of the leading organizations in the community with any interest in public health affairs. It has no operating functions and gives no direct service. The medical and dental societies should have representatives on the committee, and public-spirited practicing physicians are frequently asked to take part in the work of the council.

In a large city the public health council may have a full-time executive, often supported by the Community Chest.

In some cities the public health council combines its work with that of the hospital council, because of their closely related community functions.

Social Foundations

The beginning of the twentieth century in America was marked by the rise of great social foundations. They have met a real need in America, but probably represent a temporary phase of our national development. They have been of enormous assistance in promotion of the public health.

The foundations have been established, for the most part, from private fortunes of large industrialists for the "welfare of the people." The major purposes of the foundations in the public health field have been:

1. To give grants-in-aid to official health agencies for the demonstration of new procedures in public health. These grants have been made for only a temporary period.

2. To conduct investigations which have led to better public health procedures. Seldom has the foundation carried out the research. The work has been done under subsidy by universities or official public health agencies.

3. To furnish, through highly competent staffs, advisory and consultative services to official health agencies.

4. To aid in personnel training, so that young men can fit themselves properly to assume the responsibilities and duties of official health work.

5. Grants-in-aid for basic or applied research.

There are certain disadvantages that accrue to the whole field of voluntary health organizations. The health officer and his staff are officially responsible for all the health protection activities of the community. Sometimes the health department is not given sufficient funds to carry out the necessary work. The voluntary agencies have funds, but are often interested in specific projects rather than an over-all and comprehensive program. Thus, even though cooperation is excellent between voluntary and official health agencies, nevertheless the public health program might be developed on a basis of expediency and special interest rather than on a well-rounded, carefully planned basis.

Furthermore, there is always the danger that because the voluntary health agency has the funds, it might wish to dictate policies as to how those funds should be spent; thus the recipient is on the horns of a dilemma. The work should be done, and funds are available for the task, but he cannot carry out the work in the manner that seems most appropriate to him, because the funds are available only if the work is done in accordance with a preconceived formula of a foundation director. Hans Zinsser once called this "one of the perils of philanthropy."

The National Red Cross

The Red Cross is in a somewhat different category than other nation-wide voluntary public health agencies because it has a semi-official status. The President of the United States is always its national president, but it receives no funds from the national treasury. It is chartered as a disaster relief agency by the federal government.

It has three primary functions in an emergency:

1. Nonmedical: This consists primarily of providing the necessities of life (food, shelter, and clothing) to the refugees from disaster.

2. Medical: The Red Cross provides medical, nursing, and hospital care of the sick and injured in a disaster, and also protects the rest of the community from the hazards produced by disaster conditions.

3. Rehabilitation: The Red Cross aids in rehabilitation of the devastated area, as rapidly as circumstances permit. Often the stricken area is benefited by installation of much better permanent sanitary facilities than existed before the disaster occurred.

The Red Cross has developed a program of public health nursing in sparsely settled areas, and in many other ways has aided in health promotion of the whole nation. This work is carried out through local chapter aid and initiative. Stimulus and guidance come from the national headquarters, but the actual work is done by and through the local chapters.

The National Red Cross has its offices in Washington, D.C., and organizes local chapters in all the various communities. In case of a disaster, the local Red Cross chapter is in charge of the relief. The National Red Cross sends supplementary aid upon the request of the governor of the state.

The Red Cross does not supply medical and nursing care to the military personnel, but supplements the activities of the Medical Corps of the Army, Navy, and the Air Force, particularly in caring for the needs of the civilian population that is disturbed or perhaps rendered destitute by war conditions.

SPECIAL REFERENCES

CARTER, RICHARD: *The Gentile Legions*. Doubleday & Co., Garden City, N.Y., 1961.

GUNN, S. M., and PLATT, P. S.: *Voluntary Health Agencies. An Interpretive Study*. The Ronald Press Company, New York, 1945.

See also: "Medicine and the Changing Order." Report of a Special Committee of the New York Academy of Medicine. The Commonwealth Fund, New York, 1947.

New York Academy of Medicine: "The Role of Voluntary Public Health Agencies." Chap. XLIV of *Preventive Medicine in Modern Practice*. Paul B. Hoeber, Inc., New York, 1942.

43. HEALTH EDUCATION

One of the most important functions of the practicing physician is that of a health educator. Most doctors are not conscious of this fact. They consider health education to be the function of a specially trained technician in public relations, who uses various publicity methods out of keeping with the dignity of serious scientific medical practice.

It is true that "health education," as the term is usually applied, is a special technique which requires a highly trained and skilled personnel. Its purpose is to inform the mass of the people concerning the principles of preventive medicine and public health.

Necessity for Health Education

Health education has been developed as a special activity of official health departments because of our way of life. The democratic principle requires that there be no introduction of new administrative policies, such as establishment of full-time local health services, without the consent of the majority of the people. Compulsory vaccination against smallpox, a most effective epidemiologic measure, cannot be made a part of community regulations unless the people so desire. Thus, before each new step is taken in health promotion of the people, it becomes necessary to inform the public fully, so that the purpose of the measure is understood and the necessity for its enforcement is accepted.

Under this plan, health protection can move only as fast and as far as public opinion permits. The great mass of the population must understand and be convinced of the benefits to be derived and be aware of the sacrifices that must be made. It is a slow process — often a very discouraging procedure to the leaders in the field who see the need so clearly but who cannot act because public opinion does not permit.

The plan has other great disadvantages. The techniques of health education lend themselves to exploitation and to abuses by quacks, charlatans, promoters of spurious remedies, and the vaporings of sincere but misguided crackbrained enthusiasts.

This type of health education — perhaps better called health propaganda — is only one part of the subject.

Methods of Health Education

Three major methods are employed in health education. In two, the physician has little part; the third is his almost exclusive province. Each is discussed briefly.

Health Education as a Systematic Part of Teaching in the Schools and Colleges. This method is a function of the department of education. The subjects taught are:

1. Personal hygiene: protection and promotion of individual and family health.

2. The elements of epidemiology and preventive medicine, as a corollary of 1.

3. Community responsibility for health protection.

Thus when the student who absorbs this information becomes an adult, he can take an active and intelligent part in community affairs relating to the public health and also take appropriate measures to protect his own health and that of his family. Experience has shown that health teaching in the public schools is the most important and fundamental technique to be employed in promotion of the health status of the whole nation. A complete new generation of people might be required in order to have a change in public opinion and to secure the establishment of new public health principles, with the abandonment of old practices. With patience and persistence, the change can finally be made.

Health Information to All the People. This activity is the responsibility of the official health department, aided by various voluntary health agencies and other official agencies with an interest in this field.

This method utilizes radio, television, newspapers, lectures, motion pictures, exhibits, pamphlets, and all facilities that may be employed in securing public attention and in giving sound instruction. It requires great skill, special aptitudes, and special training.

Health Teaching by Those Who Are Actually Engaged in Giving Medical Care to the Sick. This is one of the great responsibilities and privileges of the practitioner of medicine.

Every bedside that is visited and every house that is entered by a physician, gives an opportunity for effective health education.

The major purpose of this text has been to point out the opportunity of every physician to incorporate health education as an integral part of his medical practice. The greatest opportunities of the clinician and the most productive services a doctor can render his patients are:

1. To correct misunderstanding and confusion concerning illness.

2. To instill sound knowledge concerning prevention of illness and protection of health in the minds of all his patients.

3. To carry enough conviction with his teaching so that his patients are motivated to take the necessary steps to protect themselves and their families from unnecessary illness.

4. To provide for an understanding of the influences of social and economic factors upon illness and to clarify the functions of the physician, the nurse, and other agencies in health protection of the family.

This is true health education in its best sense. It is the responsibility of the family physician, the visiting nurse, and others who give direct care and relief to the sick. The teaching is presented in the hospital, the clinic, the office, and in the homes of individuals and families. This type of health teaching is not spectacular, but its results are sound and most effective.

SPECIAL REFERENCES

ACKERMAN, LLOYD: *Health and Hygiene.* Jaques Cattel Press, Lancaster, Pa., 1943.

BAUER, W. W., and HULL, THOMAS G.: *Health Education of the Public,* 2nd ed. W. B. Saunders Company, Philadelphia, 1942.

BUCHER, C. A., and WEBSTER, L. E.: *Accent on Health.* The Macmillan Company (in press).

DIEHL, H. S.: *Healthful Living.* McGraw-Hill Book Company, Inc., New York, 1949.

NYSWANDER, D. B.: *Solving School Health Problems.* The Commonwealth Fund, New York, 1942.

TURNER, C. E.: *Community Health Education Compendium of Knowledge.* C. V. Mosby Co., St. Louis, 1951.

44. THE PUBLIC HEALTH NURSE

Public health nursing is a changing and evolutionary concept. The activities of a health department of the last century had no place for a nursing service, no interest in individual health promotion.

In America public health nursing originated in 1877, when the Women's Branch of the New York City Mission organized a service of trained nurses who were sent into the homes of the sick poor. This voluntary activity had a slow but steady growth. The pioneer visiting nurses who gave bedside nursing care in the slums of the large cities became interested in preventive medicine because they realized their inability to get at the fundamental causes of illness; they were dismayed by the futility of their efforts in meeting the real needs of the people. These young women recognized the influence of social and economic factors upon illness. They understood the necessity of preventive services, particularly for mothers and little children, and they saw the effect of poor nutrition and bad housing upon health. Visiting nurse service was combined with welfare and social services at the Henry Street Settlement in New York under Miss Lillian Wald, and this great leader initiated the concept of official community responsibility for nursing care. In 1902, the first health department nurses in the United States were appointed to the New York City Health Department: one in school health, and one to the division of child hygiene. These nurses were assigned to the city from the Henry Street Settlement by Miss Wald as a social experiment.

The value of this type of community service became apparent immediately, and two types of nursing service, official public health nursing and bedside nursing care, grew up side by side in most municipalities. Theoretically they had different functions. One service was planned to prevent illness. It used the statistical approach of the health department in its case load intake. The other service was organized to care for illness in the home after it had occurred, and used this as the point of departure in family health teaching. Both groups considered themselves "public health nurses," with a basic responsibility for health teaching. There was much overlapping of activity, of course, since there is no clear-cut point where prevention ends and treatment begins; as community health programs have developed through group planning, this duplication of work has decreased. In rural areas, bedside nursing care was sponsored by the Red Cross and other voluntary health associations, but for the most part, official public health nursing has predominated in rural communities, with little or no bedside nursing care, on either an official or unofficial basis.

The Social Security Act of 1935 was a great stimulus to public health nursing throughout the nation, particularly in rural areas and in other areas that were in greatest need of this type of service. Public health nursing has now increased to such a degree that more than one half the budget of most local health departments is allocated to this service.

The great gain during recent years had been an increase of official nursing service in rural areas and an increase in industrial nursing, with a tendency toward diminution in the number of nurses employed by nonofficial agencies.

Functions of a Public Health Nurse

As public health nursing has evolved, the concept of the functions of a public health nurse has changed markedly. It is still changing. Certain broad principles have been developed, however, which give a general idea of the scope of her work.

The major function of the public health nurse is educational. Everything she does, including the bedside care, is an educational measure as well as a direct service to the family. It is her duty to aid each of the families in her jurisdiction to prevent disease and to promote health in all members of the family. Special attention is given to mothers, to young children, and to rehabilitation in chronic illness.

The public health nurse secures early medical diagnosis and treatment for those who are sick; she renders or secures nursing care for the sick, teaching the patient and the family by demonstration and by supervision. The nurse aids the family in making adjustments of social conditions affecting the health of its members; she helps create positive attitudes in the home toward the acquisition and maintenance of health. The nurse also has the responsibility of keeping before the citizens of the community the needs and requirements of an adequate program in public health.

Case Finding. Case finding is a public health nursing function of utmost importance to the success of the total medical service plan of the community.

The visiting nurse enters more homes than any other community worker. If she has a well-developed sense of public health values and works under competent direction, she can be a very important factor in finding the early cases of illness and in getting them under early treatment.

The birth injury, the case of idiopathic scoliosis, or of tuberculosis, the unrecognized syphilitic, the woman with early cancer, as well as many other conditions, are encountered and recognized (or at least suspected) in the home by the well-qualified public health nurse as she makes her daily rounds. Part of her duty is to secure immediate and adequate treatment for these patients.

Case Holding. The public health nurse not only finds new and unrecognized cases of illness and gets them under treatment, but she is also an important factor in case holding.

She has the confidence of her people and can interpret to them the necessity for certain medical and surgical procedures. She can explain the importance of continuous and prolonged treatment, as for example in tuberculosis or in paralysis from poliomyelitis; thus she is able to convince the patients of the need for continuance of their therapeutic procedures.

Activities of the Public Health Nurse

The various activities of the health department in which the nurse participates have been described elsewhere in this text. To recapitulate briefly:

Maternity Service. The major part of this community-wide program is the responsibility of the public health nurse. She aids in the prenatal instruction, assists the prospective mother in preparing for the baby, carries out the physician's instructions concerning nursing features of prenatal care, aids in the prenatal clinic and in postnatal care.

Infancy. In certain areas the public health nurse assists in home delivery service. Customarily, she makes the necessary postnatal nursing visits, and has special responsibility for home nursing care of premature infants. She assists in the well-child conferences and instructs the mother at home in the care and hygiene of the baby. She assists in communicable disease control and in securing correction of remediable defects of infants.

Preschool and School Health. Preschool and school health work has been described in detail in Chapter 24. The nurse plays a major role in this part of the health program. She not only assists the school physician in the examinations of the children, but she also takes most of the burden of persuading families to secure correction of the physical defects that are encountered. In many instances, she actively aids the indigent family in obtaining proper treatment. Control of contagion in school children, particularly abatement of the minor and most troublesome skin diseases, such as scabies, impetigo, pediculosis, and ringworm of the scalp, is included in her daily routine.

Communicable Disease Control. The home visiting and clinic services in tuberculosis and syphilis are among the most important and effective activities of the public health nurse. She not only gives instruction in the home concerning prevention of further spread of all communicable disease, but she aids also in tracing contacts, finding sources of infection, and securing more complete reporting of these conditions. She also teaches her families the simple principles of epidemiology, and demonstrates home techniques in concurrent and terminal disinfection.

Nutrition. Instruction in the principles of nutrition, family purchasing of food, and family budgeting for a well-balanced dietary is an important activity of the nurse. She has access to low-income families and families with foreign or different backgrounds from those of the community as a whole; she has the confidence of the mothers and can talk their language. In this way she augments the work of the family physician, the clinic, and the nutritionist.

Mental Hygiene Activities and Orthopedic Service. These and the broad field of adult health services are part of the nurse's program, entering into her family health work as a part of her generalized service.

Chronic Illness. The public health nurse has become an important asset in the rehabilitation of patients suffering from chronic illness. Through her knowledge of the community, she is an effective "case finder" for those not receiving adequate care.

Her home visits, conducted under physician supervision, are invaluable to the patient and to the family. In organized home-care programs, with rehabilitation as a primary objective, the nurse is the key person around whom the program revolves.

In many areas, official health services are assigning more of their nursing facilities to health promotion of the chronically ill, particularly those of the older age groups confined to their homes by their incapacities.

Industrial Nursing

Industrial nursing has become a special public health field. The nurse is usually employed by a company to carry out the nursing program of preventive medicine and health education among the employees. Part-time service for small plants is being purchased from visiting nurse associations in increasing amounts. The nurse works under the direction of the industrial physician, who is employed either on a part-time or full-time basis. Frequently she is delegated to give emergency care for minor surgical conditions (see Chap. 30 on industrial medicine).

Qualifications for Public Health Nursing

The National Organization of Public Health Nursing has set standards of qualifications for public health nurses of different grades. These standards are revised every five years. The public health nurse must not only be a graduate of a recognized school of nursing, but she must also have special professional education and experience under supervision in the field.

Organization of a Public Health Nursing Service

An excellent public health nursing program, along the general lines outlined here, can be conducted with about one nurse per 5,000 population. If bedside nursing is included in the over-all plan, one nurse per 2,500 population might be required. The most satisfactory arrangement devised thus far is the generalized plan of nursing services. Under this plan, the official public health nurse is assigned to an area or district where she carries out all the public health nursing activities of that area. Under such a plan there are no special nursing assignments, such as full-time school nursing service, infant welfare nurses, or services for tuberculosis control; the approach to all problems is that of family health service.

Public health nursing is usually organized as a service division of the health department, with a director of nursing and one supervisor of the nursing service for each eight to ten of the nursing staff.

In many communities, the school nurses are employed by the department of education, and not by the health department. This results in a health program with divided responsibility and specialized nursing service, which is unsatisfactory from all points of view.

The nursing services are integrated with all the other health department activities by the health officer. The state health department has a division of public health nursing which acts in an advisory capacity, aiding all the local health departments in the state. The state director of nursing can aid local communities in planning nursing programs and in selection of personnel. The provision for in-service training of personnel is often an activity of the state department of nursing.

Bedside Nursing Care

Nursing care of the sick in their homes has been developed as a special community activity, chiefly under the direction of voluntary organizations (see Chap. 42).

Thus two systems of home visiting by nurses have grown up side by side. The people as a rule do not understand the distinction between the official public health nurse, who limits her work to a preventive service, which is free, and the voluntary service of bedside nursing care of the sick, for which a nominal charge is made to those who can afford to pay for the service.

The theory is clear, and it is consistent with other policies of public health work, in relation to medical care and to hospitalization of the sick. The difficulty, of course, is that often there is no real distinction between a preventive and a curative nursing service. Thus there is an inevitable overlapping of activity in the two types of nursing care. However, the leaders in the public health nursing profession believe that a community program, with a merging of the two services, is possible and essential. At present, interesting experiments are developing under joint leadership. In these tests, one nurse is assigned complete responsibility for the total public health nursing program for all families in her area.

The Future of Public Health Nursing

The unification of community nursing services is an obvious and inevitable development. In the rural areas it seems most probable that all the nursing services will be centered in the health unit. In all probability, there will be a community medical center which will include hospitalization as well as a home visiting service by physicians and nurses. The nurse who makes a home visit in prenatal and postnatal care will have her headquarters in the health center; she will have responsibility for the prenatal clinic and could be the delivery nurse in the hospital as well. In other words, the service will be offered as a unit of medical and nursing care.

Prepayment plans for complete medical care must obviously include home nursing care of families, which will be provided on an hourly instructional basis.

In the larger municipalities, the health department activities may be maintained as a separate function of government, and the health officer may not administer the community-wide plans for distribution of medical, hospital, and nursing services. It is clear, however, that the nursing services must be organized on a *unit basis,* with wide utilization by physicians of professional nurses for home visits to the patient. Many of the tasks that are now performed by the physician in the home in care of the sick can be done just as effectively by a nurse under medical direction, thus releasing the time of the physician for more suitable activities. For example, simple therapeutic procedures such as giving of insulin, the care of patients in convalescence, the diagnostic routines such as the taking of blood pressure, the securing of a blood culture or a blood film, or taking blood for biochemical assay, tests for basal metabolism, and a great many other technical procedures can be done adequately in the home by a well-prepared nurse who functions under medical direction. As time passes, her usefulness as a complement to the practice of medicine will be utilized more and more by physicians. It is probable that the hospital will utilize the nurse through home visits to those patients who have been discharged to their homes as convalescents. Such a plan should shorten the period of hospitalization and give more satisfactory care than do existing plans.

Already, in a few forward-looking communities, a plan is being developed, under medical leadership, for a system of continuous public health nursing care of patients who are referred directly from a hospital to the community nursing agencies. Certain types of patients are referred to the visiting nurse associations as they leave, or even before they leave, the hospital. Examples of situations that profit by this service are: families with a premature baby, children with rheumatic fever who have cardiac complications and are sent home for convalescence, adults with cancer or heart disease, patients with diabetes or other types of chronic illness that require continuous home nursing supervision.

Private physicians can participate in this plan for nursing care and education of their patients. The nursing service is furnished by the nursing association at cost, or, when necessary, is given free to indigent patients.

The evolvement of this type of community nursing service will probably be dependent upon all-inclusive prepayment plans for medical care, and will result in bringing the advantages of an hourly nursing service in the home to all classes of society rather than limiting these benefits to the sick poor.

Most plans for prepayment of medical care have carefully omitted nursing service from their benefits. This is a very serious mistake, since home nursing care is an increasingly important part of complete medical service. Provision for proper care in convalescence is one of the weakest links in our plan for medical service. Thus every effort should be made to integrate and incorporate home nursing in a comprehensive, continuous community plan for adequate medical care. It is obvious also that preventive services in nursing care, which at present are provided by health department nurses, will be consolidated with the instructional home nursing visits which are given to the sick. This concept of an adequate community nursing plan will require a skilled and intelligent corps of nurses who will receive more comprehensive education and better compensation than the public health nurse of today.

SPECIAL REFERENCES

FREEMAN, RUTH B.: *Public Health Nursing Practice*, 2nd ed. W. B. Saunders Co., Philadelphia, Pa., 1957.

FROST, HARRIET: *Nursing in Sickness and Health*. The Macmillan Company, New York, 1939.

GARDNER, M. S.: *Katharine Kent*. The Macmillan Company, New York, 1946.

GILBERT, RUTH: *The Public Health Nurse and Her Patient*. The Commonwealth Fund, New York, 1940.

NEWTON, KATHLEEN: *Geriatric Nursing*. The C. V. Mosby Company, St. Louis, 1950.

Nursing in Commerce and Industry. The Commonwealth Fund, New York, 1946.

Public Health Nursing Care of the Sick at Home. National League for Nursing, New York, N.Y., April, 1953.

SHEPARD, W. P., and WHEATLEY, G. M.: *J.A.M.A.*, 1952, 149:554.

WENSLEY, EDITH: *The Community and Public Health Nursing*. The Macmillan Company, New York, 1950.

45. MEDICAL SOCIAL WORK

Medical social work is an essential service in the field of preventive medicine. It is one of the important techniques devised for the purpose of securing a better understanding of the influence of economic and social factors upon prevention of disease and promotion of health of the individual and the family.

Medical social work was initiated by Dr. Richard Cabot in the outpatient clinics of the Massachusetts General Hospital in 1905. Dr. Cabot had great originality and a strong social consciousness. He realized that the outpatient clinic was not functioning effectively because the physicians were diagnosing and treating *disease* in an individual, without a real knowledge of the *person* they desired to help. The family practitioner of medicine usually has a complete understanding of all the social elements that affect the lives of his patients, since he may carry the same families through several generations. The physician in a large hospital or clinic might see the patient only once, when the patient is entirely removed from the environment in which his illness initiated, and to which he will return when he leaves the hospital.

The medical social worker was introduced first into the outpatient clinic services, and then added to the hospital staff as part of the medical team. It is not her sphere to diagnose disease nor to administer therapy. She is trained to understand and to help the patient solve personal and family problems. She is also trained to observe and interpret the relationship of social and economic conditions to disease, and to recognize the particular social problems produced by illness.

The medical social worker has now established herself as an invaluable person in the over-all comprehensive plans for care of the sick. She aids also in the prevention of recurrence of illness, and she is of great assistance in promotion of individual and family health and stability. Her main concern is the social situation of the patient. She studies his family relationships, his whole economic status, and his home and work environment, and makes an estimate of the manner in which these factors relate to his illness. With those facts at hand, she aids in making plans for carrying out his treatment and for his subsequent rehabilitation. Those factors that impinge on his life and that might be affected by his illness are reviewed, as well as the influences of his home environment that might have an effect upon his recovery.

Medical social workers conduct their activities in the hospital, in the clinic, and in the home. They help the physician understand the particular situations and problems of the patient, and they also help the patient to meet and solve those situations which to him often seem hopelessly insurmountable.

The social worker often accomplishes her results on the basis of individual case studies. Each person and each situation must be handled in accordance with its particular needs. The most important tools that the medical social worker uses are:

1. Material relief, in which actual funds are provided to assist the patient through an emergency, or until the patient is aided in securing material assistance through his own resources.

2. The medical social worker is familiar with all the resources of the community, and assists the patient in choosing the particular agency or facility that will be of greatest use to him. She also explains the benefit he can expect to receive from each source of assistance.

3. The social worker aids the patient in understanding his illness and in adjusting his life to the actual situation. Often it is necessary to discuss matters with the family, in order to help them understand the situation, and perhaps to change the family attitude toward the patient and his illness or handicap. Often the social worker contributes to the medical care of the patient by helping him understand the urgent necessity for following his treatment exactly as recommended by his physician.

A simple case history illustrates the way in which all these tools were applied in solving a single family situation:

M. H., a 48-year-old white day-laborer, came to the clinic in a weak and emaciated condition. His speech was hesitant. There was a marked tremor of his hands. He was depressed, worried, and seriously upset emotionally. He had not worked for a year because of the increasing weakness. He had a wife and a 15-year-old son, dependent upon him for support. The wife was not working; the boy was in high school. All his savings had been spent.

There was no money left at home for food or for rent, and he was sure that he would not recover from his illness. He had been under treatment for some time with a private physician, but his funds were gone and he was in despair.

The immediate problem was the diagnosis of the condition. The man proved to be suffering from early general paresis. The patient had had syphilis some 20 years previously and had been inadequately treated. His wife and son were not infected with the disease. A recommendation was made that immediate hospital treatment was essential, and the patient was referred to medical social service.

The social service worker first arranged for hospitalization of the father, in order that he should receive early and adequate treatment. Since he had no funds, the resources of the hospital, which were available for inpatient treatment of indigent patients, were drawn upon, and thus this matter was arranged satisfactorily.

An interview by the medical social worker with the wife showed a nervous, almost hysterical woman, overwhelmed by the seriousness of her husband's illness, with no funds, no food in the house, and no resources upon which she could draw.

Social service provided her with a loan of $25, to tide her over this emergency. The mother had worked as a silver polisher before her marriage and had developed some skill in this trade, but had lost all contact with her former employer. Social service soon was able to obtain a position for her in her special trade, but she was unable to do her work properly because of defective eyesight. The medical social service worker then arranged for ophthalmologic tests, and the mother was fitted with proper glasses. With this encouragement and assistance, she became self-supporting. The son in high school was able to supplement the family income by part-time after-school work secured through the suggestion of social service. The father's treatment was prolonged but successful, and on discharge from convalescence, the medical social service worker aided him in securing a position which was commensurate with his physical limitations.

This resumé of the handling of a family situation is a cross section of the day-by-day work of the medical social worker in any large hospital or clinic. It will be noted that a variety of methods was employed, including: (a) direct material aid, (b) utilization of various community resources in rehabilitation of the family, thus aiding the mother to pull the situation together and return the family to a sound financial footing, and (c) opportunity for the patient and his wife to discuss their fears and anxiety which were related to the man's illness and subsequent incapacity.

In recent years with the development of public medical care programs, the medical social worker has found a place in organizations outside the hospital, in such health agencies as federal, state, and local divisions for the care of crippled children, for the tuberculous, and for those with chronic illness of various types. She has been used as a consultant on the social aspects of these programs as well as for giving direct service to patients. Here particularly she is as much concerned with the prevention of disease as with its treatment.

SPECIAL REFERENCES

BUEL, BRADLEY: *Community Planning for Human Services.* Columbia University Press, New York, 1952.

CANNON, M. A., and BARTLETT, M. M.: *Medical Social Work. Committee on Medicine and the Changing Order, New York Academy of Medicine.* The Commonwealth Fund, New York, 1947.

ELLEDGE, C. H.: *The Rehabilitation of the Patient; Social Casework in Medicine.* J. B. Lippincott Company, Philadelphia, 1948.

Widening Horizons in Medical Education. The Commonwealth Fund, New York, 1948.

ZIMAND, SAVEL: *Public Health and Welfare. Selected Papers of Homer Folks.* The Macmillan Company, New York, 1958.

SECTION V

Comprehensive Medical Care

46. COMPREHENSIVE MEDICAL CARE

The term "comprehensive medical care" may be defined as a systematic organization of all personal services by members of all the various health professions as well as all hospital and related clinical facilities necessary to attain the highest level of health for all the people. It is planned to prevent disease, provide for diagnosis and treatment of illness, and to prevent or mitigate the disability that might be related to the ravages of chronic disease.

An ideal program for comprehensive medical care available to all the people requires careful planning and foresight, with proper assignment of responsibilities so that all services are provided at as high a quality as is consistent with reasonable cost.

The pioneer concept of medical care in the United States was that all medical care was the responsibility of the physician. He was a true general practitioner, carrying out the functions of internist, surgeon, pediatrician, the more difficult obstetrical services, and even dentistry. His major work was in diagnosis and treatment. He treated the sick poor without charge. With the exception of emergency "pest houses," utilized during epidemics, there were no hospitals. Later, institutions for custodial care of the indigent sick were established and called hospitals. The community provided the hospital, the physician gave free care to the poor.

Gradually, medical care became more complex, with emergence of specialists in various fields. The concept of trained nursing care was developed along with the initiation of various ancillary services. The official community organizations, local and state, gradually (often reluctantly) assumed some responsibility for prevention of disease, and health departments were formed; thus the concept of organized public health services was born.

In some areas the municipality assumed responsibility for free hospitalization of the indigent. The state developed institutions for custodial care of the insane. For the first time, physicians were employed *by the community*, on a full-time basis, to administer

561

custodial institutions for care of the indigent sick (usually the chronically ill) or to administer official public health services.

A strong tradition still persisted. Medical care was the responsibility of the physician. He was the key. He determined medical care policies in the community. His work was carried out on a fee-for-service basis; usually the rates varied in relation to ability of the patient to pay. The indigent were given care without charge.

This pioneer concept of medical care persists in the minds of many physicians today. It is a personal service performed by physicians, with all ancillary facilities, such as hospitals, clinics, nurses, and technicians, serving simply as aids to enable the doctor to practice medicine more effectively. In many instances the physician resents the intrusion of the public health officials in the domain of clinical medicine, and he is opposed to laymen interfering in matters relating to community-wide medical care policies.

Through voluntary or public funds, the community provides the hospital, and thus the hospital board of directors usually determines hospital policies. This often results in an antagonism between the hospital administrator, who carries out hospital policies, and the physicians who provide the medical care of the hospital.

Who Is Responsible for Medical Care?

One of the most striking recent social advances in community life has been the improvement in measures that promote health and prevent disease. It is advantageous, therefore, to review objectively the entire field of medical care and to define the responsibilities for the organization, as well as the administration, of medical services. It is most important to plan a community organization for the medical care of the future, which each year will function more effectively.

The previous discussions have indicated that the community has certain vested interests in the individual, and is, therefore, vitally concerned with the protection and promotion of his health. We have considered, at some length, the responsibilities and activities of the local, state, and federal governments in the protection of the health of the people. It has been stated that the community has the responsibility of protecting the individual and his family against the hazards incident to communal life.

We have suggested that the community could also have the responsibility of providing those facilities required to promote the return to health of those who become ill.

The Committee on Medicine and the Changing Order of the New

York Academy of Medicine has outlined the national status of medical care succinctly(1):

The situation in medicine today (in America) is not entirely satisfactory, either to the public or to the conscientious physician, medical educator, investigator or administrator. Our social order has been undergoing far-reaching and profound alterations; these changes will continue and will probably be accelerated as time passes. The practice of medicine, indeed the whole of medicine, is directly affected by the *changing order*. It in turn must help to guide and direct these changes toward the human values so long cherished by medicine.

Certain definite objectives are paramount in any plans that may be made for medical and health care:

1. To maintain and continually to improve the quality of medical services.
2. To extend medical care as rapidly as possible and to provide the best known practices and facilities of medicine to the whole population.
3. To reduce the per capita or individual cost of medical services while increasing the total expenditures for medicine.
4. To provide adequate compensation to all physicians, to utilize more fully the service of younger physicians, and to maintain medicine as a profession, not as a business.

COMMUNITY VIEWPOINT IN DEFINING "ADEQUACY"

Before undertaking a study of the adequacy of facilities for the care of the sick in any given community, it becomes necessary to define, as exactly as possible, the community's obligations and responsibilities in these matters.

On any given day in any community, the prevalence of illness severe enough to require medical, hospital, and nursing assistance is a variable matter; often it is an individual matter, dependent upon the nature of the prevailing disease, the temperament of the sick person, the economic status of the family, and the standard of living, as well as the customs and mode of life of the community. A service that is quite adequate for one person or one community is inadequate for another. Many authorities, in discussing this field, have not defined adequacy, but have assumed that adequate medical care is that type of service provided, at the present time, in the most prosperous communities. If this standard is used, then it is obvious that this represents luxury care for many communities and that a heavy subsidy must be provided to the poorer communities by the richer areas to provide this type and quality of community service for the entire nation.

Furthermore, the term "adequacy" is not static. The demands

for diverse types of medical facilities increase year by year. The pattern of medical care is changing constantly. As our population ages, increasing attention must be paid to chronic illness. Increased emphasis must be given to early detection of various types of chronic illness. Rehabilitation of the disabled becomes of growing importance.

In all our discussions, one fact cannot be forgotten: Medical services must be furnished within such limits as the people can afford to pay. These services have been and will continue to be dependent upon the standards of living and per capita income of the community.

Health is purchasable, it is true, but the costs cannot be made *prohibitive*.

Thus, we see at the very onset, that there is no comprehensive, all-embracing definition of adequacy of medical care. *Adequacy* is a flexible and not a fixed term.

The Health Organization of the League of Nations once defined adequate medical care as follows:

In the larger sense, effective medical assistance may be considered as indicating a medical service that is organized in such a way as to place at the disposal of the population all the facilities of modern medicine, in order to promote health and to detect and treat illness from its incipiency. Medical assistance must be concerned with the promotion and the preservation of health as well as the treatment and cure of disease.

At first this seems a succinct and clear definition of adequate medical care. However, on second thought one realizes that it has a very serious defect, in that it says "medical service organized in such a way as to *place at the disposal* of the population. . . ." This is the definition of the idealist, who assumes that if the medical facilities are only placed at the disposal of the people, they will be used forthwith. But experience has shown that a long period of many years may be required to teach the people the personal value and utility of medical services that may be quite adequate and readily available.

PROGRESSIVE PATIENT CARE

What are the basic elements of progressive patient care and how can they be provided most effectively?

Before the community can make provision for such medical care, it is necessary to make an estimate, at least, of the degree, extent, and types of service that need to be provided.

Types of Illness

Illness can be divided into three simple categories:

1. Acute illness.
2. Convalescence.
3. Chronic illness.

Each of these categories requires an entirely different type of physician care and of hospital and nursing care. We are at once confronted with the need for a definition. What do we mean by acute illness? When does acute illness end and convalescence begin? When does convalescence end and chronic illness begin?

The attempt has been made since the fourteenth century to clarify these distinctions. As a matter of fact, our term "quarantine" evolved from such a distinction. At the end of 40 days it was believed that the ardent spirits of the disease left the body; the illness then became chronic. If at the end of 40 days the individual had not recovered, he had chronic illness and could be discharged from quarantine.

The administrative definition frequently accepted is: illness becomes *chronic* when it lasts more than three months. Administratively, *convalescence* from illness is that period when the patient who has been acutely ill no longer requires careful medical supervision although still unable to resume his normal activities. *Invalidism* represents a state of ill health in which an individual is incapacitated for a year or more.

Types of Care

Different types of care must be provided for various types of illness. This care can also be divided into three categories:

$$\text{Ambulatory care} \underset{\longleftarrow}{\longrightarrow} \text{Domiciliary care} \underset{\longleftarrow}{\longrightarrow} \text{Hospitalization}$$

This diagram represents the flow of illness from one administrative category to another.

Here again there is wide fluctuation, depending on the standards of the family and of the community as well as upon the peculiarities of the patient. Some individuals might consider that ambulatory care for a certain type of illness was quite sufficient for their needs. Others, with the same degree of illness, would insist that the doctor call at their homes. Some patients will not go to the hospital. They insist on domiciliary care even when illness is severe. Others would feel that it is necessary to be hospitalized at the slightest illness. Furthermore, an individual progresses from one stage to another, rapidly or slowly. The ordinary course in acute illness is in the direction of the arrows of the diagram, from left to right, and back again, right to left. There is often a rapid progression in the direction of hospitalization, with a somewhat slower regression of the equation as the patient recovers.

Different types of illness require different types of care, or different combinations of these types of care, as illustrated by the accompanying diagram:

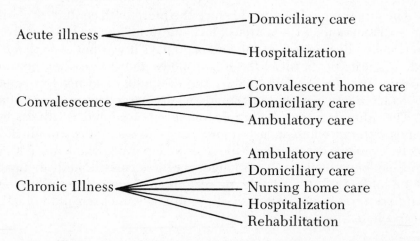

Acute illness requires provision for domiciliary care; should the patient become seriously ill, hospitalization is required. Convalescence requires no hospital care. There is a special type of care given to convalescence which is intermediate and is called "convalescent home" care. These patients progress to domiciliary care and, eventually, to ambulatory care.

Chronic illness requires a variety of facilities, ranging from hospitalization to nursing home care, which is quite different from convalescent home care; these patients might require domiciliary care also. For the chronic patient, domiciliary care is generally for nursing rather than physician care. Finally, the chronically ill might require ambulatory care, usually in the clinic where facilities are available for special therapy. Rehabilitation is an essential part of medical care in chronic disease.

Young people may have chronic illness but, more and more, chronic disease has become centered in the older age groups.

Provisions for the Care of the Acutely Ill

Provisions for the care of acute illness are dependent upon the economic status of the patient and of the community. Formerly, the standard terms used were: (a) the free patient, (b) the part-pay patient, and (c) the full-pay patient, but these terms are meaningless unless properly interpreted. The full-pay patient could be paying more than his share of the actual cost of his care, in order to subsidize the free patients. The free patient might not be given free care at all; it might cost him nothing, but the cost of his care must be borne by a voluntary or by an official agency. Since the patient might pay one tenth, one third, or three fourths of his care, the term "part-pay" means little.

In general, the expense of the care of acute illness is met, in great part, by the patient himself. Hospital revenue from the Blue Cross and payment for medical care from voluntary health insurance plans are, of course, in the category of direct patient payment. Therefore, he is almost always in the full-pay class or the part-pay class. The indigent patient who is acutely ill must have free care from the onset; usually it is provided at governmental expense.

Provisions for the Care of Convalescents and of the Chronically Ill

Convalescence from a serious illness produces a definite strain on individual and family resources, so that more provision for free care must be made by the community for this type of illness. When chronic illness occurs, it is almost essential that the great proportion of the expense be met by some official agency. In future years, the accrual of funds from Social Security will aid to some degree in meeting the cost of this type of illness.

The most expensive type of service from the community point of view is, of course, hospitalization, and the most expensive hospitalization for the individual is that for chronic disease because of the duration of this type of illness. The per capita, per day cost of hospitalization of acute illness is greatest because of the multitude of services required; but in the long run, chronic illness is more expensive, both for the individual and for the community, than acute illness.

Facilities for the Care of Illness

The community must provide proper facilities for the care of the sick, but only at a cost which the community can afford to pay. Thus, each community must give consideration first to quality of service and, equally important, to cost of service. Every effort must be made to reduce costs but not interfere with the quality of the service. In acute illness, for example, the community has the responsibility of improving domiciliary care in order to reduce the cost of hospitalization. This could be done by providing for home nursing service. The community also should improve the facilities for convalescent care outside the hospital, in order to lower the total costs of hospitalization. Furthermore, it should improve the facilities for domiciliary care of the convalescent in order to reduce convalescent home costs. Finally, the community should improve the facilities for the care of the ambulatory sick, and thereby reduce the cost of domiciliary care. Thus, in the whole gamut of illness, from hospitalization through convalescent care, domiciliary care, and finally ambulatory care, it should be possible to transfer the patient *more rapidly* from one category to the next, and thus reduce the cost of his care.

In chronic illness, emphasis must be placed on the improvement of facilities for ambulatory care, with arrangements for nursing service and physician visitation in the home, to reduce the necessity for institutional care and hospitalization.

Facilities Necessary for Progressive Patient Care

1. The Community Hospital.

a. The Short-stay Facility. This is planned for care of acute illness and is intended primarily for diagnosis, prognosis, and initial treatment of illness. It is by far the most expensive and elaborate facility. Since its activities include primarily personal services, we can anticipate increasing costs annually. (In 1962 costs of care in short-stay hospitals averaged from 20 to 30 dollars a day. Authorities agree that this cost will increase 5 per cent annually for at least five years.) The average patient stay is 6.7 days. Approximately 4 beds per 1,000 population will meet average community needs.

b. Convalescent Care. A rehabilitation facility is required for the care of the chronically ill. Preferably, it should be a division of the short-stay hospital, under the same administration and under the same roof. Rehabilitation is the focus of this facility. Period of stay can be 15 to 90 days, and per day costs should approximate 60 per cent of the short-stay facility. The average community having an aging population which will reach 10 per cent over 65 years of age by 1985, will need 2 beds per 1,000.

c. Ambulatory Patients. These patients are convalescing at home but are able to go to a physician's office or to a clinical facility for observation, therapy, and particularly rehabilitation. This service could be organized as a section of the convalescent division of the community hospital.

d.   Organized Home Care. This type of progressive patient care is planned for patients discharged from the hospital for convalescence at home but who remain under the supervision of the community hospital. Facilities are taken from the hospital to the bed patient at home by an organized team of skilled personnel, e.g., nurses, physiotherapists, and social workers. The hospital records, techniques, and equipment are utilized for rehabilitation purposes. Organized home care costs about one quarter of the patient-day cost of the short-stay hospital.

Throughout this course of progressive care, the patient is under the direct supervision of his family physician. All responsibility for preventive, diagnostic, therapeutic, and rehabilitation measures rests upon the physician of the patient. The physician in turn calls upon community facilities (including the health and welfare department) to aid him in his work.

2. The Nursing Home. In simplest terms, a nursing home is a facility in which patients with chronic illness receive long-term skilled nursing care, under medical supervision, as well as other essential personal services. The care that is required could not be rendered satisfactorily in the patient's home.

The function of the nursing home is quite distinct from a "home for the aged." The latter is planned for an elderly person with a chronic disability, requiring limited personal services and, perhaps, no nursing care.

At least 30 patients are necessary to operate a nursing home effectively, but it should not contain more than 60 to 80 beds. Daily costs per patient should be less than one half the costs of care in a hospital for acute illness.

Nursing home care should provide facilities for rehabilitation. A physiotherapist is an important staff asset. Smaller homes can share the services of one physiotherapist. The most important objective is to make the patient as self-sufficient as possible. Experience has shown that continuous efforts work wonders in getting the apparently hopelessly bedfast patient on an ambulatory basis. An excellent study on the value of rehabilitation in nursing homes was made by Park and Moe(2):

	Per Cent No Change	Per Cent Better	Per Cent Much Better
78 treated	51.3	28.2	20.5
71 controls	81.7	15.5	2.8

Approximately one attendant is required for each five or six patients. A professional nurse should be in charge of the services, but qualified practical nurses carry the nursing load; they constitute about one fourth of the total personnel.

Nursing home service has grown rapidly in recent years in order to fill a great need. Most of them are proprietary; many are located in renovated, fire-hazardous frame houses, too small and poorly equipped to be run efficiently.

Strong efforts are being made throughout the United States to develop state-wide standards for construction and operation of nursing homes, with a suitable system of periodic inspection and accreditation.

It is agreed that nursing homes should be an integral part of the community plan for adequate care of the chronically ill. These homes should be closely affiliated with the general hospital of the community. In some communities, the nursing home is on the same grounds and under direct administrative supervision of the community hospital.

County Infirmaries

These public welfare institutions are an outgrowth of the old "county poor farm." They are intended for care of the indigent person with chronic illness. Many county infirmaries have provided little more than custodial care, but the trend is to up-grade these institutions. Many of the best infirmaries now provide excellent nursing care, social service, and rehabilitation facilities as well as an outpatient service. The cost is about the same as care in a good nursing home.

Adult Foster Homes

Some communities provide foster home care for ambulatory elderly persons with chronic illness, but who are not bed-ridden and have no serious loss of mobility. Usually the patients are welfare clients. Physician and nursing care is minimal. The cost is about one half of nursing home care.

Public Health Nurses

Many communities have organized a system of public health nursing on an hourly home-visit basis. The nurses work under the supervision of the patient's physician. In large cities, this service is often provided by a voluntary nursing organization. More and more, the official public health nurses, particularly in rural areas, are providing for hourly home nursing care visits. The cost in the past has been about three dollars per hourly visit.

Ancillary Services

In many communities, voluntary agencies have organized special services to supplement the professional services required for care of the sick.

Vocational training has been planned both by official and voluntary agencies.

"Home-maker service" is a community plan which aids the family in time of stress. It provides trained home workers to assist the convalescent patient in domestic affairs.

Other ancillary devices are "meals-on-wheels," which bring adequate meals to the home of the convalescent or disabled patient.

"Loan closets" consist of a central depot of equipment for the disabled, such as crutches, wheelchairs, and hospital beds. These and many other ancillary services are organized by voluntary agencies in the community and meet a real need.

In summary: all the above facilities are needed in a community — large or small — to provide for progressive patient care. As in pioneer days, the physician is the cornerstone, but adequate comprehensive medical care can be provided only by means of an effective organization with interrelation of all the professional services and suitable facilities that are required.

EXTENT OF SICKNESS IN A COMMUNITY

How much sickness is there in a community? How many illnesses must we provide for in various categories? How serious are they? Obviously, we cannot provide medical facilities sufficient to meet every possible emergency, but we must know and provide for the probable average community morbidity. We know that the extent of illness varies with the age of an individual. Thus the age distribution of any given population will affect the morbidity rate. Industrialization modifies the type and extent of illness; furthermore, the income of the family, and the economic status of the whole community, bears an inverse ratio to the amount of illness. The poorer the family or community, the greater the amount of sickness. There are seasonal variations, epidemic variations, climatic factors, and many other influences that affect the extent and types of disease in the community and in the whole nation.

We have no completely satisfactory index of the extent of illness in the community. What do we mean by illness? How severe must it be to receive our attention? How incapacitating must it be? Everyone has minor ills and ailments at all times. An illness that is disabling to one person will be ignored by another. A variety of estimates has been made of extent of illness from various points of view, all of which have some validity.

For example, it has been estimated that:

1. On any given day, a cross section of the whole population will show 2 per cent disabled by illness.

2. The work time lost each year from illness in a large study of industrial workers is 8+ days for men and 10+ days for women.

3. Twenty per cent of persons are sick enough during any given year to require the services of a physician.

4. The average American spends about 4 per cent of his earnings on all types of medical care. About three fourths of this sum is expended for physician and hospital services.

5. Wage loss from illness and medical outlay amounts to about 6 per cent of the workers' income.

All these indices, each of which is determined by approaching the problem from different angles, give some consensus, at least, of the amount of anticipated illness in any community.

Variation in Family Illness

An estimate(3) showing variation in family illness in any given year is as follows:

60 per cent of families had little illness — cost less than $60
30 per cent of families had some illness — cost less than $250
10 per cent of families had much illness — cost over $250

The last 10 per cent group paid 40 per cent of the total costs of illness for the whole group.

This study demonstrated, as have all other similar surveys, that sickness and disability increase in inverse ratio to the income of the family. Invariably the lower the income group, the higher the rate of disability and illness.

Hospitalization

How many hospital beds are required?

The standard usually presented is four general short-stay hospital beds per 1,000 population, with two beds for patients requiring prolonged care. The number of beds provided for the mentally ill about equals the total number required for all other hospital patients.

Hospital costs are rising steadily. Authorities state that the rise will continue at the rate of about 5 per cent a year. This will require more careful utilization of hospital beds. In general hospitals, many beds have been occupied for long periods by patients with chronic disease. Obviously these patients must be transferred as rapidly as possible to an adequate but less expensive facility.

Rehabilitation Unit

Many community hospitals have constructed a convalescent unit (or rehabilitation unit), which is an integral part of the acute-care section. The patients do not require intensive nursing or physician care. Here a rehabilitation program is initiated, with plans for organized home care, so that the patient can return home much earlier than was formerly possible.

Institutions for care of tuberculosis often have empty beds because of the decline of tuberculosis as a hospital problem. Many communities have utilized these facilities to serve for rehabilitation of patients with various types of chronic disease.

New concepts of treatment of mental illness have shortened the length of hospital stay of mental disease patients. For the first time in many years, the demand for increased mental hospital beds has diminished; there is reason to believe that the standards formerly set for hospital bed requirements for mental illness will decline.

In brief, the rising costs of hospital care for acute illness make it quite evident that we must utilize existing facilities to better advantage and plan more carefully to meet the changing medical care needs. Per capita costs of medical care must not continue to increase at a more rapid rate than the national economy, yet economies in medical care must not curtail adequate service.

This is a challenge to all physicians as well as to leaders in the community who have a vital interest in the public welfare. In the past, the busy practicing physician has devoted little interest or time to the administration of medical care. He has assumed that the community provides the necessary facilities and he furnishes the essential physician care on a fee-for-service basis. It is now quite obvious that the physician must become informed on the economic and social aspects of medical care and assist in the community planning for adequate services.

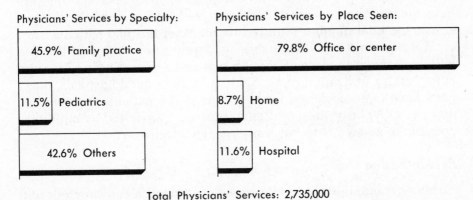

Physicians' Services by Specialty:

45.9% Family practice

11.5% Pediatrics

42.6% Others

Physicians' Services by Place Seen:

79.8% Office or center

8.7% Home

11.6% Hospital

Total Physicians' Services: 2,735,000

Figure 43. Services provided by medical groups in 1959 (estimated). Operations in hospitals: 18,500; deliveries: 6,600; laboratory: 1,450,000. (Basic data from Health Insurance Plan of Greater New York, *Annual Report, 1960.*)

How Much Physician Care Is Required?

The Health Insurance Plan of Greater New York has developed a program of comprehensive medical care for an industrial population of over 600,000 people. The utilization of medical services under a prepayment plan should give a good index of the extent and type of medical services needed, or at least desired, by the average family.

Services provided included general practitioner care, consultation with all the various specialists, and hospitalization under a Blue Cross contract.

The average person received five services a year. Eighty per cent of all physician care was given in the doctor's office, and only 8.7 per cent in the home. Physician service in the hospital totalled 11.6 per cent. Services by specialty were: family practice, 50 per cent; pediatrics, 11.5 per cent; and other specialist service, 42.5 per cent (see Fig. 43).

How Many Physicians?

It is frequently stated that there is a "shortage of physicians" in the United States, and efforts are being made continuously to increase the number of admissions to existing medical colleges and to build new schools of medicine. It is true, of course, that as population increases, a larger number of physicians, hospital beds, nurses, and other facilities for medical care are needed.

We have ample evidence, however, that we do not utilize our existing medical personnel to best advantage. Physician concentration might be 1 per 600 population in one area and 1 per 2,000 in another. If we analyze the number and quality of physician services demanded in a prepayment plan of comprehensive medical care, we learn that a maximum of 70 physicians are able to give a high quality of diversified service to 100,000 people. This requires a system of well-organized group practice with full utilization of ancillary personnel and full complement of necessary facilities.

Smaller communities and rural areas have discovered that they can secure adequate medical care through interrelated joint planning. The Bingham Foundation has done notable planning in this field in rural Maine. The plan, in essence, consists of:

1. A university medical center as the nucleus, with expert personnel, special services, well-equipped hospital, rehabilitation facilities, training opportunities, and consultant service.

2. Affiliated hospitals in the smaller outlying cities. These community hospitals vary from 60 to 200 beds. All qualified physicians in the area are elegible to staff membership. Continuous improvement in quality of medical facilities and service is secured by consultants who come out on invitation from the university center. Training is also provided in the center for physicians and other professional personnel from the affiliated hospitals.

3. Cottage Hospitals. These small institutions serve the villages and remote rural areas. Each cottage hospital is affiliated with the district hospital. Services rendered by general practitioners in the cottage hospital and through his office and home visits take care of at least 90 per cent of all medical ills. Less than 10 per cent need be referred to the district hospital; only 1 per cent will require the highly specialized care of the university center, e.g., brain surgery or heart surgery.

This type of organization of medical care is being developed in many parts of the United States. Under the plan, all physicians are actually in "group practice," since each practitioner is constantly in touch with his colleagues and can call on the pathologist, radiologist, or any other specialist when required. (Frequently the smaller rural hospitals share the services of an "itinerant" radiologist or pathologist.)

The utilization of federal Hill-Burton grants-in-aid for construction of hospitals in rural areas and the tremendous growth of Blue Cross and other health insurance plans have resulted in great improvement in extent and quality of medical care throughout the United States. Young physicians who formerly remained in the large cities (because the rural areas lacked the facilities with which they had been trained to practice medicine) now find it most advantageous and highly satisfying to practice medicine on a group basis in the smaller communities now providing the ancillary requirements for adequate medical care.

Under a well-organized plan of this type, it is possible for 70 doctors to give adequate physician care to 100,000 population. The various specialists that experience has shown would be needed are about as follows:

Adequate distribution of specialists for a community of 100,000 persons.

Specialty	Number of Physicians
General practice	28---30
Pediatrics	6---7
Obstetrics and gynecology	5---6
General surgery	4---5
Radiology	4---5
Neuropsychiatry	4---5
Ophthalmology	3---4
Allergy	2---3
Orthopedics	2---3
Otolaryngology	2---3
Dermatology	2---2
Urology	1---1
	63---74

This allocation does not make provision for industrial health services, public health physicians, or medical teachers, nor for full-time research workers.

It does provide a month's vacation a year for each physician and a weekly work load which gives ample time for recreation, community activities, and professional self-improvement.

The total physician services rendered per annum will be between

500,000 and 600,000 or an average of 5.5 services per person. This varies, of course, in epidemic years and as the population ages.

Federal Subsidy for Hospital Construction

The federal government attempted to meet the need for more hospital facilities in rural areas through the Hospital Survey and Construction Act, Public Law 725, Seventy-ninth Congress.

The act assisted each of the states in making use of its existing hospital and related facilities, and in surveying need for additional facilities.

Grants-in-aid were made to each of the states for hospital and health center construction where needed—for the most part in rural areas. The local community was required to meet appropriate standards in planning for a local hospital and to provide at least 50 per cent of the total cost.

The act proved to be a great impetus for hospital construction in rural areas. The plan was most successful in those states that took an active leadership and provided for an additional subsidy from the state funds toward rural community projects.

The great difficulty encountered was that in the areas of greatest need, the local community was unable, from its own resources, to provide for its share of the construction costs.

Costs of Medical Care

Medical care expenditures are increasing each year in the United States. In 1959 the per capita estimate of all services was $105.00. This was an increase of 7 per cent over 1958 and 14 per cent over 1957. The distribution of costs is shown in Table 47:

TABLE 47

**Distribution of Medical Care Expenditures
in 1959 per Capita**

Hospital services		$ 31.59
Physician services		28.57
Dentistry		11.25
Drugs and medicines		20.65
Appliances		6.79
Nursing home care and other professional services		6.08
	Total	$104.93

Insurance benefits covered 25 per cent of the total medical care. Hospital benefits provided 58 per cent of the cost, and physician service insurance provided 31 per cent of costs.

Table 47 is an index of future costs. In areas with an aging population, increasing medical care will be required for those 65 years and older. Where hospitalization is available to a population, the age variations have been noted in Table 48.

TABLE 48

Hospital Admissions per 1,000 Insured Persons per Annum

Years of Age	Hospital Admissions	Days in Hospital per Admission
15 to 44	93.2	6.5
45 to 64	79.1	11.0
65 +	121.2	13.2

Formerly, the average family paid for costs of illness from current income. Sickness insurance provided only for disaster, i.e., hospitalization and extensive surgery. There was no provision for the costs of prolonged chronic illness and disability. Thus, care of the chronically ill became a community burden and was met by state-supported hospitals for mental illness, city and county custodial institutions for care of chronic illness, and low-grade nursing homes.

As medical care has become more complex and as the age distribution has shifted to the older age groups, it becomes quite clear that the only way in which an average-income family can provide adequately for the costs of illness is through a systematic plan of prepayment. These payments can be made during the productive years, thus covering not only costs of current illness but also providing insurance against costs of chronic illness and disability during old age.

In the previous discussion of chronic illness, we have noted the conclusions of the White House Conference of 1961. This Conference recommended that a nation-wide plan should be formulated to give the wage earner an opportunity to provide for the emergency costs of chronic illness in later years by a system of prepayment insurance. This system would be an integral part of the existing Social Security System. (The White House Recommendation is currently [1962] under consideration by the National Congress.)

Provision for Payment of Medical Care

In general, every family and every person desire to pay for medical services from their own resources. In the United States, this is not considered a government obligation but as much a personal responsibility as paying for other life necessities, such as food, shelter, and clothing.

As already noted, however, medical care has become increasingly expensive. Thus the family of average income has found that the extensive serious illness can result in a great drain of income. This situation has been met by insurance plans against disastrous illness, particularly hospitalization.

Plans for Sickness Insurance

One of the suggestions for improvement in the system of fee-for-service care in illness has been the utilization of the "insurance" principle for payment of medical care.

Life insurance has been established firmly in the United States for more than a century, but sickness insurance did not follow suit. By 1920 the concept of a nation-wide compulsory sickness insurance plan became important enough to arouse organized opposition by commercial insurance companies, employers' associations, and the organized medical profession. Meanwhile, workmen's compensation for injury made great advances and became a part of the social structure. At first the worker was reimbursed for costs of medical care and for time lost because of injury due to occupation. Later, actual illness resulting from the worker's job was also compensated.

Workmen's compensation resulted in development of industrial health services, organized at the cost of industry for the purpose of:

1. Preventing illness and injury.
2. Promoting the health of the worker, and thus lowering the costs of the compensation act.

The activities of an industrial health service and benefits derived therefrom are described in Chapter 30.

Although no medical services are given to families in most of these plans, and only emergency medical care is provided to employees, nevertheless, the plans do give a suggestion of the value of organized care in prevention of illness, and workmen's compensation has indicated the importance of a prepayment plan for care of illness or injury.

The Report of the Committee on the Costs of Medical Care(4) brought out the defects of the fee-for-service system of medical care, and the majority of the committee recommended: (a) a system of group practice centering around a community hospital, (b) a sound system of sickness insurance under government sponsorship.

Voluntary Health Insurance*

The payment for medical care that has evolved through the years in the United States has been, basically, payment in "cash or kind" for individual medical services. This has included physician, dental, and nursing care, hospital expenses, and the like. During the last century the physician's pay was, not infrequently, farm produce — a pig, a horse, hay, or potatoes. As medical science improved, surgery developed and hospitals began to be a commonly accepted adjunct to medical care. The costs of medical care rose precipitously. Often, in fact, the costs of unexpected illness resulted in a severe drain on the family budget.

The American people had long been accustomed to group insurance coverage, on a prepayment premium basis, to provide for such disasters as death of the breadwinner, destruction of home or business by fire, or marine disaster. A logical development, therefore, was a voluntary plan for prepayment premiums on a group coverage basis, to insure against the severe financial loss caused by disastrous illness.

Another quite different development was the plan by isolated industries of compulsory payment for comprehensive medical care; a good example is a coal-mining community. The mine authorities, in order to conserve labor and to provide for accident care, would establish, near the mine, a small emergency hospital and a medical service. The physician was selected by the company and was on a salary, or rather a retainer fee, with rights to collect fees for special services such as obstetrics, pediatrics, and care of venereal disease. Part of the costs of this service was paid by the company, but each miner was compelled to pay a specified amount each month for medical service. The miners seldom liked the plan, as they had no

---

*This term is a misnomer. The plans as they have developed are, in reality, insurance against the financial hazards of severe acute illness.

part in selection of the doctor, but on the whole the method met a real need.

Thus the germ of two separate plans for prepayment for medical care on a group basis was established: (a) a compulsory plan rendering comprehensive care, and (b) a voluntary insurance plan for indemnification of the family in case of a disaster.

The Blue Cross. The Blue Cross developed as a voluntary cooperative plan of insurance against financial hazards of illness that required hospitalization. At first it provided for specified services which included practically all the costs of an average hospitalized illness. It did not pay for costs of prolonged hospitalization (usually two to three weeks was the limit). The plan received the enthusiastic support of the voluntary hospitals and soon found favor with the public. After a precarious infancy of about ten years, the Blue Cross really began its phenomenal growth. In 1940 it had some 5,000,000 subscribers. By 1950 nearly 40,000,000 people in the United States were enrolled in the Blue Cross.

Since 1950, the Blue Cross plans, which vary somewhat in different communities but which are basically alike, have grown to include a large proportion of the total population as subscribers.

In 1960, the Blue Cross estimated that 132 millions of people in the United States held some form of health insurance. More than 120 millions had surgical insurance and 86 millions had medical insurance. Blue Cross also estimated that 5.6 billions of dollars were paid out in health insurance benefits during the year 1960.

In addition to Blue Cross, other group insurance contracts that are sold by private insurance companies to meet the costs of hospital illness increased from 1940 to 1960 from about 5,000,000 to more than 20,000,000 persons under coverage. The Blue Cross plan provided for none of the costs of physician care.

The Blue Shield. This organization is a voluntary association which provides for insurance against the costs of physician care, both surgical and medical, for hospitalized persons. It does not pay for costs of domiciliary or ambulatory care in the physician's office. This plan was a logical development, since the average man has felt that he can meet the costs of routine illness from the current family budget, and thus the insurance principle does not apply to this need. Surgical fees for hospitalized illness, however, represent to him a real disaster.

In addition to the above plans, state and local medical societies have organized programs for prepayment for physician services.

Limited Coverage. Originally the plan of the Blue Cross was to provide for comprehensive service benefits, but unpredicted increased costs of hospitalization occurred during the period subsequent to World War II. Rather than increase premiums, the trend has been to limit benefits and to provide for specified cash payments toward hospital room and board, together with certain additional specified benefits. The Blue Shield also has tended to provide for a specified indemnity against costs of physician care, and particularly surgical care in hospitalized illness. Coverage for home calls and visits to doctors' offices have not been popular because of high premium costs. Thus the whole trend of voluntary sickness insurance has been away from comprehensive medical care and toward *indemnity*, largely to meet a part of the high costs of hospitalized illness.

From the point of view of preventive medicine this development is unfavorable. The real problems of adequate medical care cannot be met under these plans. Here the element of time enters, for a long period of time is required to convince the average man that the costs, even on a periodic prepayment basis, for comprehensive medical care are a necessary and essential charge against current family budgets.

The plans that have been developed so far, fine as they are, do not meet our needs. The real need is for the development of a prepayment plan for comprehensive medical care with a broad coverage, at a cost that the average man is willing to pay. Most important of all, these plans must include facilities for suitable preventive services. It is quite obvious that we have not yet reached the stage of development in our national thinking which will provide for these plans on a voluntary association basis. Social development is a slow process. Advancement of mass consciousness toward a desirable goal, the approach to which is quite obvious and simple to the statesman or sociologist, is a long tedious road, full of obstacles and hazards, but it is the road that must be traveled if we are to maintain the sound and basic principles of democracy upon which our nation is founded.

Voluntary Insurance Plans for Comprehensive Medical Care. The logical development of insurance plans against disastrous illness has been family or group insurance plans to pay for *all the costs* of comprehensive medical care.

The group plans have been most successful in industrial areas. Organized labor has developed plans for payment of medical care for union members and their families as a fringe benefit. It has been estimated that more than 70 per cent of all workers under collective bargaining agreements with employers have at least one type of health insurance. These benefits have been extended to dependents of the workers, and more recently the health insurance benefits have been continued for retired employees.

Numerous plans have been organized for provision of comprehensive medical care through prepayment premiums. One of the most notable is the Health Insurance Plan of Greater New York, with an enrollment of over 600,000 persons (in 1962). It is not an accident that this plan developed in a large city, for the plan requires the cooperation of large groups. For example, all the employees of the municipally owned transit system are given comprehensive medical care under the plan. The medical care is given by organized physician groups which provide specialist care as well as general medical service. The plan contracts with the Blue Cross for hospital care of its clients. Specified services are given which are broad in scope but not all inclusive; for example, dental care is not included.

Numerous other experiments in comprehensive coverage for medical care are being developed in various parts of the nation. There can be no question that if this general plan of social experimentation continues, whereby (using the technique of the "pilot plant" of industry) lessons are learned and mistakes made on a small scale, eventually, slowly, and with infinite patience and judicial, unbiased consideration, there will evolve a program that will be applicable to our system of local self-government, our traditions, and our social philosophy.

Dental Health Service Prepayment Plans. Prepayment plans for dental care are eliminated from most plans of health insurance. This is an anomalous situation, since dental care is one of the most predictable of all the insurance risks. Furthermore, early care is truly preventive since it can obviate subsequent costly correction of dental defects.

No data are available concerning costs of dental care if the service were to begin at infancy and be continued on a preventive and continuous basis throughout life.

The American Dental Association in 1944 proposed a plan(5) for a prepayment dental service for family groups which provides for a monthly subscription of $1 for an individual and $2.50 per month for a family. There are some limitations in the contract, but the provisions are quite liberal. The plan is proposed on a trial basis and undoubtedly will be modified as experience indicates.

By 1960, approximately 600,000 persons in the United States had prepayment contracts through the Dental Insurance Plan, Inc., Group Health Dental Insurance, and other organizations. About one half of the beneficiaries were in New York State.

Compulsory Health Insurance

This policy has been advocated for the industrially employed, particularly by the American Association for Labor Legislation. The social principles that are involved are:

1. Cash benefits during periods of illness.
2. Adequate medical care during illness and incapacity.
3. Promotion of extensive programs of preventive medicine to lessen incidence of disease.

The program would be paid by: (a) salary deductions from workers, (b) an equal contribution by the employer, and (c) an additional partial contribution by government. Various plans of this general type have been presented to legislatures or to actual plebiscite in several states, but as yet (1962) no state-wide plan has been adopted.

NATION-WIDE MEDICAL CARE INSURANCE

For many years there has been an interest in, and agitation for, a nation-wide improvement in the system of provision of medical care to the American people. Many authorities have felt that best results could be secured through the organization of a federally administered medical plan. The advantages that are usually presented(6) for a federally administered medical and health service are:

1. A federal program would assure equality and uniformity of health service throughout the country.
2. The costs of health services in relation to family income could be made uniform throughout the nation.
3. Medical care of persons who move from one state to another could be handled more easily under a federal administration.
4. The quality of administration under federal auspices is generally superior to that of state or local agencies.

Most of the stimulus for a national medical service has initiated with sociologists and economists. The organized medical profession has felt, for the most part, that the existing system was satisfactory. Public health officials and voluntary health and welfare organizations, as well as official welfare departments, have seen the problem from the point of view of community-wide need, and have been active in the study of these matters.

In 1935 the report of the Committee on Economic Security recommended to President Franklin D. Roosevelt that a nation-wide public health program be established which should be aided financially and technically by the federal government. The program should be administered by state and local health departments. This plan represented no change in national policies but was simply an extension of existing practices. It resulted directly in the national Social Security Act, which was passed in 1935.

The Social Security Act

This important act has been discussed elsewhere in the text. It has provided not only for tremendous expansion of purely public health services, but also has made provision for remedial care of the blind, the crippled, and for needy mothers and children, in all parts of the United States.

The Social Security Act met with general approval and only slight opposition. Public health was developed along well-established lines. Physicians and hospitals were paid for remedial services rendered under the various provisions of the act. The national health agencies — the Children's Bureau and the U.S. Public Health Service — formulated the general program, in conjunction with the Association of State and Territorial Health Officers, and gave grants-in-aid to all the states. The funds were allocated to the various states on an equitable basis and administered by them. Each state in turn allocated funds for direct services to local official health and welfare agencies, which administered the grants under state supervision.

The Situation since 1935

The Committee on the Costs of Medical Care made the report[4] of its nation-wide study in 1932. The committee agreed that:

1. Promotion of public health facilities should be undertaken on a nation-wide basis.
2. Government should assume control of measures relating to medical, nursing, and hospital care of the indigent.

The majority of the committee recommended that measures should be taken to improve distribution of medical care throughout the nation by initiating:

1. Some system of sickness insurance under government sponsorship.

2. A system of group practice centering in community hospitals.

The report caused great opposition and initiated a large amount of general interest. The net result was the development of an extensive and very popular plan of hospital insurance, with limited benefits.

President Roosevelt then called a national health conference to consider this report in 1938. This conference reported that:

1. Preventive health services for the nation are, as a whole, grossly insufficient.

2. Hospital and other institutional facilities for the care of the sick are inadequate in many communities, especially in the rural areas. Financial support for hospital care and other professional services in hospitals is both insufficient and precarious, especially for services to people who cannot pay the costs of the care needed.

3. One third of the population, including persons with or without income, is receiving inadequate or no medical care.

4. An even larger fraction of the population suffers from economic burdens created by illness.

This startling and condemnatory report of inadequacies of the existing system for provision of medical care caused a tremendous furor. The conference recommended:

1. Nation-wide expansion of the public health and of maternal and child health services.

2. Expansion of national hospital facilities.

3. A national program for the medical care of the indigent, with one half the total annual costs to be met by the federal government.

4. A suggestion that federal government aid be granted to states to study their own problems and develop their own plans in regard to sickness insurance.

5. A plan for insurance against loss of wages during sickness.

The cost of recommendations 1, 2, and 3 to federal, state, and local governments was estimated to be about $80,000,000 annually.

The essentials of this report were embodied in the Wagner bill, which was submitted to Congress in 1939.

This bill was extensively opposed by the organized medical profession, which felt that there should be "a continued development of the private practice of medicine, subject to such change as may be necessary to maintain the quality of medical services and to increase their availability."

The medical profession as a whole did not desire to become civil servants, working under a nation-wide plan for distribution of medical care, which it feared would be organized and administered under federal auspices. It preferred the present plan of local determination of needs, and local administrative control, in any extension of plans for provision of medical service to the indigent and to the "medically" indigent.

Proposed Plan of the Conference of Twenty-nine

The objectives of a nation-wide medical care plan have been set forth in detail by the Health Program Conference of the Committee on Research in Medical Economics(7). A brief summary of this report follows:

1. **Aims.** The aim of a nation-wide health program is good medical care to all people in proportion to their needs and regardless of their ability to pay for these services.

2. **Scope.** This care should be comprehensive and coordinated. It should not be limited to hospitalization, to reimbursement for accident, or to other types of "catastrophic" and unpredictable illness.

3. **Financing.** The plan should provide for equal distribution of costs. Provision should be made for prepayment, at regular intervals and over long periods, by those who have adequate incomes, with a system of general taxation to meet the costs of service for the poor, and for others who are unable to meet the periodic assessments.

4. **Grouping of Facilities.** Facilities for care of the sick should be coordinated and administered in such a manner that they may be utilized to fullest advantage to the community. Preventive services should be incorporated in the everyday activities of curative medicine, rather than as a separate unit of activity.

5. **Results.** The committee postulates that a nation-wide plan of this type should become a completely comprehensive medical service which would be available to all, which would be scientifically efficient, economical in cost, of a high quality, securely financed, with assurances of adequate income to physicians and other personnel. There would be assurance also of professional opportunity, commensurate with individual training and ability.

The committee insists that such a nation-wide system should be administered on a federal, or on a "federal-state" basis. The federal government should make provision for a nation-wide collection of funds through a compulsory, prepayment, contributory plan of sickness insurance, which should be combined with a system of general taxation to meet full costs of the service. No individual should be assessed more than the actual costs of his share of service, as actuarially adjusted. Those who cannot meet these actual costs will be provided for from general taxation.

The unit of administration of the national system should be the local community, but the local administrative unit would function under a national standard of procedures. The federal government would assume the responsibility for distribution of funds and for unification of administration of the medical services.

Under this plan, the local administrative unit could have a very limited autonomy and almost no prerogatives in relation to determination of policy.

Limitations of Federal Functions

Each state is a sovereign power, and the federal government possesses only those governmental functions that are expressly granted to it by the states. Many states are unwilling to sacrifice the principle of local self-government concerning provision of medical facilities to all for the obvious advantages of a centrally administered nation-wide plan.

Each type of governmental authority—federal, state, or local— has certain functions which it is best fitted to administer. For example, the federal government is obviously best fitted to administer public health matters that are of international significance or of interstate concern, but other governmental services are supplied best by the local community. For example, the local community in which the author resides supplies his family with an adequate and excellent supply of water. It is true that the local water supply system is under the supervision of the division of sanitary engineering of the state board of health, and the quality of the water conforms to the national standard for interstate carriers, but the administration of the service is a local responsibility. If the state board of health should attempt to administer our local water supply system, it would be both costly and inefficient. If the federal government were to assume responsibility for administration of the water supply service of our town, I am perfectly certain that my family would be thirsty a good part of the time.

Many physicians believe that the most satisfactory system for development of adequate medical services for the United States as a whole is the much less comprehensive, but much sounder, system of slow evolutional development on a local community basis, of state-wide programs that are framed to meet the needs of each local and state situation. Minimum standards of adequacy of medical care could be provided by the federal government, and federal government subsidy could be provided as grants-in-aid, during the developmental stages of the plans.

This system was used with success in the gradual development of full-time local health departments under the Social Security Act, in order to meet each particular need in each area in the country. This plan is still growing. It will require many years before all parts of the nation have equal provisions, but the plan has the great advantage that each unit is locally sponsored and locally administered.

A comprehensive master plan for adequate medical care might be formulated by each state, so drawn as to meet its own requirements. The advice of the U.S. Public Health Service and other federal agencies should be sought in drawing up these plans, but the basis of each state plan would be that primary responsibility for administration of the program should rest with the local community. It would be anticipated, as a matter of course, that each local community would develop its plan under state guidance.

The financing of each plan should be a local responsibility, with supplementary aid from the state, where the particular situation required such assistance.

It must be admitted that the evolution of plans for improvement in medical services on a local autonomy basis is discouragingly slow. It does not keep pace with advances in medical science nor with improvements in techniques of administration. It must be remembered that the evolution of social structure under the principles of democratic government is a slow, tedious, discouraging, painful process, yet somehow, despite all its faults, we like it.

RELATIONSHIP OF PREVENTIVE MEDICINE TO ADEQUATE MEDICAL CARE

Preventive medicine is completely dependent, for its future development, upon a proper provision for a satisfactory type of local, comprehensive, community-wide medical care. As has been pointed out in previous pages, the great advances in the field of preventive medicine, particularly in geriatrics, must be developed on the basis of prevention of disease in the individual, rather than by mass methods. This can only mean that preventive medicine of the future will be carried out by those who give direct medical, nursing, and hospital care. Those direct services in preventive medicine rendered for community benefit—as, for example, immunization clinic service—will be carried out by the practicing physician, who will be paid by the community for rendering this type of service.

Opportunities for Physicians in the Field of Administration

The advances made in formulation of comprehensive and co-ordinated plans for provision of adequate medical care to all the people are developed on a unified nation-wide basis or evolved under a system of local autonomy with state and federal aid.

In any case, those facilities that are to be provided must be administered by capable, well-trained medical officers, with a competent staff.

Under such a plan, each community will have its health center, and the activities of this local community-supported medical unit will encompass all official medical functions, both preventive and curative. The community hospital and all public clinics will be administered by the local public health service. Laboratory diagnosis, roentgenologic diagnosis, and home nursing care will be directed through the health center under the administration of its director. The well-accepted health department activities, such as general sanitation, vital statistics, health education, school health work, infant and maternal hygiene, and communicable disease control will, of course, be fused with the other activities of the health center.

This is not an impractical, idealistic conception. It is being worked out successfully in many parts of the United States, particularly in the rural areas. It is so flexible that it lends itself to a great many types of communities and to a great variety of cultures.

The administration of this type of official medical service requires a physician who possesses administrative talent and training of no mean order. It requires a man with vision and a high degree of social consciousness as well as a sense of community responsibility.

This type of man is already emerging to meet the growing needs. Foresighted leaders in medical education have furnished the facilities for proper training of these men.

Thus the future for the field of preventive medicine and public health is most promising. It will require men of courage, tenacity, and real ability; men who are willing enough and farsighted enough to make the necessary sacrifices in order to secure the proper training to carry on this work successfully. It is a real challenge and a great opportunity to the young physician of the next generation.

REFERENCES

1. *Preliminary Report of the Committee on Medicine and the Changing Order.* New York Academy of Medicine, New York, 1945.

2. PARK, W. E., and MOE, M. I.: *Pub. Health Rep.*, 1960, **75**:605.

3. *Preliminary Report on National Program for Medical Care, Committee on Administrative Practice,* American Public Health Association, *Am. J. Pub. Health*, 1944, **34**:984.

4. *Medical Care for the American People; the Final Report of the Committee on the Costs of Medical Care.* University of Chicago Press, Chicago, Ill., 1932. (This committee was self-appointed and consisted of distinguished sociologists, economists, businessmen, physicians, and educators. Dr. Ray Lyman Wilbur was its chairman.)

5. *Report of the Committee of the American Dental Association on a Proposed Plan for Prepayment of Dental Insurance.* American Dental Association, Chicago, 1944.

6. HEGE, J. R.: *Am. J. Pub. Health*, 1944, **34**:1234.

7. *Report of the Health Program Conference of the Committee on Research in Medical Economics, New York, Dec., 1944.* Committee on Research in Medical Economics, 1790 Broadway, New York 19, N.Y., (This conference was a self-appointed group of 29 physicians, economists, educators, federal officers, and hospital superintendents.)

SPECIAL REFERENCES

ANDERSON, O. W., and SHEATSLEY, P. B.: *Comprehensive Medical Insurance.* Health Information Foundation, Research Series 9, New York, 1959.

BLUESTONE, E. M.: *J.A.M.A.*, 1954, **155**:1379.

DAILY, E. F.: *J.A.M.A.*, 1959, **170**:272.

DURSEN, P., BOLAMUTH, E., and SHAPIRO, C.: *Hospital Utilization and Prepaid Medical Care. Hospital Monograph Series 3,* Am. Hosp. Assoc, 15 East Division St., Chicago, Ill.

COLDMANN, F., and FRAENKEL, M.: *J. Chron. Dis.*, 1960, **11**:77.

COLDMANN, F.: *Am. J. Pub. Health*, 1960, **50**:1274.

Health and Insurance Plans: U.S. Dept. of Labor, Bureau of Labor Statistics, Bull. No. 1199-2., page 186, Oct., 1956.

Progressive Patient Care: Symposium on Progressive Patient Care. J. Am. Hosp. Assoc., Jan. 1959.

SHAPIRO, S., and EINHORN, M.: *Pub. Health Rep.*, 1958, **73**:687.

SOMERS, H. M., and SOMERS, A. R.: *Doctors, Patients, and Health Insurance.* Brookings Institution, Washington, D.C., 1960.

Finis

We do not suppose that the time will ever come, let our sanitary regulations be ever so well matured, when no human being will die of any other cause than old age — the wearing out of the human machine. But what we anticipate is, a gradual sanitary improvement, a gradual removal and avoidance of the causes of disease, a gradual diminution of human suffering, and a gradual reduction of the number of premature and unnecessary deaths. And there can be no objection to aiming at abstract perfection, and to continuing our efforts at reformation until it is attained.

LEMUEL SHATTUCK

INDEX

595